As homelessness becomes an increasingly visible problem, the health care of homeless people is beginning to appear on the agenda of politicians, health care workers and policy makers. In contrast with the popular stereotype of elderly alcoholic males or bag ladies that the word homeless tends to trigger, homelessness affects families as well as young single people. The health needs of these various groups are not homogeneous.

This book brings together the experience of mental health care teams around the world in addressing the problems of mental illness in the homeless. The difficulties in assessment and service delivery are discussed at length with an emphasis on application of existing knowledge in health care. In addressing social policy implications as well as clinical management, models and definitions of homelessness in different cultures, this volume will offer a practical support for all those working with the homeless on a day-to-day basis.

Homelessness and Mental Health

STUDIES IN SOCIAL AND COMMUNITY PSYCHIATRY

Volumes in this series examine the social dimensions of mental illness as they affect diagnosis and management, and address a range of fundamental issues in the development of community-based mental health services.

Series editor
PETER J. TYRER
Professor of Community Psychiatry, St Mary's Hospital Medical School, London

Homelessness and Mental Health

edited by

DINESH BHUGRA

Institute of Psychiatry
London, UK

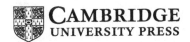

CAMBRIDGE
UNIVERSITY PRESS

CAMBRIDGE UNIVERSITY PRESS
Cambridge, New York, Melbourne, Madrid, Cape Town, Singapore, São Paulo

Cambridge University Press
The Edinburgh Building, Cambridge CB2 8RU, UK

Published in the United States of America by Cambridge University Press, New York

www.cambridge.org
Information on this title: www.cambridge.org/9780521452021

First published 1996
This digitally printed version 2007

A catalogue record for this publication is available from the British Library

Library of Congress Cataloguing in Publication data

Homelessness and mental health / edited by D. Bhugra.
      p.   cm. – (Studies in social and community psychiatry)
      ISBN 0 521 45202 3 (hc)
      1. Homeless persons – Mental health.   2. Homeless persons –
Mental health services.   I. Bhugra, Dinesh.   II. Series.
      [DNLM: 1. Homeless Persons – psychology.   2. Mental
Disorders – therapy.   3. Mental Health Services – organization
& administration.   4. Health Services Needs and Demand.
WA 305 H7655 1996]
RC451.4.H64H66   1996
      362.2′08′6942 – dc20
DNLM/DLC
      for Library of Congress   96–3407 CIP

ISBN 978-0-521-45202-1 hardback
ISBN 978-0-521-03773-0 paperback

Dedicated to
Suman and Rajesh and their families

Contents

Part IV POLICY AND EVALUATION

Contributors

PROFESSOR LEONA BACHRACH
Maryland Psychiatric Research Center, Department of Psychiatry, University of Maryland School of Medicine, Catonsville, MD 20879, USA

DR DINESH BHUGRA
Department of Psychiatry, Institute of Psychiatry, De Crespigny Park, Denmark Hill, London SE5 8AF, UK

DR PREBEN BRANDT
Shelter for Homeless People, 'Sundholm', Sundholmsvej 6–14, DK 2300, Copenhagen S, Denmark

PROFESSOR WILLIAM BREAKEY
Department of Psychiatry and Behavioral Science, The Henry Phipps Psychiatric Service, 600 North Wolfe Street, Meyer 4-181, Baltimore, MD 21287-7481, USA

PROFESSOR CARL COHEN
SUNY Health Science Center at Brooklyn, 450 Clarkson Avenue, Brooklyn, NY 11203, USA

MAUREEN CRANE
SUNY Health Science Center at Brooklyn, 450 Clarkson Avenue, Brooklyn, NY 11203, USA

DR DAVID EL-KABIR
Wytham Hall, 117 Sutherland Avenue, London W9 2QJ, UK

DR JOSEPH FERNANDEZ
Programme for the Homeless, St Brendan's Hospital, Dublin 7, Eire

PROFESSOR HELEN HERRMAN
St Vincent's Hospital, Fitzroy, Victoria 3065, Australia

DR PHILIP JOSEPH
Paterson Wing, St Mary's Hospital, Praed Street, London W2 1NY, UK

DR DAVID KINGDON
Department of Psychiatry, Bassetlaw General Hospital, Kilton, Nottinghamshire S81 0BD, UK

DR JANE MARSHALL
Addiction Sciences Building, 4, Windsor Walk, London SE5 8AF, UK

'DR MAX MARSHALL
University of Manchester, Department of Community Psychiatry, Academic Unit, Royal Preston Hospital, Sharowe Green Lane, Fullwood, Preston, Lancashire, PR2 48T, UK

DR ALAN MCNAUGHT
The Maudesley Hospital, Denmark Hill, London SE5 8AZ, UK

DR POVL MUNK-JØRGENSEN
Institute for Basic Psychiatric Research, Department of Psychiatric Demography, Psychiatric Hospital in Aarhus, Skovagervej 2, DK-8240 Risskov, Denmark

DR CECILY NEIL
CSIRO-Division of Construction and Engineering, Graham Road, P.O. Box 56, Highe H, Victoria 3190, Australia

DR SIMON RAMSDEN
Wytham Hall, 117 Sutherland Avenue, London W9 2QJ, UK

DR WULF RÖSSLER
Mental Health Services Research Unit, Central Institute of Mental Health, J5, D-6815, Mannheim, Germany

Dr Hans Joachim Salize
  Mental Health Services Research Unit, Central Institute of Mental
  Health, J5, D-6815, Mannheim, Germany

Dr Philip Timms
  Mental Health Team for Single Homeless People, Fourth Floor,
  156–164 Tooley Street, London SE1 2NR, UK

Preface

'I had a home once – I had once a husband –
I am a widow, poor and broken-hearted!'
Loud blew the wind, unheard was her complaining.
On drove the chariot.

The Widow
Robert Southey 1774–1843

Homelessness is a universal phenomenon. Virtually all countries around the globe will experience some degree of homelessness. The numbers will depend upon several political, social and economic factors. The traditional stereotype of a homeless individual as a Skid Row alcoholic has given way to homeless individuals, young and old, black and white, male and female with homeless families and sheltered accommodation of variable quality. Not all mentally ill are homeless and neither are all homeless mentally ill. However, there is a very clear association between the two.

The temptation to look at only one module of homelessness and singular linear causality leading to homelessness must be resisted. Different countries have different experiences of homelessness and have devised different methods of dealing with the problems of mentally ill homeless individuals, but whether all models can be transported and used across cultures remains to be seen. However, the need to learn from others' experience, their good models and mistakes makes it possible to see the problems of mentally ill homeless in a completely different light.

This is the first volume to bring together authors from different countries with a great deal of clinical and non-clinical expertise on the double helix of homelessness and mental illness. I have been very fortunate in gathering a group of dedicated authors who have not only offered advice but have delivered their contributions in a way that made putting this book together a pleasure. I am particularly indebted to Drs Jane Marshall, Max Marshall and Philip Timms for their advice and support. I am grateful to Dr Richard Barling and Dr Jocelyn Foster of Cambridge University Press for their patience and guidance.

Dinesh Bhugra

PART I

INTRODUCTION AND SPECIAL GROUPS

1

Introduction

DINESH BHUGRA

Homelessness and its consequences have become much more visible on the streets of big cities as well as villages across the globe in the last few years. In the UK this has been linked with the policy of closing psychiatric hospitals because there is often a clear association between mental illness and homelessness, though the direction of such an association may not always be very obvious. Across the world, experiences of poverty, homelessness and mental illness are universal. However, the definitions of homelessness, expectations from the government of the day and the availability of mental health services all play a role in the visibility of the homeless mentally ill on the streets. A large volume of literature on the homeless mentally ill exists in the USA. The availability of information from our European partners remains somewhat limited, especially in English. The work on urbanization and mental illness focuses on the internal migration to big cities in the developing countries. However, the impact of rapid industrialization, increasing populations and limited availability of land and cheap housing make overcrowding with its resultant problems a real issue. The impact of these factors varies across nations and societies. Even though the ideas and reality of homelessness are not entirely new, their increased visibility in the bright lights of the city means that across the globe similar experiences are beginning to emerge. The universal confusion about the definitions of homelessness makes it essential to try to get an international perspective. Internal migration, unemployment, closure of casual accommodation and disinvestment in public housing appear to be some of the international themes. Furthermore, within the UK definitions of homelessness vary as do housing conditions across different parts of the country, which makes direct comparisons on the level of homelessness difficult.

The relationship of poor housing, available housing at affordable costs, unemployment and increasing rates of repossession due to economic factors on the one hand and on the other hand mental illness resulting from all these factors and often leading to loss of 'home' turns into a vicious spiral. The factors are complex and often very difficult to tease out. In a survey of homelessness in London carried out in 1961–2 only one London Borough did not advance the view that the housing shortage was a significant factor in homelessness (Greve *et al.*, 1971). These authors acknowledged that the Victorian notions of the deserving and the non-deserving persisted and the judgemental approach continued to flourish in conditions of general housing shortage. Unfortunately these views still persist certainly with politicians, and to a lesser degree with the public.

Temporary accommodation – regarded as halfway or intermediate housing by the Councils – reflects substandard housing in which people wait until normal standard council housing is available or until they are judged fit or eligible to have it. There may be a complex procedure of moving people from temporary accommodation to intermediate housing before moving them on to more permanent placement. However, with the rapid reduction in the housing pool and lack of availability of council properties more and more people are staying in unsuitable temporary accommodation for longer periods.

The relief of the poor, including the homeless, began as a form of charity, with government interest arising very gradually (Glastonbury, 1971). The workhouses were the central provision for the homeless and even then their numbers were not sufficient to cater for the levels of homelessness prevalent at the time. The separation within the workhouse was initially according to sex but it changed according to physical ability as well as age. The major responsibility for the care of homeless families has largely remained with health and welfare interests. After the Second World War, there was a massive upsurge in house building with the local councils leading the way. However, changes in government policy and political dogma meant that although the initial aim was to provide cheap, affordable, low rent accommodation, the properties were sold to owner-occupiers who were then caught in the vicious grip of wanting to get out of low quality multi-storeyed tower blocks but there were limited options.

Observing the Skid Row and its occupants in the USA, Bogue (1963) reported that Skid Row men shared three conditions in that they were homeless, poor and had a multiplicity of personal problems, which included poor interpersonal relationships that led to daily heavy drinking and in withdrawal from conventional family living. Bogue (1963) went on to outline various problems in identifying numbers of homeless individuals and their needs in physical, psychological and social spheres. He pointed out that Skid Row residents are a divergent and depressed group with high rates of unemployment, incredibly low incomes, irregular employment and low educational status, and contrary to their reputation they were not migratory individuals. These residents could be grouped into disabled, resident working men, 'bums', migratory workers, criminals and workers in illegal enterprises and chronic alcoholics. Runaways and adventurers, vacationers, young veterans, sexual perverts and mentally ill were excluded from the data collection. Over the years the conventional stereotype of the Skid Row homeless individual has given way to a variety of complex images.

Homelessness through its definition focuses on home or roof or shelter and ignores other aspects of individual's social functioning including job, social support, finances etc. (Lipton *et al.*, 1983), although Wright (1989) defines homelessness as a lack of customary regular access to a conventional dwelling unit. All components of this definition can be challenged. The literal homeless with no access at all to any kind of accommodation need to be differentiated from those living in temporary housing or marginal housing.

The range of psychiatric morbidity among the homeless population varies according to diagnosis, method of diagnosis and methods and sources of collection of samples (for a review, see Bhugra, 1993). Craig *et al.* (1995) suggested that prevalence of functional psychoses amongst the users of night shelters could vary between 30% to 50%. The barriers to effective health care for homeless people according to these authors were as follows:

1. The major emphasis of modern psychiatric practice has been the provision of intensive but brief treatment for the acute phase of a mental illness.
2. Psychiatric services are organized to serve specific geographical sectors.
3. A shift in overall health care resources away from people with chronic severe mental illness.
4. Failure to recognize the high care needs of homeless mentally ill people who formerly resided in the large direct access hostels.

With an increasing emphasis on care in the community in spite of the existence of various legislations, identification and management of mental illness in the homeless population is a problem.

The recommendations put forward by Craig *et al.* (1995) are useful for the service providers as well as the clients and government departments. The political will to bring about a more stable and permanent change is paramount in providing accommodation that is affordable and reliable. The provision of services will vary according to the local needs and the pace at which shift to the community services occurs (for details, see Bhugra *et al.*, 1995). This volume offers a snap-shot view of the relationship between homelessness and mental illness across the globe. This is not a comprehensive view taking in all nations or cultures, but a selected few where the literature and experience of dealing with homelessness is widely available.

The history of homelessness is discussed by Timms in Chapter 2. His caution that the history of homelessness is affected by the silence of the homeless themselves is an important one. Access to legislative historical material can offer only one perspective. Although the monasteries and houses of religion may have sheltered some who may have been classified as homeless in other times, the lunatic pauper was not an unknown figure. Homeless people, as well as the mentally ill homeless, have been around for several centuries – the lesson being that their needs may not have changed but both the resources available and the public perception have changed.

McNaught and Bhugra discuss at length in Chapter 3 the definitions and problems associated with such definitions as well as pathways into homelessness. Employment, social support and family set-up together with social security regulations all play a role in the process of homelessness, as well as in keeping the individual in the state of homelessness. Health and social policies impact upon the process and state of homelessness. The causation of and influence on the homelessness of the young male will differ from that seen on the married or single mother with young children or infants (Chapter 4). The dangers of homelessness vary according to the age, gender and ethnicity of the individual. The specific gender role expectations as well as mothering styles and techniques along with public mothering produce incredible pressures on the young single mother who may have very temporary or marginal housing, no social support, no economic benefits and poor role models for mothering. The young homeless boy may move to the metropolis attracted by the bright lights and then be forced to earn money as a prostitute with inherent sexual and physical dangers. The spread of HIV infection may work as a further complicating factor. The relationship between being placed in care and subsequent homelessness is fairly well described. The runaway and throwaway youths may have their own different sets of problems and worries. Associated sexual, physical and emotional abuse complicate the picture even further. Physical illness in the homeless may act as co-morbidity with psychiatric illness, but it may also encourage the homeless individual to seek help. Orodental problems in both sexes and gynaecological problems have been well demonstrated and in Chapter 5, Jane Marshall explains the pathways into homelessness of these women. In spite of the age and gender similarities, these groups are still heterogeneous and their restlessness with services along with a degree of rootlessness needs to be taken into account when planning services. A further complication is the complex interaction between homelessness, mental illness and criminal behaviour. Those homeless individuals who have no mental illness also have a low level of criminal convictions, whereas with personality disorders and alcoholism the rates go up tremendously. Although in at least one sample violence was less likely it was still higher than expected for the general population. The emphasis on general materialism can only add to the misery and frustration of the homeless individual who may resort to criminal activities. As Joseph suggests in Chapter 6, the involvement of the police simply because of their availability also means that they are more likely to be involved in the compulsory detention of mentally ill homeless individuals. Even court assessments and court diversion schemes pick up elements of criminal activity among the homeless. As both primary and secondary care may be blocked in this group the response to the treatment may be affected too. Long term follow-ups are difficult due to geographical mobility of the homeless individuals.

The service needs have to take into account the problems associated with sectorization and catchment areas. Although money is supposed to follow the patient the purchaser–provider split on the one hand and fund-holding general practices on the other in the UK make it almost impossible for a needs led service. Furthermore, co-morbidity and dual diagnosis complicated with homeless characteristics make it difficult to access sympathetic services. In Chapter 7, Jane Marshall and Bhugra propose that innovative service provisions are needed, which will include outreach and engagement in non-traditional settings, long-term case management at an intensive level, wide ranging health and housing options and closer links between non-statutory and statutory mental health services. Similar suggestions are put forward in Chapter 8 by Breakey with the American experience behind his team. He proposes that an Assertive Community Team with the inclusion of 'consumer advocates' is one of the many innovative approaches. This coupled with Critical Time Intervention focusing on medication adherence, money management, substance use management and crisis management show encouraging results. There are further innovative strategies that Breakey recommends.

Max Marshall points out in Chapter 9 that the needs of those living in shelters and those living in hostels are relatively different even though a degree of confusion may occur in defining these accommodations and describing their functions. There is an element of hostels being used as stop-gap arrangements initially, but then ending up as 'semi-permanent' placement, but also the findings that earlier rates of schizophrenia in the hostels may have been reported higher than some recent ones. Schizophrenia remains the commonest diagnosis among the mentally ill hostel residents and Max Marshall argues that this group also shows high levels of socially unacceptable behaviour including self-harm, violence and sexually offensive behaviour. All these factors have to be studied and their management added to the package for the individual's needs management.

Another innovative outreach for the mentally ill homeless patients is that of Great Chapel Street where the general practitioners provide an assertive outreach service. In Chapter 11, El-Kabir and Ramsden emphasize that the reasons for consulting doctors are complex and are often not taken lightly in spite of multiple social and physical handicaps. If this consultation process is taken as an enabling process the help-seeking becomes much more acceptable and the response to help itself becomes much more useful and workable. The diversity of the group and the diversity of help available and models available have to be taken into account. To this end the American, the Australian and the European experiences outlined in Chapters 12 to 14 provide outstanding models for learning. It is clear from the Danish example that even in societies with highly developed welfare systems the problems of homelessness among the young, accumulating severely mentally ill in lodging houses and direct discharge of patients from psychiatric hospitals to hostels is not unknown. The impact of political factors is demonstrated by the unification in Germany, which has been associated with an increase in the numbers of homeless individuals. While comparing the needs of homeless mentally ill old individuals across London and New York, Cohen and Crane observe in Chapter 10 that the pathways into homelessness are different – the first episode of homelessness may have been triggered by a specific event although complicating factors related to homelessness may differ in this age group compared to the younger homeless. Economic downturn in both countries in the early 1980s with the loss of manufacturing jobs and the shift to service economies produced similar results. Other welfare factors and deinstitutionalization may have contributed to the absolute numbers of homeless individuals. These differences, as well as similarities, need to be remembered when planning for services for different age groups. Bachrach quite rightly suggests in Chapter 13 that even after mentally ill individuals have been provided with housing they may still be mentally ill. They will require more than a mere residential assignment to deal with their disabilities (which may be multiple) and multiple interventions at multiple levels may be needed. The interaction of sociological and clinical factors may exacerbate restlessness and situational instability and the clinician will have to plan both types of management activities. The Australian experience (Chapter 14) suggests that integration of a state funded mental health care system along with comprehensive health insurance may lead to the promotion and support of primary medical practitioners. The use of life charts enables the clinicians to identify risk factors as well as levels of disaffiliation – both of which play a role in the prevention and management of homelessness as well as mental illness. Although the Melbourne Study defined a substantial core of relatively stable people, these findings are by no means universal. Very few mental health facilities have the resources to provide appropriate housing facilities and similarly very few housing facilities have the resources to provide appropriate care and support for people with psychiatric illness especially if the illness is not under control.

This remains a universal observation and only changes in the social policy may produce changes in the field. Kingdon argues forcefully in Chapter 15 that housing policies, police legislation and the development of appropriate care facilities are crucial in successfully managing people who may have mental illness as well as being homeless. These services have to be evaluated to justify their existence and any improvizations that are made. In Chapter 16 we see that the various methods of evaluating these services have to be more specific for the mentally ill homeless individuals.

This volume begins the dialogue on the clinical, social and psychological needs of homeless individuals in this country with specific examples from various developed countries. The multiplicity of needs means that services need to be sensitive in providing multi-dimensional culturally sensitive services that will also enable the clinician to stop the revolving door phenomena for patients who are chronically severely mentally ill.

References

Bhugra, D. (1993). Unemployment, poverty and homelessness. In D. Bhugra & J. Leff (eds.), *Principles of Social Psychiatry*, pp. 355–84. Oxford: Blackwell Scientific Publications.

Bhugra, D., Bridges, K. & Thompson, C. (1995). *Caring for a Community*. College Council Report. London: Gaskell.

Bogue, D. (1963). *Skid Row in American Cities*. Chicago: University of Chicago Press.

Craig, T., Bayliss, E., Klein, O., Manning, P. & Reader, L. (1995). *The Homeless Mentally Ill Initiative*. London: Department of Health.

Glastonbury, B. (1971). *Homeless Near a Thousand Homes*. London: George Allen & Unwin.

Greve, J., Page, D. & Greve, S. (1971). *Homelessness in London*. Edinburgh: Scottish Academic Press.

Lipton, F. R. M., Sobatin, A. & Katz, S. E. (1983). Down and out in the city: the homeless mentally ill. *Hospital and Community Psychiatry*, **34**, 817–22.

Wright, J. (1989). *Address Unknown: Homeless in America*. New York: Aldine de Gruyter.

2

Homelessness and mental illness: a brief history

Philip Timms

The issue of psychiatric disorder and homelessness is widely believed to be a contemporary phenomenon without historical precedent. Discussion characteristically revolves around the twin topics of hospital closure and 'care in the community' policies. However, there are historical antecedents to the contemporary situation, albeit poorly documented. To limit discussion to the provision or non-provision of psychiatric services is to divorce in an arbitrary and artificial way the history of the homeless mentally ill from the wider context of poverty and homelessness in the UK.

However, the homeless of past centuries were, in the main, without a voice and so all that is left to use are details of legislation, court proceedings, crude occupancy statistics and contemporary mythologies of vagrancy, with the mentally ill mentioned usually only in passing. There have, however, been two common threads running through the centuries. One has been the visibility of the street homeless, leading to the construction of strange mythologies about Mafia-like underworld societies of vagrants (Beier, 1987, pp. 123–45). The other has been the institution established by the state to deal with the poor and indigent – the workhouse.

The evolution of the workhouse

Both homelessness and society's responses to it are products of social conditions. They have been part of the make-up of British society since the late thirteenth century. The first statutes concerned with the issue of homeless people, or vagrants, were passed in 1349, 1351 and 1388.

Of course, during this period, there still flourished large numbers of monasteries and houses of religion that provided a widespread system of relief to the poor. However, the theological landscape was changing. The teaching of St Francis, that total renunciation of possessions was part of a spiritual ideal, had produced a relatively benevolent view of both poverty and of the reliance on others through begging (Southern, 1970). The subsequent growth of the Franciscan order and its acquisition of more worldly elements of wealth and power had produced a more cynical view of this teaching.

The nature of the wandering homeless had also changed. Prior to this period, charity had been extended to the old, the infirm and those on pilgrimages. Now large numbers of destitute industrial workers appeared on the scene and the combination of rising population and falling wages was driving peasants off the land. This had become possible because the feudal contractual relationship between land-lord and villein, which tied the peasant to his land and his lord, had begun to break down. This social dislocation was exacerbated by the profound social disruption of many areas of the country caused by the Black Death (Trevelyan, 1986).

So, the wandering poor came to be seen, at best, as immoral idlers, at worst as a threat to the very fabric of society. Punishment was the mainspring of policy set out in these acts, with the penalty of the stocks for able-bodied beggars. However, the numbers of homeless people increased in spite of the rigours of the legal sanctions. With Henry VIII's dissolution of the monasteries in the first half of the sixteenth century, even the limited provision of religious charity disappeared. The problem, however, remained and so, from 1531 to 1601 the Tudors and Elizabeth I initiated a system of local relief in which the main provider of care was the local parish rather than a religious foundation. New institutions, 'Houses of Correction', or bridewells, were established, the first being chartered in London in 1553. An act of 1576 ordered their establishment in all counties and corporate towns (Power & Tawney, 1924, pp. 307–8). Some of the sentiments of this act are current here and in the USA.

> to the intent youth may be accustomed and brought up in labour
> and work, and then not likely to grow up able rogues, and to the
> intent that such as already be grown up in idleness and so rogues at
> this present, may not have any just excuse in saying that they cannot
> get any service of work
>
> (De Schweinitz, 1943).

These were, in fact, the first workhouses, institutions that persisted up until this century and the descendants of which still survive today in the shape of Department of Social Security (DSS) resettlement units. As the extract from the act suggests, they were supposed to train and rehabilitate through work. However, the aim of punishment was also stated within this and subsequent acts.

The advantage of devolving responsibility to the local level was that any response would be responsive to local need and be locally accountable. On the other hand, no allowance was made for the ability of a given parish to respond to the demands placed upon it. The funds available were insufficient to provide a satisfactory service and by the seventeenth century most were little better than gaols. The workhouses built in the eighteenth century faced similar problems and became similarly squalid and punitive.

The next major development of this service was the Poor Law Amendment Act of 1834, which combined all but the larger parishes into Unions. This reduced the number of workhouses from 15 000 to 650 and resulted in the building of institutions such as the Camberwell Spike, closed in 1985. The test of destitution was merely the willingness to enter the workhouse and it was specified that no resident should be better off than any independent labourer. Conditions were, therefore, made as unpleasant as possible. The works of Dickens and Hardy are eloquent testament to the rigour with which this policy was applied and the dread of the workhouse became a fixed part of the psychological landscape of the English working classes. It was originally recommended that separate institutions should be set up for children and the ill. However, with a few exceptions, General Mixed Workhouses were the rule (Leach & Wing, 1980, pp. 2–4).

In 1864 the Metropolitan Poor Act ordered the unions to provide separate casual wards to segregate the vagrant, mobile poor from the local poor of the parish. In 1982 a 2 day detention system was introduced, whereby the vagrant inmate was obliged to give 1 day's labour for 2 nights' board.

In spite of this statutory provision for the destitute, the rapid urban expansion of the mid-nineteenth century overwhelmed the system that had, after all, originated in a predominantly rural period. Organizations such as the Salvation Army, spurred by the appalling conditions of the workhouses (Booth, 1890), began to see themselves as providers of superior accommodation for the poor that was supportive rather than punitive. Commercial providers, such as Rowton Hotels, saw a niche in the market and developed dormitory-style hostels.

Punitive attitudes towards those of no fixed abode began to change, at least in legislation, in 1909 when the Royal Commission on the Poor Law accepted the principle that society's duty was to help the vagrant rather than to punish him (or her). In 1919 the new Ministry of Health assumed responsibility for supervising Poor Law adminis-tration but the individual institutions remained under the direct control of the local Boards of Guardians. In spite of the legislative changes, conditions in the Casual Wards continued to be grim and punitive. It was not until the Poor Law Act of 1930 that the administration of poor relief was taken over by local authorities. A Department Committee that preceded this act estimated that a quarter of the users of casual wards were suffering from mental illness, mental handicap or alcoholism. Separate facilities were recommen-ded for some groups such as women, the sick and the young but none for the mentally ill (Tidmarsh & Wood, 1986).

The advent of the Second World War in 1939 proved to be a watershed for the casual wards. Able-bodied men were recruited for the war effort and the occupancy of casual wards dropped to a few thousand from a peak of 16 911 in May 1932. Post-war social optimism led to the belief that 'vagrancy' could be eradicated, leading to the establishment of the National Assistance Board (NAB) in 1948. Its aim was 'to make provision whereby persons without a settled way of living may be influenced to lead a more settled way of life'. The Casual Wards were taken over so that the NAB could 'provide and maintain centres, to be known as reception centres, for the temporary board and lodging of such persons'. However, by this time occupancy had dropped to levels that rendered most of them redundant. This was presumably due to high levels of employment at the time and to the welfare state's newly introduced provisions for ameliorating poverty and preventing destitution. Thus, the NAB promptly closed 136 of the 270 centres it had taken over, the number declining to just 17 in 1970. However, echoes of the workhouse remained. Instead of a day's work there was a 'work task' that had to be completed before an individual could leave after an overnight stay. A study published in 1964 revealed that men dependent on reception centre food had suffered from severe malnutrition (Ollendorff & Morgan, 1968).

Sick bays were established, visiting medical officers appointed, and referrals increasingly made to local services (Tidmarsh, 1972). However, this seemed to make little impact on the high levels of psychiatric morbidity in such establishments (Edwards *et al.*, 1968).

The 'lunatic paupers'

A stock character of the Elizabethan and Jacobean period was the wandering lunatic, the Tom O'Bedlam or Abram Man. Shakespeare gives Lear a short speech bemoaning the fate of those with 'houseless heads and unfed sides' and chastises himself, as sovereign, for having 'ta'en too little care of this'. Edgar then enters, disguised as a madman who calls himself 'poor Tom ... whom the foul fiend vexes' (King Lear, Act III, Scene IV). However, the documentary evidence is scant and contradictory concerning the real-life patterns for this archetypal character. The names seem to have derived from the Bethlehem hospital, Abram possibly referring to the name of one of the wards. By the early seventeenth century it only had between 20–30 beds to serve the whole country (MacDonald, 1981), so it is perhaps not surprising that ex-patients were to be found wandering the highways and byways of the land. According to different accounts they either made marks on their arm or carried a tin plate on their arm to identify them as ex-patients. This has been interpreted as amounting to a licence to beg, and there is a recorded case of a false licence having been bought to facilitate begging in 1598. However by 1675 the practice had presumably died out as the governors of Bethlehem made a public announcement that people presenting themselves in this way were frauds (Beier, 1987, pp. 115–17). Licence or not, in Elizabethan England the standard method of dealing with them seems to have been that described by Edgar in King Lear: 'Whipped from tithing to tithing, and stock-punish'd and imprison'd'.

One of the first specific legislative mentions of the homeless mentally ill is to be found in an Act of Parliament of 1714 concerned with the management of vagrancy in general (Allderidge, 1979). The 'Act for ... the More Effectual Punishing of such Rogues, Vagabonds, Sturdy Beggars, and Vagrants, and Sending them Whither They Ought to be Sent'. It specifically forbade whipping for lunatics. The objects of this act were 'Persons of little or no Estates, who, by

Lunacy, or otherwise, are furiously mad, and dangerous to be permitted to go abroad'. It empowered two or more Justices of the Peace to confine such persons 'safely locked up in such secure place' while 'such lunacy or madness shall continue'. The costs for any such confinement for paupers would be met by the parish concerned – as today, the funding was supposed to follow the patient. Failing this, the act also empowered Justices to return anyone so confined who did not belong to the parish or town in which they were arrested. An amendment in 1744 (Porter, 1989, p. 118) was only notable in providing for 'keeping, maintaining and curing' – cure being mentioned for the first time.

There is little evidence of the numbers confined as a result of this act, or of the situations in which they were to be confined. There was, after all, only one asylum in the whole country, Bethlem (Parry-Jones, 1972). Some workhouses, such as St Peter's in Bristol, separated the 'pauper lunatics' from those of sound mind (Porter, 1989, p. 118). Others did not. In 1812, the philanthropist Sir George Onesiphorous Paul (Paul, 1812) found individuals deemed mad 'chained in the cellar or garret of a workhouse'. More often they would be 'fastened to the leg of a table, tied to a post in an outhouse, or perhaps shut up in an uninhabited ruin; or if his lunacy be inoffensive, left to ramble half naked and half starved through the streets and highways, teased by the scoff and jest of all that is vulgar, ignorant and unfeeling'. It is perhaps worth remembering that his observations formed part of an argument for the establishment of separate institutions for the mentally ill.

A House of Commons committee of 1807 reported that there were 1765 pauper lunatics in Poor Houses, Houses of Industry and Houses of Correction (Porter, 1989). Further evidence that workhouses continued to serve as repositories for the mentally ill comes from a comment in a Poor Law Commissioners report of 1842.

> From the express prohibition of the detention of dangerous persons of unsound mind in a workhouse ... combined with the prevalent practice of keeping insane persons in a workhouse before the passing of the Poor Law Amendment Act, it may be inferred that persons of unsound mind, not being dangerous, may be legally kept in a workhouse. It must, however, be remembered that with lunatics, the first object ought to be their cure by means of proper medical treatment. This can only be obtained in a well-regulated asylum; and therefore the detention of any curable lunatic in a workhouse is highly objectionable on the score both of humanity and economy.

Again, the possibility of cure is mentioned, with the optimistic premise that what could not be achieved by the workhouse could be achieved by the asylum.

This disapproval of the use of the workhouse as accommodation for the mentally ill was echoed 17 years later by the Lunacy Commission (1859) who stated 'stringent conditions (to deal with able bodied paupers of sound mind) are not only unnecessary for the insane but are obviously very unjust and detrimental to them'.

A further tangential reference is found in the observations made by a foreign visitor in 1871 on the functions of the workhouse:

> The workhouse purports at one and the same time to be: (i) a place where able-bodied adults who cannot or will not find employment can be set to work; (ii) an asylum for the blind, the deaf and dumb or otherwise incapacitated for labour; (iii) a hospital for the sick poor; (iv) a school for orphans, foundlings, and other poor children; (v) a lying in home for mothers; (vi) an asylum for those of unsound mind not being actually dangerous; (vii) a resting place for such vagabonds as it is not deemed possible or desirable to send to prison
>
> (Webb & Webb, 1929).

The general feeling that the workhouse was not a good place for the mad resulted in 1875 in a weekly grant to all unions in England and Wales from the Poor Law Board. Four shillings per person per week was to be paid towards the extra cost of maintaining pauper lunatics in county asylums (Cochrane, 1988). As the entire cost would otherwise fall upon the local parish rates, this was a powerful inducement and could result in the saving of 60% of a local metropolitan union's expenditure on such people. However, in 1889 14% (11 827) of pauper lunatics in England and Wales outside London were still confined in workhouses, 8% at home and 78% in county asylums. However, in London only 2% (275) were accommodated in workhouses, 2% at home and 96% in London City Council (LCC) asylums. This can be related to the LCC's vigorous programme of asylum-building, prompted by the expense of paying for placements outside the LCC area. So, outside London at least, the workhouse continued to be a substantial provider of shelter for the mentally ill up until the First World War.

From then until the Second World War very little seems to have been written on the subject. Even George Orwell does not seem to have noticed any madness in his perambulations through the world of the destitute in the London and Paris of the 1930s. To be fair, he was at pains to stress the ordinariness of the men who found themselves destitute, to portray them as the casual victims of a callous economic system. However, he does seem to have noticed that 'there is an imbecile in every collection of tramps' (Orwell, 1933) – presumably those who would today be regarded as having learning difficulties.

The hostel closure 'programme'

Much has been written both for and against the closure of mental hospitals over the last 40 years although the decline in psychiatric bed numbers began in 1955. Over the last 15 years a parallel series of institutional closures has been in train, the closure of the traditional hostels for the homeless. These included not only the DHSS reception centres/resettlement units but also Salvation Army Hostels, Rowton Houses and night shelters. There was never any overall, co-ordinated plan and the closures took place for a variety of reasons, similar in many ways to those leading to the closures of mental hospitals. Three of the Rowton hotels precipitated a crisis in 1983 (GLC, 1986), when local authorities, Camden in particular, started to pressure the owners into improving the conditions in their squalid establishments. The company owning the Rowton hotels promptly threatened to evict all the residents. The situation was resolved by the local authorities responsible buying the three hostels, with the objective of closing them within 5 years.

Nationally, the DHSS had a policy of closing resettlement units for some time in 1975 (Hewettson, 1975), having contracted from 215 in 1948 to 21 in 1970. It was felt that centrally-funded institutions were inappropriate in view of the responsibilities incumbent on local social service and housing departments. In addition, large institutions were viewed as unsuitable places for influencing people 'to lead a more settled way of life'.

A policy was decided on the closure of all resettlement units and their replacement by local initiatives, spear-headed by the closure of the Camberwell reception centre in September 1985. A system of capital and revenue grants was to be made available to alternative providers, who were expected to include the voluntary sector and local authorities. Perhaps significantly, the word 'community' was used to describe these new hostels. There was to be no overall reduction in funding, but potential service-providers were slow in coming forward. Eight such schemes had been approved by 1989, but none had sufficient bed-spaces to replace the units due for closure. The resettlement agency thus found itself double-funding and the closure policy stalled (The Resettlement Units Executive Agency, 1991). There now remained 1796 beds in resettlement units, 670 of which were in London, the national focus of the homelessness problem.

In London in 1981 there were 9751 bed spaces in direct access hostels, 6000 in large, traditional hostels for the homeless. A report by the London Boroughs Association (LBA) described them as 'at once a resource and a problem' (GLC/LBA, 1981). A resource because of the shelter provided, a problem because of the often appalling physical conditions and catastrophically inadequate staffing. This same report recommended the opening of 600 beds yearly to replace the old hostels, but noted that such schemes were facing financial and planning difficulties. Belated enforcement of fire regulations led to the contraction of some hostels and the closure of others, most recently the 280-bedded Salvation Army hostel in Blackfriars Road in 1991. By 1985 the numbers of direct access bed-spaces had declined to 4885 (SHIL, 1986) and by 1990 to around 2000 (Harrison *et al.*, 1992). The closure of the Camberwell Spike alone, the largest of the old NAB reception centres, resulted in the loss of 900 bed-spaces. Direct access reprovision for this institution amounted to only 62 bed-spaces, the result being in specialist referral-only units.

The Spicer initiative hostels and cold-weather shelters pushed the number up to 2533 in 1991, but this still meant that there had been a 75% loss of direct-access hostel spaces over the previous decade.

Psychiatry and the homeless mentally ill

The first psychiatrist to address the issue directly was a German psychiatrist, K. Wilmanns, (1906). At this time in Germany, vagrancy was an offence and those who could not demonstrate that they had a home to go to could be arrested and confined in the police workhouse. He noticed that many of the homeless so detained were transferred to his hospital from the local workhouse. In his survey of these patients he found 120 homeless men and women who had been committed with a diagnosis of schizophrenia. American workers Faris & Dunham (1959) suggested in 1939 that the prevalence of mental illness was higher in what they called 'the disorganised community'.

Two roughly-equivalent descriptive classifications of the homeless were constructed, both breaking down the population into itinerant workers, itinerant non-workers and non-itinerant non-workers. Anderson, an American sociologist writing in the 1920s (Anderson, 1922) called these respectively hobos, tramps and bums. Thirty years later Henri Ey, a French psychiatrist (Vexliard, 1953), used the terms errants, vagabonds and clochards to label equivalent groups.

Neither of these served to clarify matters to any degree. More significantly Bogue, a sociologist, looked at the inhabitants of Chicago's Skid Row in 1956 (Bogue, 1963). Although alcoholism was his main focus (and indeed he found a very high rate of alcoholism) his non-psychiatric researchers noted that roughly one in five of the men he interviewed were suffering from 'mental illness' or 'mental and nervous trouble' of some description. He commented that voluntary agencies should be able to 'recommend a psychiatric examination' in order to provide this section of the destitute population with an appropriate service.

Post-war interest in this country started with Stuart Whiteley's 1955 review of a series of acute male admissions to a South London observation ward. He noted that 8% were of no fixed abode, a much higher proportion than would be expected from the numbers of homeless men in the local area. He diagnosed around a third as suffering from schizophrenia, mostly with delusional ideas. He noted that, compared with homeless men with other diagnoses, those suffering from schizophrenia tended to be living in the most impoverished circumstances, such as night shelters, rather than common lodging houses. His view was that, for his patients, 'the main cause [of homelessness] is the personality defect which does not allow him to form relationships'. He went on to recommend that

> When he falls ill, the down and out should, ideally, be treated in a separate institution ... where his environment was as near his normal habitat as possible. He would then be more likely to stay ... it would be an advantage if he could be committed to the institution for a definite period, and as so many appear in court, this should be possible.
>
> (Whiteley, 1955).

By the time Birmingham psychiatrists Berry and Orwin conducted a survey of admissions in 1966, 23% of their acute male admissions were of no fixed abode. In addition, this proportion was rising fast compared with non-urban hospitals in their region. Of these homeless patients, 74% had previous hospital admission and the authors commented that 'Their plight is evidence that the initial enthusiasm evoked by the new act [1959 Mental Health Act] for the discharge of psychotics into the community was premature and has resulted in the overwhelming of community services'. They also recognized a housing issue: 'Redevelopment of the centre of Birmingham has resulted in a reduction in the number of lodgings available for persons of no fixed abode'.

Their identification of the themes of inadequate community care and lack of low-cost housing was prescient, but their recommendation of further investigation into this phenomenon did not bear fruit. These first studies of those who had actually managed to come to the attention of hospital services were followed by more epidemiological surveys of hostel populations. Griffith Edwards in London was the first to survey a hostel, interviewing (with a team) the entire population of the Camberwell Reception Centre on one night in 1968 (Edwards *et al.*, 1968). He found that the proportion of those who had been admitted to mental hospital, 25%, equalled the proportion of those with alcohol problems. This was the first epidemiological evidence to challenge the almost universal stereotype of the homeless man as drinker.

This evidence for a high prevalence of mental illness in the homeless population was confirmed by Ian Lodge Patch's 1970 doorstep survey (Lodge Patch, 1971) of two Salvation Army hostels for men. He diagnosed 15% as suffering from schizophrenia and an astounding 50% as being personality disordered. As his evaluations were based on one-off interviews, it seems highly likely that many of these men were actually suffering from schizophrenia. He again commented on community care: 'The small number of schizophrenics who were receiving treatment suggests both a failure of community care and inappropriately early discharge'. These sentiments were echoed by Crossley & Denmark (1969) in another survey of a Salvation Army hostel which demonstrated a high prevalence of psychotic illness – 'It is surely not right to unload onto a voluntary organisation, whose function is not to act as a therapeutic agency, patients who still need community care?'

Robin Priest's 1976 Edinburgh survey approached the problem in a more sophisticated fashion, comparing a general survey of the homeless population with those who were actually admitted to

Table 2.1. *British hostel surveys*

Reference	Schizophrenia (%)	Alcoholism (%)	Affective disorder (%)	Personality disorder (%)
Edwards *et al.* (1968)	24	25	N/K	N/K
Crossley & Denmark (1969)	20	N/K	N/K	66
Priest (1976)	32	18	5	18
Lodge patch (1971)	15	N/K	8	51
Tidmarsh (1972)	~25	25	~5	17

N/K, not known.

hospital. He again confirmed a very high prevalence of schizophrenia in the homeless population (32%), but not surprisingly found that this prevalence was greater than in the subgroup of the homeless population presenting to psychiatric services for treatment. The population outside hospital were more likely to suffer from schizophrenia than those in hospital. This finding suggested that, compared with men with alcohol-related problems or those with personality disorders, those with a diagnosis of schizophrenia tended not to find their way to treatment services (see Table 2.1).

In fact, over the majority of the post-war period, successive surveys in British hostels, night shelters and prisons (Coid, 1988) have demonstrated the presence of large numbers of homeless men with schizophrenia and alcohol problems. There has been a curious absence of those less-severe anxiety and depressive disorders that characterize the bulk of the psychiatric symptomatology presenting in a general practice setting. This may have been due to more extreme psychopathology tending to mask more affective complaints.

Conclusion

Homeless people, and thus the homeless mentally ill, have been a constant feature of the English social landscape since the fourteenth century. The mechanisms for dealing with the problem have been moulded by the changing tempers of the times. Throughout the centuries, societal attitudes towards the homeless and the homeless mentally ill have been characterized by a cycle of vacillation between ideas of punishment and ideas of help.

Although sparsely documented, the presence of the mentally ill in those institutions set up to deal with the homeless and indigent has been a recurrent theme since the latter part of the seventeenth century. Disquiet about this situation was intermittently expressed by various committees from the mid-nineteenth century. Even at this time, the heyday of the Victorian asylum, it appears that substantial numbers of the mentally ill were still accommodated in Poor Law institutions rather than psychiatric ones. What evidence there is suggests that the essentials of the situation have remained substantially unchanged over the last 150 years, straddling the period of the asylum's ascendancy, the era of psychiatric deinstitutionalization and latterly the era of 'community care'. Even when its resources were apparently greater, certainly in terms of bed numbers, psychiatry had never really got to grips with the substantial numbers of people with severe, long-term psychiatric illness who were accommodated in institutions for the indigent and homeless (Craig & Timms, 1992).

The action taken by government in the 1980s and 1990s in setting up the Central London Homeless Mentally Ill Initiative was prompted by the new visibility of the homeless mentally ill on the streets. In many people's minds that was a consequence of the closures of psychiatric units. However, the evidence suggests that it had more to do with the hostel deinstitutionalization of the 1980s than the decline in psychiatric beds, which had been going on for 35 years. This suggests the depressing idea that, in spite of recent rhetoric about community care, society at large has always been intimidated by the sight of the homeless mentally ill and has always been quite happy to lock them away. Whether it is in an asylum, a workhouse or a prison does not really seem to matter. There have been recent efforts to bring psychiatric and social care to some of these milieux. Only time will tell if these enterprises can produce a significant shift from the low-cost, no-care solutions of the past.

References

Allderidge, P. (1979). Hospitals, madhouses and asylums: cycles in the care of the insane. *British Journal of Psychiatry*, **134**, 321–33.
Anderson, N. (1922). *The Hobo: The Sociology of the Homeless Man.* Chicago: University of Chicago Press.

Beier, A. L. (1987). *Masterless Men: The Vagrancy Problem in England 1560–1640*. London: Methuen.

Berry, C. & Orwin, A. (1966). No fixed abode: a survey of mental hospital admissions. *British Journal of Psychiatry*, **112**, 1019–25.

Bogue, D. J. (1963). *Skid Row in American cities*. Chicago: Community and Family Study Centre, University of Chicago.

Booth, C. (1890). *In Darkest England and the way out*. New York: Funk & Wagnalls.

Cochrane, C. (1988). *The Asylum and its Psychiatry*. Routledge: London.

Coid, J. W. (1988). Mentally abnormal prisoners on remand. I. Rejected or accepted by the NHS? *British Medical Journal*, **296**, 1779–82.

Craig, T. & Timms, P. W. (1992). Out of the wards and onto the streets? Deinstitutionalisation and homelessness in Britain. *Journal of Mental Health*, **1**, 265–75.

Crossley, B. & Denmark, J. C. (1969). Community care – a study of the psychiatric morbidity of a Salvation Army hostel. *British Journal of Sociology*, **20**, 443–9.

De Schweinitz, K. (1943). *England's Road to Social Security*. Pittsburgh: University of Pennsylvania Press.

Edwards, G., Williamson, V., Hawker, A., Hensman, C. & Postsyan, S. (1968). Census of a reception centre. *British Journal of Psychiatry*, **114**, 1031–9.

Faris, R. E. & Dunham, H. W. (1959). *Mental Disorders in Urban Areas: an Ecological Study of Schizophrenia and other Psychoses*. Chicago: University of Chicago Press.

GLC (Greater London Council) (1986). *Four Victorian Hostels*. London Borough of Havering: GLC.

GLC/LBA (Greater London Council/London Boroughs Association) (1981). Report of a Joint Working Party on provision in London for people without a settled way of living. *Hostels for the Single Homeless in London*. London: LBA.

Harrison, M., Chandler, R. & Green, G. (1992). *Hostels in London: A Statistical Overview*. London: Resource Information Service.

Hewettson, J. (1975). Homeless people as an at-risk group. *Proceedings of the Royal Society of Medicine*, **68**, 9–13.

Leach, J. & Wing, J. (1980). *Helping Destitute Men*. London: Tavistock.

Lodge Patch, I. (1971). Homeless men in London. I. Demographic findings in a lodging house sample. *British Journal of Psychiatry*, **118**, 313–17.

Lunacy Commission (1859). Supplement to Twelfth Report of the Commissioners in Lunacy. London: House of Commons.

Macdonald, M. (1981). *Mystical Bedlam*. Cambridge: Cambridge University Press.

Ollendorff, R. J. V. & Morgan, A. (1968). Survey of Residents in Camberwell Reception Centre. Unpublished report to the National Assistance Board.

Orwell, G. (1933). *Down and Out in Paris and London*. London: Penguin.
Parry-Jones, W. L. (1972). *The Trade in Lunacy*. London: Routledge.
Paul, G. O., Sir (1812). *Observations on the Subject of Lunatic Asylums*. Gloucester: private publication.
Porter, R. (1989). *Mind-forg'd Manacles: A History of Madness in England from the Restoration to the Regency*. London: Penguin.
Power, E. & Tawney, R. H. (eds.) (1924). *Tudor Economic Documents*, vol. II.
Priest, R. G. (1976). The homeless person and the psychiatric services: an Edinburgh survey. *British Journal of Psychiatry*, **128**, 128–36.
SHIL (Single Homelessness in London) (1986). A Report by the Single Homelessness in London Working Party. London: SHIL.
Southern, R. W. (1970). *Western Society and the Church in the Middle Ages*. Harmondsworth: Penguin.
The Resettlement Units Executive Agency. (1991). Annual Report and Financial Statement 1990/91. London: HMSO.
Tidmarsh, D. (1972). Services for the destitute: Camberwell reception centre. In J. Wing & A. M. Hailey (eds.), *Evaluating a Community Psychiatric Service. The Camberwell Register, 1964–1971*, pp. 73–6. Oxford: Oxford University Press.
Tidmarsh, D. & Wood, S. (1986). Report to DHSS on Research at Camberwell Reception Centre. London: Institute of Psychiatry. (Unpublished).
Trevelyan, G. M. (1986). *English Social History*. London: Penguin.
Vexliard, A. (1953). *Le Clochard: Étude de Psycholgie Sociale*. Paris: Desclee de Brouwer.
Webb, S. & Webb, B. (1929). *English Poor Law History: Part 2: The Last Hundred Years*. London: Longmans, Green & Co.
Whiteley, J. S. (1955). Down and out in London: mental illness in the lower social groups. *Lancet*, **2**, 608–10.
Wilmanns, K. (1906). Zur psychopathologie des landstreichers: eine klinishe studie. Leipzig: Johann Ambrosius Barth.

3

Models of homelessness

ALAN MCNAUGHT AND DINESH BHUGRA

Introduction

There is no single definition of homelessness accepted by all who use this term. Homelessness exists throughout this and other nations as will become extremely clear in the accounts in this book, and the homeless population is diverse.

In the UK, the National Assistance Act of 1948 requires every local authority to provide 'temporary accommodation for persons who are in urgent need thereof, being need arising in circumstances that would not reasonably have been foreseen'. Hence, local authorities have a statutory obligation to provide accommodation to individuals who are roofless, and have not placed themselves in this state. In practical terms, this definition of homelessness is probably the most important one for individuals living in the UK. When these conditions are fulfilled, local authorities have a statutory obligation to act and provide shelter to the homeless person.

Whether individuals have been 'blameworthy' in becoming homeless, or not, remains an arbitrary decision made by local authorities. Because resources are scarce, a narrow working definition of homelessness tends to be used. Local authorities are more likely to embrace the needs of homeless families, rather than the single homeless, hence the latter group are more likely to be excluded, under the terms of the Act.

Voluntary agencies working with homeless people have tended to use a far broader definition of homelessness. The charity Shelter working for the homeless, for instance, extends the definition of homelessness to those living in very bad housing conditions. Thus people living in very poor quality housing, or sleeping over with friends on a temporary basis, or squatting in a derelict flat would also be defined as homeless. The emphasis is on 'home' rather than the conditions. The limits of such a definition remain unclear.

It emerges that there remains no single consensual definition of homelessness and that any definition will lie somewhere on a spectrum between 'not deliberately roofless' to 'all roofless and all those resident in bad housing'. It is important to bear this debate in mind while assessing any models of homelessness.

Wright (1989) has stated that to be homeless is to lack 'regular and customary access to a conventional dwelling unit'. He goes on to draw a distinction between the literally homeless (those individuals who live and sleep on the streets), and the marginally homeless (those 'who have a more or less reasonable claim to a more or less stable housing situation of more or less minimal adequacy, being closer to the "less" than the "more" on one or all criteria'.) In attempting to define homelessness, we have, therefore, concentrated on only one aspect of homeless peoples' lives – their residential situation. Bachrach (1984) has stated that 'most current definitions appear to agree, either implicitly or explicitly, that for homelessness to be present, the absence of physical residence must occur under conditions of social isolation or dissatisfaction'. Lipton *et al.* (1983) have made a similar point stating that the term 'homeless' is a misnomer, a catchword that discounts other aspects of individuals lives (e.g. their employment status, health, social ties). Pointing out that social isolation is a part of homeless peoples' lives, does not, however, help us to arrive at a clear definition of the term.

One question that needs to be considered, if one wishes to define homelessness is 'how long is someone roofless before they are homeless?' If someone is without accommodation for one day, are they homeless? If not, when do they become homeless? Is it a week or a month or longer? It is obvious that there is no one definition that is universally accepted, or likely to be acceptable. This is because different terms reflect, in part, the needs of those giving the definition. This disagreement and difficulty do hamper research on homelessness (Bachrach, 1984). Without a single agreed definition, it is difficult to compare different bodies of research. Often a relatively accessible group of homeless people (e.g. hostel dwellers) are defined as 'the homeless' and their characteristics generalized to other groups of homeless people. It is, therefore, particularly important with any research or discussion of homelessness to ask who is included and who excluded by the definition being used, and avoid generalizing findings to other groups of homeless people to whom they may not apply (see also Chapter 8).

Classification

Within this diversity of homeless people there are, however, sub-groups of homeless individuals who share characteristics and may also share certain needs. Classifying homeless people is of use if identification of a subgroup of homeless people leads to greater understanding of how individuals in that group became homeless and how they can be helped. Classification can be based on aetiology (how individuals became homeless), on current impairment or on socio-demographic factors. Classification of any group of people should, ideally, include all members of the group, in discrete and readily recognizable subgroups of individuals.

Leach (1979) proposed that homeless people should be divided into 'intrinsics' and 'extrinics'. 'Intrinsics' were homeless people whose mental or physical disability was the cause of their homelessness, and had therefore predicted their homelessness. 'Extrinsics', by contrast, were homeless because of situational factors (e.g. job loss, poverty etc.). He stated that the two groups would require different services. Their needs and priorities will differ as will their management.

Morse et al. (1991) proposed a system that focuses on current psychiatric or physical impairment, regardless of whether such impairment was the original cause of the homelessness, or not. They demonstrated that both systems identified subgroups with different needs, but that their system was superior at identifying groups of individuals with high levels of service needs. Cohen (1994, and Chapter 10) suggests that the characterizations of homelessness as a trait rather than a state reflect the tensions between social justice and public concepts as well as economic resources.

The UK Royal College of Psychiatrists Working Party Report on Homelessness and Mental Illness (Bhugra, 1991) recommended that three categories of homeless people be recognized: the single homeless, young single homeless and homeless families. The single homeless have been the most extensively investigated group, to date. The group consists of single men and women over 25 years of age. Wright

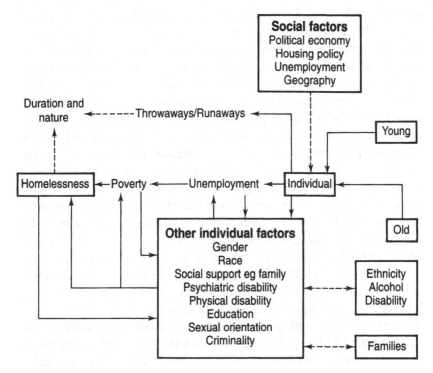

Figure 3.1. Pathways into homelessness and types and interaction of various factors.

(1989) argues that subgroups of homeless are very different and they can be divided according to social origins, background characteristics and needs. The portrait can be of a pathway into homelessness along with uniqueness of each group. In addition he challenges the concepts of deserving and undeserving homeless people. These remain moral judgements. He classified homeless as homeless families, lone homeless (which were further subdivided into men, children and women), and then those with special factors like disability, ethnicity, education, geography, criminality, extreme poverty and nature and reasons for homelessness. In the study conducted by Wright & Weber (1987) 16–26% belonged to homeless family groups and the rest were defined as lone homeless. Furthermore, 6% were children or adolescents below 19 years of age, 20% were adult women and 74% were adult men (see Figure 3.1 for pathways into homelessness and types of homelessness). This is not a clear, linked pathway and various factors influence it along the way. The vast majority of the single homeless are males. The level of psychiatric morbidity in this group is known to be high. Weller *et al.* (1989) reported that 41% of a group of single homeless attending a Christmas shelter gave a history of psychosis and 72% were psychotic at the time of interview. Previously published estimates of what Wright (1989) calls ADM disorders (alcoholism, drug abuse and mental illness) among the homeless have varied from 10–55% (see also Bhugra, 1993 for a review). It is worth emphasizing once again that the subset of homeless people who have addiction problems may need very specialized housing and social service needs. Substance abuse may be a consequence of homelessness as observed by Winkleby & White (1992). Alcohol, Skid Row and single male homeless are inextricably linked in the public conscious- ness. As Wright (1989) points out this stereotype is not entirely without foundation and citing data from his studies in New York, where alcohol abuse among homeless men dropped from 49% in 1968–72 to 28% in 1981–84 suggests that alcohol abuse is not that unimportant a factor in homelessness but that other factors have become far more important. As with most of the studies on homeless- ness, the role of alcohol abuse and definition of alcoholism also varies and Wright (1989) sets this figure around 40%. It is difficult to know how these rates measure up to the control (let us say 'normal') population when the exact rates of alcohol abuse are not clear in this group. Of a subsample of 204 homeless persons who had an alcohol problem, among the total of 979, it was observed that they were male, white and old with more troubled marital histories along with social isolation, transiency and longer periods of unemployment (Roth & Bean, 1985). Similar findings emerged from the work of Wright *et al.* (1985) as well as from Winkleby & White's (1992) survey. In the New York survey of Wright *et al.* (1985), American Indians had the highest rates and the Hispanics and Asians the lowest – irrespective of gender. It is worth noting that homeless people may drink or use chemicals to alleviate the miseries of life and to cope as best they can in a cloud and haze of alcohol and chemicals.

Pathways

In this section of the chapter we shall attempt to define some of the pathways that lead to a person being homeless. Lamb & Lamb (1990) questioned the underlying reasons for the chronically and severely mentally ill becoming and remaining homeless. A shortage of housing of course may lead to or cause homelessness among the mentally ill. In addition problems of resources within agencies providing services, may add to the confusion in terms of identifying needs and not offering adequate and appropriate services may well lead to homelessness. Problems of youth, co-morbidity with substance abuse and laws are said to contribute to homelessness (Gelberg *et al.*, 1988; Koegel & Burnam, 1988; Koegel *et al.*, 1988; see also Figure 3.1). The question that Lamb & Lamb are addressing in their study is to find out how mental illness contributes to homelessness. Cohen & Thompson (1992) argue that the difference between homeless mentally ill and mentally ill homeless is not purely semantic. Deinstitutionalization is seen as an important factor in the increasing tide of homeless mentally ill. These authors assert that homelessness as a problem of severe mental illness emerged in the early 1980s and the biases were created by methodological weaknesses in the research. More rigorous scientific studies have reported much lower rates (see Bhugra, 1993 for a review). Lamb & Lamb (1990) studied 53 consecutive admissions of homeless people (those who were living on the streets, on the beach, in parks or public places – shelters not included) using a structured interview. Forty patients were male and 42 had had a prior psychiatric hospitalization and 87% had manifested major overt psychopathology at the point of admission. Two thirds were diagnosed as having schizophrenia. On the other hand a study by Winkleby & White (1992) reported that of 1399 homeless adults studied, 45.6% reported no impairments. They were distinguished by being younger, minority status and lower educational status. In this study injuries were the commonest physical health problem. They became homeless at an older age and most had worked full-time before the onset of the problem. Those who had a history of psychiatric hospitalization reported high rates of physical and sexual abuse and foster care placement before the age of 18. Respondents with multiple disorders on becoming homeless reported the highest prevalence of divorce and separation. Those who did not have any impairment at the onset of homelessness developed substance abuse the longer they remained homeless. This study has some methodological problems but the demonstration of pathways is interesting.

The large numbers of homeless people seen in inner cities has raised the question of their origin. One popular answer to this is that deinstitutionalization and inadequate community provisions for psychiatric patients has led to large numbers of psychiatric patients now living 'on the streets'. This remains a controversial argument. It has been demonstrated on numerous occasions that a large proportion of homeless people suffer with severe psychiatric disabilities. Various studies (Marshall, 1989; Priest, 1971) have reported levels of severe psychiatric morbidity of between 20 and 40% in homeless patients in a variety of settings (hostels, street dwellers etc.). However, it is less clear what levels of various psychiatric contact these patients have had. When the question has been posed only small numbers of patients have had prolonged previous psychiatric contact. Timms & Fry (1989) reported that 7 out of 124 homeless men using a London hostel had had psychiatric admissions for longer than a year, despite the fact that over 50% had severe psychiatric illnesses. Dayson (1993) reported on the levels of vagrancy amongst patients with severe psychiatric illnesses 1 year after these patients had been moved from psychiatric hospitals (where they had had an average stay of 15.5 years) to community hostels. Of the 278 patients discharged, only one had definitely, and a further five had possibly, become vagrants. A further one patient had been imprisoned and 6% had been readmitted to and remained in the psychiatric hospital. Susser et al. (1990) point out that various surveys reported from the USA on the prevalence of mental illness among the homeless have major problems. They suggest that these surveys should be construed as 'case surveys' of homelessness since most gathered data on homeless populations without selecting a comparison (or a control) group. These authors draw our attention not only to the problems of definitions of homelessness but also to differences between incidence and prevalence and problems of sampling. Another caveat in all of these studies is that of standardized measurement of mental disorder in these populations since a number of studies present clinical diagnoses and not operationalized diagnoses. If one was to view the homeless as a specific culture the measurement of certain aspects of mental state will be biased towards the category fallacy that anthropologists caution psychiatrists about. Susser et al. (1990) give the examples of demoralization in the diagnosis of depression. Thus the 'state-dependent' mental state needs to be borne in mind. When exposed to stressors, normal individuals may feel stress that is often reversible. However, this may lead to psychopathology, which is seen to be based on persisting traits of individuals. Susser et al. (1990) draw attention to the point that intense feelings of distress may well be the norm when a person is homeless – whether this is reversible or becomes converted to psychopathology is difficult to ascertain. Any variation in distress may of course result from heterogeneity of stressor as well as from heterogeneity in individual reactions to a similar event.

There is evidence, then, that deinstitutionalization does not lead directly to large numbers of chronically mentally ill people who were previously in institutions becoming homeless. However, deinstitutionalization may have had an impact on younger individuals with severe psychiatric illnesses who have not had long periods of time in psychiatric institutions. Clinicians working in adult psychiatry complain that it is often very difficult to admit acutely disturbed patients due to a lack of available admission beds. Such shortages arise because patients who are no longer acutely ill, remain on admission wards because of the lack of long-term facilities for them to move on to (Hirsch, 1992). One consequence of this is that there is an increased pressure to discharge patients early in their treatment, perhaps to unsuitable facilities. The Mental Health Act Commission has expressed concerns that this policy leads to patients being discharged without adequate aftercare having been organized. Weller *et al.* (1993) pointed out that cuts in social services have increased the difficulty in providing adequate aftercare for psychiatrically ill patients.

Leff (1993) has suggested that the 1983 Mental Health Act may be another reason for the apparent difficulty in admitting acutely ill patients. This Act, 'while safeguarding patients' own rights, has made many health professionals reluctant to use its compulsory powers except in extreme cases'. He further states that the burdens on families caring for psychiatrically ill relatives can lead to such 'interpersonal protection', that patients leave home without having accommodation to move into. It appears likely then that deinstitutionalization may lead to some mentally ill patients being homeless, who would previously have been cared for in long-term or rehabilitation beds of large psychiatric asylums.

Economic factors also play a large part in the plight of the mentally ill. Individuals suffering from a chronic mental illness are unlikely to be able to maintain themselves in employment, particularly at times of high unemployment. High levels of unemployment have been a feature of the UK economy over the last 10–15 years. Poverty is another regular consequence of chronic mental illness (see Bhugra, 1993 for a review). Local authorities' housing stocks have gradually diminished since tenants have bought their properties under the government's 'right to buy' scheme – and this has reduced the stock of cheap rented accommodation. This is the type of accommodation that is particularly required by impoverished individuals and families. Redevelopment and 'gentrification' of the inner cities has also decreased the availability of cheap rented accommodation. In summary, high unemployment and the lack of cheap rented accommodation have combined to make it more difficult for individuals with chronic mental illness to find affordable accommodation.

Individual factors in addition to mental illness are also important in determining the pathway into homelessness.

1. *Gender.* Males are at greater risk of homelessness than females (Rossi *et al.*, 1987). This is particularly true if one is considering the single homeless and the young homeless – but not the case with homeless families, which are usually composed of a mother and her children (Bassuk *et al.*, 1986). Local authority housing policies generally prioritize women with children over single men, and this may be part of the reason why there are more (visible) homeless men. Schizophrenia has an earlier age of onset in men than women (Lewine *et al.*, 1981). Some studies (e.g. Augermeyer *et al.*, 1989) suggest that the outcome of schizophrenia in women is better than in men. The later onset in women may mean that they have a longer period, before becoming ill, during which they have residential stability and build up a network of relationships. These factors, and the relatively better prognosis, may then lessen the likelihood of the women who develop schizophrenia becoming homeless. Furthermore, Bardenstein & McGlashan (1990) have reported that schizophrenic men are prone to express negative, defect symptoms (e.g. social withdrawal), demonstrate anti-social behaviour and misuse drugs and alcohol, all of which would increase their risk of becoming homeless.

Though males are at greater risk of being homeless than females, it should be noted that homeless females exhibit higher levels of serious psychiatric morbidity than males (Marshall & Reed, 1992). They reported that 71% of residents in a hostel for homeless women suffered from schizophrenia. An additional factor reported from Canada (Goering *et al.*, 1990) was the demoralization among the female homeless, although they recognized their needs for resources and skills and felt that they wanted to maintain their autonomy and have their rights respected. Among a sample of 300 women, Smith & North (1994) reported that those with dependent children under the age of 16 were less likely to have psychiatric illness, whereas among those with dependent children not living with them life-time psychiatric illness increased dramatically. Thus, in planning any services not only is needs assessment vital but a consumer preference study to ascertain their values and support is also essential.

2. *Substance misuse*. Wright (1987) has estimated that the rate of alcohol abuse is 3–5 times greater in the homeless. Drug abuse, too, is a common problem, particularly among younger homeless people (Stark *et al.*, 1989). These problems are likely to worsen the longer homelessness continues. The rates of substance abuse have received even less attention. Wright *et al.* (1985) estimated drug abuse rate in their sample to be around 13%. The first choice of 37% of the sample was heroin, methadone or crack and 22% used cocaine. A similar proportion used cannabis and the rest used a miscellany of street drugs. About 58% of the drug abusers were likely to be intravenous abusers. Rates were highest among younger males and the highest rate, unlike that of alcohol, was observed among black men, followed by Hispanic men then black women and then white men. It is not surprising to note that the rates of substance abuse were lower among adult members of homeless families than among lone homeless individuals. The drug problem was most pronounced for homeless men in their late teens and twenties (Wright, 1989). It is again not surprising to find that a range of problems coexists with drug abuse – these include skin disorders, liver disease, AIDS, seizure and other neurological disorders, anaemias and infections with an underlying increase in cases of tuberculosis.

3. *Marital status*. Most of the homeless are single or separated (Burt & Cohen, 1989). This lack of social ties may discourage social stability and hence increase the risk of becoming homeless. It may be that the homelessness led to change in marital status even though the reverse may be true. It is noted that women are more likely to be in shelter or sleeping on friends' floors (see Marshall & Reed, 1992) and also in hostels or bed and breakfast whereas men are more likely to be wanderers.

4. *Separated parents and social services care*. It appears that a large proportion of the homeless, particularly the young single homeless

have come from broken homes or out of social services care (Bhugra, 1993). Such children may have run away from unhappy domestic situations or have been thrown out because of anti-social behaviour. Once 'on the streets', they may become involved in illegal activities, including prostitution and drug and alcohol abuse (Ritter, 1989). The children or teenagers may be runaways or throwaways (for details see Chapters 4 and 6).

5. *Sexual orientation.* Krucks (1991) has reported that young homosexual and bisexual males have become at increased risk of homelessness. They cited prejudice, homophobia and discrimination as the reasons why young gay and bisexual men are more likely to become homeless than their heterosexual counterparts. This process of being thrown out may encourage them to becoming prostitutes.

6. *Ethnic grouping.* Traditionally the homeless in the UK have included disproportionately large numbers of men of Scottish and Irish extraction. A profile of the users of a homeless persons drop-in centre (Baron's Court Report, 1993) in London, for the month of February 1993, revealed that 10% of the users described themselves as African or Caribbean, 7% as black British, 3% as Asian and 20% were of Irish extraction. Leaf & Cohen (1982) in the USA detailed demographic changes in the population of homeless men in New York City shelters between 1970 and 1980. They reported that the proportions of Hispanic and black people amongst the homeless increased during these 10 years. Among women, Smith & North (1994) have reported on high numbers of African American women.

Severe psychiatric illness remains an important factor that may lead to homelessness. Susser *et al.* (1991) measured the prevalence of homelessness (past and present) among 377 patients admitted to a New York State hospital over a period of 3 months. Of this sample 28% had been homeless at some time during their lives. They tested for seven proposed risk factors for homelessness in this mentally ill group: male gender, age under 40 years, black race, urban residence, schizophrenia related diagnosis, alcohol abuse and drug abuse. Somewhat surprisingly, the only significant association with homelessness (revealed by logistic regression analyses) was for urban residence. They concluded that 'the risk factors for homelessness in psychiatric patients may be somewhat different from those on the general population'. This research awaits replication.

As noted above the longer an individual remained homeless, the more likely he/she is to have such impairments. It is, of course, possible that these individuals would have developed psychiatric problems or substance abuse problems anyway, however it seems likely that the stressors inherent in surviving as a homeless person were aetiologically significant. Certainly, it seems unlikely that homelessness per se is likely to be of therapeutic value to individuals suffering from severe mental illness. This having been said, however, Marshall (1989) has noted that hostels for the homeless in Oxford contain a high proportion of mentally ill individuals and tolerate 'a pattern of deviant behaviour similar to that expected in a ward of long stay psychiatric patients'. Such tolerance could be said to create a low 'expressed emotion' environment and may therefore reduce the risk of relapse in individuals with schizophrenia.

In conclusion, the pathways that lead to an individual being homeless and severely mentally ill are multiple, indeed no two people in such a situation have arrived at it by the same route. Social and macro-economic factors are important, particularly in determining the overall levels of homelessness. Policy decisions on the manage-ment of psychiatric patients are likely to play a role that particularly affects the severely mentally ill. Individual characteristics predispose people to becoming homeless. Once homeless one may be at greater risk of becoming mentally ill and developing substance abuse. The effects of severe mental illness leave some individuals at greater risk of becoming homeless. Once homeless and mentally ill, individuals may be caught in a situation that may be beyond their capabilities to alter.

In summary then, this chapter has highlighted the difficulties that exist in attempting to define the term 'homeless' and cautioned against findings on one group of homeless people being applied to others. We have reviewed some of the classification systems used for homeless people and in this book we will use a scheme proposed by the Royal College of Psychiatrists, Working Party (Bhugra, 1991). Finally, we have attempted to highlight some of the pathways that lead to individuals becoming homeless and mentally ill. Both con-clusions may make the occurrence of the other more likely, however economic factors (e.g. unemployment levels, accommodation costs), social and health policies (e.g. deinstitutionalization) and individual characteristics all play roles in predisposing people to these condi-tions.

References

Augermeyer, M. C., Goldstein, J. M. & Kuhu, L. (1989). Gender differences in schizophrenia: rehospitalization and community survival. *Psychological Medicine*, **19**, 365–82.

Bachrach, L. L. (1984). Interpreting research on the homeless mentally ill: some caveats. *Hospital and Community Psychiatry*, **35**, 914–17.

Bardenstein, K. K. & McGlashan, T. H. (1990). Gender differences of affective, schizoaffective and schizophrenic disorders: a review. *Schizophrenia Research*, **3**, 159–72.

Barons Court Report (1993). Barons Court Project – six month monitoring report. Oct 1992 to March 1993. London: Barons Court Project.

Bassuk, E., Rubin, L. & Laurant, A. (1986). Characteristics of sheltered homeless families. *American Journal of Public Health*, **76**, 1097–101.

Bhugra, D. (1991). Homelessness and Mental Illness. Working Party Report, Royal College of Psychiatrists, London.

Bhugra, D. (1993). Unemployment, poverty and homelessness. In D. Bhugra & J. Leff (eds.), *Principles of Social Psychiatry*, pp. 335–84. Oxford: Blackwell Scientific Publications.

Burt, M. R. & Cohen, B. E. (1989). Differences among homeless single women, women with children and single men. *Social Problems*, **36**, 508–24.

Cohen, C. I. (1994). Down and out in New York and London: a cross national comparison of homelessness. *Hospital and Community Psychiatry*, **45**, 769–76.

Cohen, C. I. & Thompson, K. S. (1992). Homeless mentally ill or mentally ill homeless. *American Journal of Psychiatry*, **149**, 816–23.

Dayson, D. (1993). The TAPS project: crime, vagrancy and readmission. *British Journal of Psychiatry*, **162** (Supplement 19), 40–4.

Gelberg, L., Linn, S. & Leake, B. D. (1988). Mental health, alcohol and drug use, and criminal history among homeless adults. *American Journal of Psychiatry*, **145**, 191–6.

Goering, P., Paduchak, D. & Durbin, J. (1990). Housing homeless women: a consumer preference study. *Hospital and Community Psychiatry*, **41**, 790–4.

Herzberg, J. (1987). No fixed abode: a comparison of men and women admitted to an east London psychiatric hospital. *British Journal of Psychiatry*, **156**, 621–7.

Hirsch, S. R. (1992). Services for the severe mentally ill: a planning blight. *Psychiatric Bulletin*, **16**, 673–5.

Koegel, P. & Burnam, M. A. (1988). Alcoholism among homeless adults in the inner city of Los Angeles. *Archives of General Psychiatry*, **45**, 1011–18.

Koegel, P., Burnam, M. A. & Farr, R. K. (1988). The prevalence of specific psychiatric disorders among homeless individuals in the inner city of Los Angeles. *Archives of General Psychiatry*, **45**, 1085–92.

Krucks, G. (1991). Gay and lesbian homeless/street youth: special issues and concerns. *Journal of Adolescent Health*, **12**, 515–18.

Lamb, H. R. & Lamb, D. M. (1990). Factors contributing to homelessness among the clinically and severely mentally ill. *Hospital and Community Psychiatry*, **41**, 301–5.

Leach, J. (1979). Providing for the destitute. In J. K. Wing & R. Olsen (eds.), *Community Care of the Mentally Disabled*, pp. 90–105. Oxford: Oxford University Press.

Leaf, A. & Cohen, M. (1982). *Providing Services for the Homeless: The New York City Program*. New York: City of New York Human Resources Administration.

Leff, J. (1993). All the homeless people where do they all come from? *British Medical Journal*, **306**, 669–70.

Lewine, R. J., Strauss, J. S. & Giff, T. E. (1981). Sex differences in age of first hospital admission for schizophrenia: fact or artifact? *American Journal of Psychiatry*, **138**, 440–4.

Lipton, F. R. M., Sobatin, A. & Katz, S. E. (1983). Down and out in the city: the homeless mentally ill. *Hospital and Community Psychiatry*, **34**, 817–22.

Marshall, M. (1989). Collected and neglected. Are Oxford hostels for the homeless filling up with disabled psychiatric patients? *British Medical Journal*, **299**, 706–9.

Marshall, J. E. & Reed, J. L. (1992). Psychiatric morbidity in homeless women. *British Journal of Psychiatry*, **160**, 761–8.

Morse, G. A., Calsyn, R. J. & Burger, G. K. (1991). A comparison of taxonomic systems for classifying homeless men. *The International Journal of Social Psychiatry*, **37**, 90–8.

Priest, R. G. (1971). The Edinburgh homeless. *American Journal of Psychotherapy*, **25**, 194–213.

Ritter, B. (1989). Abuse of the adolescent: New York state. *Journal of Medicine*, **89**, 156–8.

Roth, D. & Bean, J. (1985). *Alcohol Problems and Homelessness: Findings from the Ohio Study*. Ohio Department of Mental Health Cleveland, OH: Office of Programme Evaluation and Research.

Rossi, P., Wright, J., Fresher, G. & Withs, G. (1987). The urban homeless: estimating composition and size. *Science*, **235**, 1336–41.

Smith, E. M. & North, C. S. (1994). Not all homeless women are alike: effects of motherhood and the presence of children. *Community Mental Health Journal*, **30**(6), 601–10.

Stark, C., Scott, J., Etell, M. *et al.* (1989). *A Survey of the "Long Stay" Users of DSS Resettlement Units*. A research report. London: Department of Social Security.

Susser, E., Conover, S. & Struening, E. L. (1990). Mental illness in the homeless: problems of epidemiologic method in surveys of the 1980s. *Community Mental Health Journal*, **26**, 391–414.

Susser, E. S., Shang, P. & Genover, S. A. (1991). Risk factors for homelessness among patients admitted to a state mental hospital. *American Journal of Psychiatry*, **12**, 1659–64.

Timms, P. W. & Fry, A. H. (1989). Homelessness and mental illness. *Health Trends*, **21**, 70–1.

Weller, M., Tobransky, R., Hollander, D. & Ibrahimi, S. (1989). Psychiatry and destitution at Christmas 1985–1988. *Lancet*, **ii**, 1509–11.

Weller, M. P. E., Sammut, R. G., Santos, M. J. H. & Horton, J. (1993). "Who's sleeping in my bed?" *Psychiatric Bulletin*, **17**, 652–4.

Winkleby, M. A. & White, R. (1992). Homeless adults without apparent medical and psychiatric impairment: onset of morbidity over time. *Hospital and Community Psychiatry*, **43**, 1017–23.

Wright, J. D. (1987). The National Health care for the homeless program. In R. Bingham *et al.* (eds.), *The Homeless in Contemporary Society*, pp. 150–69. London: Sage.

Wright, J. D. (1989). *Address Unknown: Homeless*. New York: Aldine de Gruyter.

Wright, J. D. & Weber, E. (1987). *Homelessness and Health*. New York: McGraw Hill.

Wright, J. D., Rossi, P., Knight, J. *et al.* (1985). *Health and Homelessness*. Amherst, MA: Social and Demographic Research Institute.

4

Young homeless and homeless families: a review

Dinesh Bhugra

Introduction

The most alarming increase in the homeless population over the last 20 years has been the dramatic rise in the number of homeless families with children. The homeless youth have appeared in increasing numbers on our streets. In England, Shelter (a charity for the homeless) estimated that 58 000 people were either sleeping rough or were unauthorized tenants or squatters. Up to another 137 000 single people were estimated to be living in hostels and lodgings in addition to 317 000 insecure private tenants and 1.2 million 'hidden' homeless (Burrows & Walentowicz, 1992). In the USA in 1986 it was reported, following a survey of 25 cities, that 80% of the sample had reported an increase in the number of homeless families with children (US Conference of Mayors, 1986). A year later on average the numbers had gone up by another one third (US Conference of Mayors, 1987). Various changes in housing policies and a reduction in available housing stock available at affordable rents along with low cost new building are among some of the reasons for this increase (see Chapter 3). For homeless families stresses and coping strategies are different from those experienced by the single homeless. In homeless families in addition to individual stress, there is also the impact on the family unit along with all of the interactions that happen between the unit members. Within that unit, family homelessness can affect not only emotional growth but behavioural and nutritional status of the children.

The stereotypes of homeless youth running away towards the bright lights does not hold up to close scrutiny. There is no typical homeless family or runaway or homeless youth. These individuals

41

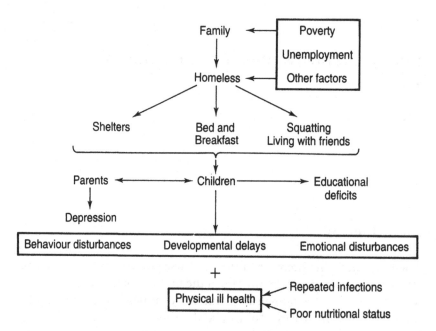

Figure 4.1. Pathways into homelessness and consequences of homelessness on the family.

come from a range of socio-economic classes, races, ages, backgrounds, and their needs, whether physical, social, economic or health, also vary.

In this chapter the needs of homeless families, homeless children and homeless youth will be addressed and suggestions for identification and management of problem areas will be made.

Homeless families

Over the past decade there has been a large increase in the number of households in England accepted as officially homeless from 53 110 in 1978 to 145 800 in 1990 (Faculty of Public Health Medicine). The number of families in London accepted as homeless under the terms of the 1985 Housing Act increased by nearly threefold.

Figure 4.1 outlines the sequelae of homelessness in families. This figure is not meant to be comprehensive but indicates many of the problems of homeless families that need to be assessed multi-axially. Homeless families in the UK can be divided into those who are roofless and those who live in bed and breakfast accommodation, the latter being a majority. Homeless families are often housed by their councils in bed and breakfast accommodation where the conditions are basic and the whole family may live in one room with access to communal cooking facilities and toilet facilities shared between up to 30 families.

In the USA McChesney (1992) carried out a study of 80 homeless mothers in five shelters in Los Angeles County over a period of 16 months from April 1985. Although shelters had been selected to broadly represent all major areas in the city the women had to agree to be interviewed. The number of refusals is not reported, therefore the sample may not be representative. Mothers, and occasionally their partners, were interviewed using loosely structured interviews and families were followed for as long as possible. The most basic problem reported with this group was their poverty, which prevented them from having 'homes'. Lack of money was an important factor in their daily existence and they had lurched from crisis to crisis, with their successes being only temporary and solutions transitory. Victor (1992) reported similar findings in England. On the basis of the source of income prior to homelessness and on the characteristics of the primary earner the following four types of homeless families emerged: unemployed couples, mothers leaving relationships, aid to families with dependent children (AFDC), and mothers who had been homeless teenagers. Although the four groups were distinct there was considerable overlap. In the first category of unemployed couples – marginal men were the main wage earners. However, their ability to support their families depended upon the economic business cycle. These couples were in their mid-thirties with two or more children and the wage earner was usually a blue collar worker. These were seen as traditional families where the husband earned and the wife looked after the children. Even within the shelter this role division was maintained. In the second group, of mothers leaving relationships – the typical mother was in her twenties with one or more children. She was more likely to have been to high school and had worked prior to having children. The proximate cause of their poverty was the break-up of a relationship with an economically successful partner. Following this break-up the mothers were left with the children and with no success in obtaining work along with limited or no access to child care. In contrast AFDC mothers were heads of households – their male companions were peripheral to the control unit. These mothers had two or more children, were less well educated and had limited work experience. The last category included women who had been abused, were younger (in their early 20's), usually with one child often an infant. They may have had a history of fostering and may have run away from this placement often because of sexual abuse. This group was described as having learnt subsistence prostitution. These mothers were also more likely to need support and rehabilitative services attached to specialized housing alternatives (Bassuk *et al.*, 1986). Making facilities for child care available along with the benefits of voluntary help and voluntary organizations are important factors in planning their management.

Bassuk *et al.*'s (1986) sample from Massachusetts included 80 homeless women and 151 children drawn from 14 family shelters. Women were young and over two thirds came from broken homes. They had poor work records, few supports and long histories of residential instability. Nearly three quarters (71%) were given a diagnosis of personality disorder. Boxhill & Beaty (1990), in a study of 40 homeless women and their children, observed that these mothers and children were building their relationships in an open personal space. The authors reported six themes to emerge from their study. These were: an intense desire to demonstrate internalized values as a way of asserting self; questioning the certainty of anything and ambiguity of everything; conflict over the need for attention and the experienced demand for independence; public mothering; unravelling of the mother role; external control being placed on this maternal role. Little wonder that an internalized confusion may arise within mothers and their relationships. Smith & North (1994) studied 300 homeless women (90% of whom were mothers) in St Louis from night shelters and day centres. Using the Diagnostic Interview Schedule/ Homeless Supplement, DSM-III R diagnoses were reached. Two third (67%) of the women had children under the age of 16 in their physical custody in these shelters. Fifty women (17%) did not have physical custody of *any* of their children under 16. Unlike previous studies this sample was predominantly (76%) African American and mothers with children were more likely to be unemployed. The authors suggest that in their sample, women with children had greater social vulnerabilities (like unemployment and dependent children) and fewer personal vulnerabilities (substance abuse and other psychiatric problems). Among those without children nearly half had a non-substance Axis 1 life-time psychiatric disorder and nearly half reported a substance abuse problem, and combining these disorders nearly three quarters had a life-time psychiatric diagnosis.

Reasons for family homelessness in this group include break-up of relationships, poor work record, unavailability of work as well as child care facilities, sexual abuse, eviction, domestic conflict and unsafe living conditions (Mills & Ota, 1989). Each family unit will thus have a different set of problems needing to be identified. Domestic conflicts also have implications for poor self-esteem and relationship difficulties (Bhugra, 1993). These may in turn produce isolation and loneliness and poor social support. Mothers may end up providing inappropriate models for children who may not, in turn, be able to form close friendships and trusting relationships. One study in West London reported that 16% of homeless women were clinically depressed and another 19% suffered from borderline depression (M. Tempia, personal communication). Using the General Health Questionnaire (GHQ-12; Goldberg, 1978), Victor (1992) found that 20% of her sample in West London suffered from significant mental morbidity. In addition to psychological problems, the physical problems of living in a cramped space with a lack of adequate personal, medical and social facilities are bound to contribute to ill-health. Nearly half (46%) of homeless people reported long-term illness or a disability lasting longer than a year (Victor, 1992). One tenth reported an acute episode of ill-health. General practice consultation rates in this group in the previous fortnight were twice the national rate of consultation, thereby indicating a large pool of ill-health. Although bed and breakfast families and sometimes those placed in hostels in the UK are technically able to register with a general practitioner not all have access to primary care facilities. In Victor's (1992) sample in London, 92% of homeless people were registered with a general practitioner, although 44% of them had registered only within the past year. Furthermore, 18% lived 8 km or more away from the surgery, thereby suggesting that some surgeries may be reluctant to take homeless people on. Some of the management issues related to this group are discussed below and in Chapter 7.

Homeless children

The literature suggests that homeless families typically consist of women on their own or with their young children who are usually under the age of 5. In studies from the USA it has been estimated that on any given night there are 6800 children and youths aged 16 or under who belong to homeless families (GAO, 1989). In addition a further 300 000 children may be counted as homeless per year. Furthermore, another 186 000 children may be doubled up in housing shared with relatives or friends. The GAO study reported that 52% of homeless children in their survey were aged 5 or younger – nearly two thirds of children aged 16 or under seen by the National Health Care for the Homeless projects were aged 1 to 5. Most of the families in the shelter belonged to ethnic minorities (Bassuk, 1987, Miller & Lin, 1988). As noted earlier, Victor (1992) reported from London that being female and young was related to being housed in bed and breakfast hotels. Of the 522 subjects, 207 (55%) had between one and seven dependent children under the age of 16, most parents having a single child of school age. Solarz (1992) emphasizes that a separate group of families and children exist who may survive by living rough. There is no doubt that in the studies reported so far the children have borne the brunt of physical and mental health problems.

Bassuk's (1986) work referred to earlier, revealed that only women's relationships with men were characterized by instability, conflict and violence. The children from this study had been administered the Denver Developmental Screening Test to test developmental milestones in four areas: language, gross motor skills, fine motor co-ordination and personal and social development. The children interviewed in the series revealed very high (47% of pre-schoolers) rates of at least one developmental delay. One third (33%) had lags in two or more areas. The school-age children suffered from serious emotional problems. On the children's Depression Inventory and the children's Manifest Anxiety Scale about half scored high enough to warrant fuller psychiatric evaluation. Almost all had thought of committing suicide. Most of the older children were doing poorly in school – one quarter were in a special class and nearly half (43%) had to repeat a year. In addition some children were ashamed of their social status of being homeless and kept it hidden from schoolmates. Furthermore, this group did not generally contact helping agencies either. Only 14% of children were involved in day care. The immediate cause of homelessness was housing related.

Whitman et al. (1990) have also reported language development delay in children of homeless families. Horowitz *et al.* (1988) compared three groups of children: 'hotel children' (i.e. those living in welfare hotels with their families); non-hotel children in an attendance improvement/dropout prevention programme and non-hotel children in the community. School environment was observed as a 'facilitator' in hotel children's adaptation to their environment. Solarz (1992) raised the question of whether these increased rates in developmental delays and emotional problems are due to homelessness, poor personal space or poverty. It would be very difficult to tease out these threads especially if research focuses on shelter populations only.

One study from Boston did not replicate Bassuk *et al.*'s findings (Lewis & Meyers, 1989) but they had looked at a sample attending a clinic, which may explain the low rates. Any minor behavioural, emotional or developmental delay may not reach the threshold to warrant clinical intervention and to therefore be seen at the clinic. However, Wood *et al.* (1991) reported that 9% of their sample from Los Angeles had failed two or more sections of the Denver Developmental Screening Test. They also reported more problems with aggression. Molnar *et al.*'s (1988) study of children aged between $2\frac{1}{2}$ and 5 reported that these children exhibited a range of problem behaviours including speech delay, aggression, inappropriate social behaviour, poor attention span and impulse control. Their relationships with their peers were 'immature'. The authors argue that this inappropriate behaviour may be one way of coping with the environment. These children are also more prone to being abused physically and sexually and to being neglected.

The rates of medical disorders in children in homeless families are about twice the rates expected for children in the general population. Homeless children are more vulnerable to infections, gastrointestinal problems, higher blood lead levels and nutritional deficiencies (Institute of Medicine, 1988; Miller & Lin, 1988; Wright, 1989). It is possible that these problems are linked with poverty and poor housing as well as material deprivation. Wood *et al.* (1991) reported that although both homeless and poorly housed families had poor dietary patterns the former were more likely to experience more periods of hunger and food deprivation. Children's dietary patterns, availability of cheap, filling, starchy or fatty foods and poor cooking environment may all contribute to poor nutritional status. Inadequate facilities for personal hygiene, poor quality of cleanliness and living in close quarters all add up to increased risks of infection.

Children from bed and breakfast families with 'an address' can theoretically be admitted to schools. However, rates of attendance are difficult to obtain. These children are likely to miss school because of poor health, looking after younger siblings and the transitory nature of their accommodation. They are likely to perform poorly and have had previous trouble with school authorities.

Adolescents

Adolescents or runaway youths are, in some ways, the most vulnerable of the 'special' groups of homeless. Unlike the lovable fictional images of Tom Sawyer, Oliver Twist, Huckleberry Finn and David Copperfield, modern day runaway youths are often running away from foster homes or parental homes, violence, neglect, physical and sexual abuse. The problems this group faces are complex and often interlinked with prostitution and the inherent risks that this life-style brings. Adolescence is a period of individuation and individual growth with the support of the family and society at large. This individuation thus becomes more complicated for runaway adolescents.

Adolescent homeless have been categorized into runaways, throwaways and the homeless. Runaways were defined as youth who remain away from home at least overnight without parent or caretaker permission. Homeless youth are those with no parental, foster or institutional home and include pushouts (urged to leave) and throwaways (left home with parental knowledge or approval without an alternative place to stay). The last group is that of street kids who feel they belong on the street and have become accustomed to fending for themselves (Robertson, 1992).

Abrahams & Mungall (1992) defined a runaway as a young person aged under 18 who has left home or local authority care without agreement and has stayed away for a 'significant period of time', the length of time regarded as significant being related to the age of the runaway. Runaway is a mode of departure and may not necessarily be equated with a young homeless person. As these authors emphasize, the essence of this definition is being away without consent, explicit or otherwise.

The UK Department of the Environment (1982), has defined single and homeless as:

1. Being without adequate shelter now.
2. Facing the loss of shelter within a month.
3. Living in a situation of no security of tenure and being forced to seek alternative accommodation within a time period that the client considers to be immediate (e.g. potential discharges from Institutions of all types; living with friends or relatives in over-crowded conditions; illegal tenancies).
4. Those living in reception centres, crash pads, derelict buildings, squats (unlicensed), hostels, lodging houses, cheap hotels and boarding houses.

In England and Wales the ages of 16 and 17 remain 'grey areas', since although parents may legally refuse to allow the youth to leave home this right is difficult to enforce. In Scotland a 16 year old may legally leave home with or without parental consent.

Abrahams & Mungall (1992) studied 4 police force areas in England along with 5 of 75 Metropolitan divisions. They monitored the lists of reported missing persons. During the study period, 6068 persons had reportedly run away – 70% from home and the rest from care. When they extrapolated these figures nationally they estimated that there were 43 000 runaways per year with 102 000 incidents in 1990. The majority of the runaways were in the 14–16 age range and those in institutional care were more likely to run away. Some institutions were vulnerable and more likely to produce runaways. Only 2% of cases went far away from their home area. The study population was predominantly white (58%) but 26% of runaways from care homes (compared to 16% from homes) were Afro-Caribbean. Asians were only marginally more likely (6% compared to 4%) to run away from home than institutional care. Common causes for running away were danger to self and other vulnerability factors such as prostitution, pregnancy, sexual abuse and learning difficulties.

More recent reports indicate that these numbers are on the increase in the UK especially among the 16–18 year olds – the age too young to be eligible for social security and too old for social services departments, and that nearly half (49%) of the group left or were thrown out of home as a result of domestic conflict (Wiggans, 1989a).

Raychaba (1989) has highlighted the close links between being placed in care and homelessness. In a sample of homeless young people in Greater Manchester, Wiggans (1989a) reported that young people were more likely to be unemployed, to come from broken homes and to have been in care. A similar picture has emerged in Ireland where the homeless youth came from the poorest sections where important factors included urban deprivation and family instability, and the group was vulnerable to drugs, prostitution and the effects of physical hardship (Simon Community, 1983). Harvey & Menton (1989) conclude that Ireland's young homeless people are being left by the wayside. In the very first year of a self-help advice and settlement service, one third of the users were under 20 (Focus Point, 1987).

There are many similarities between youth from care and homeless youth (Raychaba, 1989). The former group were more likely to abuse chemical substances and to exhibit anger, frustration, depression and self-destructive behaviour. Similar findings have been reported by Feitel et al. (1992) and Greenblatt & Robertson (1993). More than three quarters in one sample suffered from 'extreme emotional depression' and 50% had attempted or seriously considered commit-ting suicide (Covenant House, 1985). Jenkins & Stahle (1972) concluded that runaways were described most commonly as insecure, unhappy and impulsive – all attributable to poor self-image along with feelings of inadequacy and lack of self-confidence. Mowbray et al. (1985) reported that nearly a quarter of a Detroit sample exhibited violent disturbed behaviour and 10% were considered self-destruc-tive. Like the younger children from homeless families, and because of similar reasons of coming into care along with the transitory nature of accommodation and lack of constancy, this group performs badly in social and educational areas. This also means that they are unable to find and keep a job and accommodation. Another complication is that because of poor social and peer support systems the institutional 'support' ends rather suddenly and the youth are 'extruded' into appalling conditions.

Prostitution and substance abuse may become a major problem. Benjamin (1985) observed that many of those children who end up in juvenile prostitution have been failed twice – once by their family and the second time by the welfare system. The placements in care institutions may teach this group deviant values and practices associated with social isolation; low self-esteem, passivity, a sense of powerlessness and inability to develop successful, healthy relation-ships all add up to the possibility that such experiences may encourage prostitution. The young person leaving care with minimal education and little, if any, employment-related skills is dangerously prone to enter into prostitution – a specific form of homelessness (Raychaba, 1989). Male prostitution is primarily an adolescent phenomenon largely because homosexual clientele may prefer a young male. The younger a youth appears, the more tricks he can generate thereby making more money. Males may start to make less money as they become older and with this they may end up performing acts they may have refused at a younger age. As their self-esteem is often linked with the ability to make money they may become progressively more depressed, suicidal and may turn to other criminal activity (Price, 1989). Greenblatt & Robertson (1993) studied 93 homeless adolescents between the ages of 13 and 17 in the Hollywood area of Los Angeles. One third had had more than 10 sexual partners in the previous year and about a third reported trading sex for money, food or drugs. Only 31% were girls and 40% were non-white. For 44% homelessness had been episodic, while 39% were chronically homeless. A majority of the parents (57%) were divorced, and family conflicts, physical abuse, sexual abuse and pregnancy were common reasons for leaving. Boys were more likely than girls to have had sex at an earlier age (usually before the age of 13). Most identified themselves as heterosexual and 18% reported sex with intravenous drug users. Although most knew the cause of AIDS, its spread and prevention, safe sex was still not very common. For female prostitutes an additional problem may be the role of the pimps. Initial tricks may be one way of hanging on to their boyfriends who may then use violence to control them. For many female adolescents getting pregnant may become a means to escape from one kind of life-style, but at the same time it starts off yet another vicious circle. As Price (1989) pointed out, adolescent prostitutes were more likely to use denial as a form of dealing with risks and some may concede that they are not likely to live long anyway.

The causes of homelessness in this group remain multiple. Janus *et al.* (1987) interviewed 149 youths between the ages of 16 and 21. Of these, 73% reported physical abuse and 43% blamed their running away on it. Furthermore, 40% had suffered sexual assaults and rape, and more than one third (36%) had been forced into sexual activity against their will, 31% were sexually molested and 51% reported sexual abuse. The economic structures of a single parent family were more likely to contribute to their running away. Chaotic, abusive patterns of interaction and the inability of families to cope with their children's needs led the authors to comment that the dysfunction observed in these families was very prominent and serious and the family members may have higher than hitherto realized expectations of their children leading to a conflict with 'arrested' psycho-social development of the youth. Therefore a simple return to the same or similar atmosphere would never be good enough. If this expectation of higher achievement than the youths are able to achieve is shown consistently in other studies it may also raise vital points in managing these individuals in institutional settings, which lay even stronger emphasis on communal rather than individual functioning.

As noted above, the mental health of adolescents needs to be visualized in the context of normal adolescent development. Physiological, cognitive and emotional changes remain inextricably linked. Adolescence is a period of growth, experimentation and individuation. Separating from the original family and establishing a new identity, mastering new personal and social skills and forming new relationships and developing a stable set of values are all part of this growth. This may be aided by support, guidance, modelling and consistent help by adults.

Adolescents experience a deepening of their emotions, higher levels of anxiety and depression and more marked mood swings (Rutter & Hersov, 1985). Using check lists for assessing behaviour, Wolk & Brandon (1977) reported that runaways had a significantly poorer self-concept and were not only more defensive but also had poor personal adjustment. Similar findings were reported by Schaffer & Caton (1984). These authors observed that four fifths of their sample scored at a level of disturbance likely to indicate significant psychiatric disability. One third of the girls had a history of attempted suicide and 70% of the youth admitted substance abuse. In addition 37% of boys and 19% of girls in this sample had been charged with an offence – most commonly assault or robbery. Robertson (1992) argued that such high criminal rates may be a reflection of the needs for basic survival.

Feitel et al. (1992) reported that 90% of their sample from a shelter for homeless youth in New York, fulfilled the criteria for an emotional disorder. Three quarters were depressed and 41% had considered suicide and more than one quarter had attempted suicide.

Van der Ploeg (1989) studied 212 homeless adolescents in Holland. Differentiating between street youth and homeless youth (the former sleeping rough in car parks, on streets, in doorways and the latter wandering around from one address to the next) the author collected basic information on 212 young people and interviewed 86 at length. Boys were three times more likely to be homeless and foreign youth formed one third of the sample. Of the 90% that were jobless about one third had been unemployed for over a year. Van der Pleog (1989) characterized these along five dimensions:

1. *Negative family backgrounds.* Nearly three quarters (73%) came from families where parents had been divorced and 70% rarely kept in touch with their fathers.
2. *History of professional help.* Of the sample, 12% had been involved with seven or more helping organizations, 79% had been in residential institutions and 21% had been with foster families.
3. *Negative experiences at school.* Of the youth, 22% were persistent truants and 70% had changed schools more than once, while 40% had repeated one or more classes and 10% had changed school eight times.
4. *Few friends.* Defining firm friendship as lasting at least one year only 15% had friends, and 11% had no friends at all. This may reflect the mobility as well as social skills and poor access to peer groups for forming friendships.
5. *Low self-perception.* These youths had a positive opinion of themselves and the majority saw themselves as adult, clever, self assured and cheerful. Van der Ploeg argued that this was a façade and that these youths had an inadequate self-perception and a poor perception of their situation. Over 50% believed that their destinies were determined by factors outside their control. Wiggans (1989b) criticized Van der Ploeg's model on the grounds that Van der Ploeg had failed to outline the causal model that had been the original intention and, in addition, the reality of the focus was on pathology and weakness rather than the individual's strength.

Implications for service

It would appear from the above review that the experiences of homeless families and children and homeless youth are far from homogeneous although some common strands emerge. The implications for services are many. The Council on Scientific Affairs (1989) emphasized that the health care needs of homeless runaways or adolescent homeless included poor nutritional factors, substance abuse, mental, physical and sexual health and victimization. Thus, the care for these groups must research different facets to understand the true extent of the problem. Firstly, epidemiological studies are required to ascertain the exact extent of the problem in any geographical area. Secondly, the needs of such groups and individuals must be assessed and a multi-axial needs assessment programme has to be developed. The comprehensive, accessible, appropriate, sensitive and available services must be developed. Both physical and psychological needs must be documented and management offered. Reuniting adolescents with their families is highly unlikely to resolve the problems and may in reality aggravate the difficulties.

For homeless families and children

1. Strategies to decrease family poverty need to be developed. This is largely a political question, but in smaller communities developing voluntary services and working in partnership with statutory organizations may help the individual to cope better.
2. Flexibility in providing jobs and shelters will go a long way in reducing not only the numbers of homeless but also the duration of homelessness and give a sense of security to the parents and their children.
3. Flexibility in educational provisions with special emphasis on enrolling homeless children at the nearest school rather than their 'old' school may make schooling more acceptable, and may encourage child–parent participation and a sense of belonging and purpose and provide the child with an improved self-esteem through peer interaction.
4. Specially targeted programmes that enable a reduction in poverty to occur along with a reduction in homelessness are more likely to be accepted. However, this step again is a reflection of the political will. Low-cost, safe, affordable, well-managed housing even if it does not encourage families to stay put and settle down may at least make it more likely.
5. Specific help in the form of shelters and counselling for victims of domestic violence, sexual and physical abuse, is likely to help those in the most need.
6. Joint programmes and projects with support from the Departments of the Environment, Health and Education will enable

voluntary organizations to tackle the issue even more actively and strongly.

For homeless adolescents

1. Prioritization of needs at an individual level with joint projects as suggested above may enable the individual to learn skills and manage crises and reduce the duration of homelessness.
2. Ongoing evaluation of the services available and continued research into determining the exact levels of needs will enable the individual to feel part of the community and enable them to reduce their feelings of isolation and extrusion.
3. A continuum of facilities from sheltered accommodation to long-term residential housing and transitional care will enable the individual to find the support and shelter that matches up with their needs.
4. Easy accessibility and availability of a range of individual, group and family work, parenting skills, management of substance abuse and other special factors will encourage individuals to seek early and appropriate help and resolution.
5. In cases with co-morbidity and psychological problems case management may provide an ideal solution.
6. Interagency co-operation and advocacy schemes may lead to a better quality and acceptability of services.

Conclusions

The underlying causes of homelessness are varied and for the three groups of homeless families, children and adolescents the individual needs must be determined, thus allowing prioritization of care and an early response to reduce the period of uncertainty, anguish and homelessness. On the one hand homeless children suffer from a multitude of problems and the educational aspects of their life-style need to be highlighted. Homeless youth, on the other hand, are more likely to be the products of broken homes, are as likely to run away as to be thrown out and are likely to end up in prostitution with its inherent risks. It is possible that all these factors are interdependent. The situation is complex but identification of the special needs of homeless families, youth and children, followed by a clear assessment

of needs and appropriate accessible services along with working
towards cheap, accessible and appropriate housing should go some
way towards controlling stress and reducing psychological distress.

References

Abrahams, C. & Mungall, R. (1992). *Runaways: Exploding the Myths.*
London: National Children's Home.
Bassuk, E. L. (1987). The feminization of homelessness: families in
Boston shelters. *American Journal of Social Psychiatry*, **7**, 19–23.
Bassuk, E. L., Rubin, L. & Lauriat, A. S. (1984). Is homelessness a
mental health problem? *American Journal of Psychiatry*, **141**, 1546–50.
Bassuk, E. L., Rubin, L. & Lauriat, A. S. (1986). Characteristics of
sheltered homeless families. *American Journal of Public Health*, **76**,
1097–101.
Benjamin, M. (1985). *Juvenile Prostitution: A Portrait of the 'Life'.* Toronto:
Ministry of Community & Social Services.
Bhugra, D. (1993). Unemployment, poverty and homelessness. In D.
Bhugra and J. Leff (eds.) *Principles of Social Psychiatry*, pp. 355–84.
Oxford: Blackwell Scientific Publications.
Boxill, N. A. & Beaty, A. L. (1990). Mother/child interactions among
homeless women and their children in a public night shelter in
Atlanta, Georgia. *Child and Youth Services*, **14**, 49–64.
Burrows, L. & Walentowicz, P. (1992). *Homes Cost Less Than
Homelessness.* London: Shelter.
Covenant House (1985). *The Covenant Experience.* Toronto: Covenant
House.
CSA (Council on Scientific Affairs) (1989). Health care needs of
homeless and runaway youths. *Journal of the American Medical
Association*, **262**, 1358–61.
Department of the Environment (1982). *Single and Homeless.* London:
HMSO.
Focus Point (1987). *Towards a Resettlement Strategy and Annual Report.*
Dublin: Focus Point.
Feitel, B., Margetson, N., Chamas, J. & Lipman, C. (1992).
Psychosocial background and behavioural and emotional disorders
of homeless and runaway youth. *Hospital and Community Psychiatry*,
43, 155–9.
GAO (General Accounting Office) (1989). *Children and Youths.*
Washington, DC: General Accounting Office.
Goldberg, D. (1978). *General Health Questionnaire.* Windsor:
NFER-Nelson.
Greenblatt, M. & Robertson, M. J. (1993). Life styles, adaptive
strategies and sexual behaviours of homeless adolescents. *Hospital
and Community Psychiatry*, **44**, 1177–80.

Harvey, B. & Menton, M. (1989). Ireland's young homeless. *Children and Youth Services Review*, **11**, 31–43.

Horowitz, S., Springer, C. & Kase, G. (1988). Stress in hotel children: the effects of homelessness on attitudes towards school. *Children's Environment Quarterly*, **5**, 34–6.

Institute of Medicine (1988). *Homelessness, Health and Human Needs*. Washington DC: National Academy Press.

Janus, M.-D., McCormack, A., Burgess, A. W. & Hartman, C. (1987). *Adolescent Runaways: Causes and Consequences*. Lexington, MA: Lexington Books.

Jenkins, R. & Stahle, G. (1972). The runaway reaction. *Journal of the American Academy of Child and Adolescent Psychiatry*, **11**, 294–313.

Lewis, M. & Meyers, A. (1989). The growth and development of status and homeless children entering shelters in Boston. *Public Health Report*, **104**, 247–50.

McChesney, K. Y. (1992). Homeless families: four patterns of poverty. In M. J. Robertson & M. Greenblatt (eds.), *Homeless: A National Perspective*, pp. 245–56. New York: Plenum Press.

Miller, D. & Lin, E. C. (1988). Children in sheltered homeless families: reported health status and use of health services. *Paediatrics*, **81**, 668–73.

Mills, C. & Ota, H. (1989). Homeless women with minor children in the Detroit Metropolitan Area. *Social Work*, **34**, 485–9.

Molnar, G., Klein, T., Knitzer, J. *et al.* (1988). Home is Where the Heart is: The Crisis of Homeless Children and Families in New York City. Report to the Edna McConnell Clark Foundation. New York Bank Street College of Education.

Mowbray, C., Johnson, S., Solarz, A. & Combs, C. (1985). *Mental Health and Homeless in Detroit: A Research Study*. Detroit: Michigan Dept of Health.

Price, V. A. (1989). Characteristics and needs of Boston street youth: one agency's responses. *Children and Youth Services Review*, **11**, 75–90.

Raychaba, B. (1989). Canadian youth in care: leaving care to be on our own with no direction from home. *Children and Youth Services Review*, **11**, 61–73.

Robertson, J. M. (1992). Homeless and runaway youths. In M. J. Robertson & M. Greenblatt (eds.), *Homelessness: a National Perspective*, pp. 287–98. New York: Plenum Press.

Rutter, M. & Hersov, L. (eds.) (1985). *Child and Adolescent Psychiatry*. Oxford: Blackwell Scientific Publications.

Schaffer, D. & Caton, C. L. M. (1984). *Runaway and Homeless Youth in New York City*. New York: Ittleson Foundation.

Simon Community (1983). *Need for Shelter for Young People in Distress*. Dublin: Simon Community.

Smith, E. M. & North, C. S. (1994). Not all homeless women are alike: effects of motherhood and the presence of children. *Community Mental Health Journal*, **30**, 601–10.

Solarz, A. L. (1992). To be young and homeless. In M. J. Robertson & M. Greenblatt (eds.), *Homelessness: A National Perspective*, pp. 275–86. New York: Plenum Press.

US Conference of Mayors (1986). The Growth of Hunger, Homelessness and Poverty in America's Cities in 1985. Washington, DC: Conference of Mayors.

US Conference of Mayors (1987). The Continuing Growth of Hunger, Homelessness and Poverty in America's Cities. Washington, DC: Conference of Mayors.

Van der Ploeg, J. D. (1989). Homelessness: a multi dimensional problem. *Children and Youth Services Review*, **11**, 45–56.

Victor, C. R. (1992). Health status of the temporarily homeless population and residents of North West Thames Region. *British Medical Journal*, **305**, 387–91.

Whitman, B. Y., Sprankel, J., Stretch, J. J. *et al.* (n.d.). *Children of the Homeless: A High Risk Population for Developmental Delays*. St. Louis: Office of Mental Retardation–Developmental Disability Resources.

Wiggans, A. (1989a). Youthwork and homelessness in England. *Children and Youth Services Review*, **11**, 5–29.

Wiggans, A. (1989b). Critique of Van der Ploeg. *Children and Youth Services Review*, **11**, 57–60.

Wolk, S. & Brandon, J. (1977). Runaway adolescents' perceptions of parents and self. *Adolescence*, **12**, 175–87.

Wood, D., Valdez, R. B., Hayashi, T. *et al.* (1991). The health of homeless children: a comparison study. *Paediatrics*, **86**, 858–66.

Wright, J. (1989). Poverty, homelessness, health, nutrition and children. Presented at the Johns Hopkins University Institute for Policy Studies. April. Washington, DC.

5

Homeless women

E. JANE MARSHALL

Introduction

The proportion of women amongst the adult homeless population increased throughout the 1970s and 1980s and is currently estimated at between 10% and 25%. Women with children are now the fastest growing segment of the homeless population in the USA (Smith & North, 1994). Information about homeless women is limited to studies that have been carried out in accessible settings such as hostels, shelters and day centres, and cannot, therefore, be generalized. In studies where homeless men and women have been interviewed, the numbers of women are small and comparisons between the sexes have not been made (Arce *et al.*, 1983; Bassuk *et al.*, 1984; Fischer *et al.*, 1986; Kroll *et al.*, 1986).

The current situation and the specific problems experienced by homeless women in Britain and the USA can be better understood in the light of historical evidence.

Homeless women in the nineteenth and twentieth centuries

Britain

After the Industrial Revolution in Britain, people moved to the cities and towns to look for work. The increased demand for accommodation caused a housing shortage. Women worked in factories, mills and shops but their wages were low and their accommodation options limited. Until the 1880s, when social reformers began to intervene in the housing crisis, working women could either rent rooms, lodge or board with a household, stay in common lodging houses or in accommodation provided by their employer (Watson & Austerberry, 1986). Living-in was a condition of employment in the drapery and allied trades and in domestic service. Many women resorted to prostitution in order to earn a living, or to supplement meagre wages (Higgs & Hayward, 1910), but then had difficulty finding accommodation because landladies were unwilling to let rooms to prostitutes.

The lack of housing provision led to homelessness in both men and women. Accommodation for homeless women was provided in common lodging houses, charitable refuges and casual wards. There was a great range in the lodging houses available. At one end of the spectrum were establishments that only took in 'respectable' working women and at the other end were mixed common lodging houses where men and women were crowded together. An inquiry in 1886 revealed that of a sample of 597 people in common lodging houses, 176 (30%) were women (Ribton-Turner, 1887). A census of charitable refuges in London in 1891 revealed that 21% of the residents were women (Tillard & Booth, 1924). The casual wards, administered under the Poor Law Acts, supposedly catered for those out of work and seeking employment. Anyone taken in for one night was obliged to stay the next day and night in order to work for their board by oakum-picking. They then had to move on. Conditions in the casual wards were unacceptable to most women, who preferred the lodging houses. In 1886 the ratio of men to women in the casual wards was 79% to 21% (Ribton-Turner, 1887).

The social reform movement of the late nineteenth century and early twentieth centuries provoked interest in the plight of the homeless and led to an increase in provision for homeless women. The Salvation Army, one of the voluntary organizations founded at this time, took a sympathetic and less punitive attitude to homeless women than other organizations and set up shelters for homeless women, and homes for prostitutes and unmarried mothers.

A London census on 15 January 1909 revealed that 1483 women were in common lodging houses and 184 in casual wards, many fewer than the men in either type of accommodation. These figures, however, were considered to be an underestimate (Higgs & Hayward, 1910). Homeless women found it difficult to find accommodation in common lodging houses because there was a common perception that they were more difficult to manage than men. Common lodging house managers would therefore either raise their prices beyond what the women could afford or would refuse accommodation (Higgs & Hayward, 1910). Homeless women also eschewed the casual wards because of the punitive treatment meted out and only used them as a last resort (Higgs & Hayward, 1910).

During the interwar period, homeless women could be divided into one group that was temporarily stranded and two larger groups that were permanently homeless (Menzies, 1927). The temporarily homeless included young women who had run away from home or who had drifted up from the country in search of work, and older women with a history of 'drink and drug addiction, pilfering, evil temper or some mental twist to account for their plight' (Menzies, 1927). These temporarily stranded women usually found accommodation in facilities run by charities. The permanently homeless consisted of (1) unskilled workers, vagrants and down-and-outs and (2) prostitutes. The unskilled workers and prostitutes largely stayed in the common lodging houses, which remained a major source of provision for homeless women. The casual wards were a less important source of accommodation for homeless women and were used mainly by older women, vagrants and down-and-outs.

In 1925 there were 17 310 places in London County Council licensed lodging houses, but only 1630 (9.42%) were available for women and conditions were worse for women than for men (Chesterton, 1926). This was another ploy to turn women away based on the perception that they were more difficult to manage! For instance, there was a general lack of washing facilities in womens' lodging houses, whereas in mens' establishments there were baths. A 1930 census reported that the casual ward population on one night in London and several other provincial poor law unions was composed of 2472 men, but only 110 women (Watson & Austerberry, 1986). Of these women, 56 were aged between 40 and 60 years and a further 25 were over 60 years.

Mrs Cecil Chesterton lived as a destitute woman on the streets of London for a short period of time and recorded her experiences in a book entitled '*In Darkest London*' (Chesterton, 1926). Her vivid description of what it was like to stay in Salvation Army and other shelters, in licensed and unlicensed lodging houses, in doss houses, the casual ward and also on the streets is still relevant. As a homeless woman, her life came to be 'governed by an obsession for food and sleep' and she understood how the destitute experience 'effaces individuality, weighs down the will, clogs the instinct to do battle which is the heritage of man'. 'One instinct only remains vital, apart from the desire for food and shelter, and that is the passionate determination not to be trapped into an institution', by which she meant the casual ward. She concluded that women became homeless because of 'poverty, ... the shortage of housing ..., illness, bad luck, increase of rent', not because of 'moral delinquency' and that the accommodation provided for the destitute woman was inadequate and generally of a low standard. When she returned home she set up the Cecil Houses (Inc.) Public Lodging Houses Fund and later houses for homeless single women that were financed by voluntary donations.

After the Second World War the only statutory provision for single homeless women was the casual ward. These were renamed 'reception centres' and were administered by the new National Assistance Board. Conditions were less punitive and the aim was to help the single homeless to 'settle down'. That homeless women did not use the reception centres was confirmed in a 1952 census, which reported that numbers rarely exceeded 100 women on any one night (Watson & Austerbery, 1986). Common lodging houses were declining in number and importance and one study reported that most women in Glasgow's lodging houses were over 60 years of age and widowed (Laidlaw, 1956). Privately rented accommodation was the most important option for single people.

In the 1950s, legislation decontrolling rents and property development, particularly in cities, led to an increase in the cost of privately rented accommodation and the closure of many common lodging houses and hostels.

A census of single homeless accommodation carried out by the National Assistance Board (1966) reported that 29 798 men and 1905 women were living in reception centres, common lodging houses or hotels, or sleeping rough. The report did not consider why there were so few homeless women, compared with men, nor did it assess their characteristics. The 'concealed homeless' were ignored. This census was updated in 1972 (Digby, 1976) when it was estimated that 23 300 single homeless men and 2200 single homeless women were living in hostels and lodging house accommodation nationally. But during the intervening years bed numbers for women had decreased, so that by 1972 the voluntary sector (e.g. Salvation and Church Armies) provided almost 75% of the total beds for women and the private sector provided only 14%. There is evidence that many of the women living in such hostels had a history of psychiatric illness and previous convictions. A survey of the records of 200 women admitted to the Southwark Reception Centre in London over a 6 month period prior to its closure in 1962 revealed that 76 were overtly 'mentally disturbed' (London County Council, 1962). Of these women, 54 had a history of psychiatric hospitalization and of this group 21 were schizophrenic. After the centre was reopened in 1967, the high psychiatric morbidity again merited comment by the Visiting Medical Officer (McEwan, 1967).

United States of America

There is scattered evidence that homeless women lived on Skid Rows across the USA in the nineteenth century, many working in brothels. In Philadelphia, between 1790 and 1870, white women constituted a substantial minority of those arrested for Skid Row type offences such as vagrancy, public drunkenness, idleness and disorderly conduct (Blumberg *et al.*, 1978). However, by 1880, the proportion of white women began to decline, and by 1920 less than 10% of whites arrested for such offences were women. This was due to the social reform movement of the late nineteenth and early twentieth centuries, which also occurred in the USA. Women were treated as victims and were more acceptable as objects of charitable giving to social welfare agencies and church organizations. Although their numbers dwindled, women did not disappear from Skid Row in the USA, but they were generally ignored by researchers.

By the mid-1950s two thirds of homeless women in New York were reported as having severe alcohol problems and high rates of psychiatric and physical illness (Chase, 1956 and Myerson, 1957 cited in Garrett & Bahr, 1973). Little changed over the next decade (Garrett & Volk, 1970). Garrett & Bahr (1973) interviewed 52 of the 61 women admitted to the Women's Shelter in New York's Bowery district over a 2 month period in 1969. The women were younger than a comparative sample of homeless men and more women than men were black (44% versus 25%). Thirty three (63%) women had a drinking problem, but these women did not participate in the drinking institutions of Skid Row in the same way as men, and were extremely isolated and disaffiliated.

Blumberg *et al.* (1978) examined the differences between 4 Skid Row women, 20 Skid Row-like women and 60 non-Skid Row women with alcohol problems seen at a Diagnostic and Rehabilitation Center in Philadelphia between 1963 and 1972. The Skid Row women were mostly over 50 years, had no families, lived on the street and were described as 'inadequate persons'. The Skid Row-like women differed from the Skid Row women only in degree; they were younger, had no contact with their families and lived in cheap rooms. A few were prostitutes. All had alcohol problems and the black women also had drug problems. The non-Skid Row women were mainly divorced and separated housewives with serious alcohol problems, who lived with their children and had intact family relationships. Blumberg *et al.* (1978) also described other groups of women living in the slum area near Philadelphia's Skid Row. These included an 'invisible' group of alcoholic Skid Row-like women in the 35–55 age range, living with men as 'housekeepers'; older residentially stable women in cheap accommodation, living on savings and social security; landladies of Skid Row tenants eking out a living and not far removed from a Skid Row-like life-style themselves.

Types of homeless women

Homeless women, like homeless men, are a heterogeneous group. Some attempt at classification may be helpful, in that it highlights the presence of subgroups within the population, but it is artificial because some women fit into many subgroups. The presence or not of children identifies three subgroups: women without children, mothers with children present and mothers without children present. Classification can also be according to type, to location or by using a temporal system (Scott, 1993). Typological classification divides homeless women into the young single homeless, older single homeless and homeless women with children. Classification according to location divides homeless women into those sleeping rough, residents of hostels, residents of shelters, residents of bed and breakfast hotel accommodation (largely homeless families in Great Britain) and other situations (Watson & Austerberry, 1986). Women often manage to conceal their homelessness for as long as possible, either by staying with friends or by remaining in unsatisfactory relationships with men. Watson & Austerberry (1986) found that younger, employed women were more likely to stay with friends or to remain in unstable relationships when they lost accommodation, but that older,

Table 5.1. *Age of homeless women compared with homeless men: British studies*

Study	Men:Women	Men	Women
Digby (1976)	1821:172	43% <50	51% <50
Drake *et al.* (1982)	398:122	29% <30	62% <30
Herzberg (1987)[a]	62:48	40.5	36.3
Fernandez (1984)[b]	15:28	40.5	37.0
Marshall & Reed (1992)[a]	0:70		52.1
Adams (1991)	0:64		45% <44
Scott (1991)	0:46		70% <40
James (1991)[a]	0:43		32.7

[a] Mean age.
[b] Median age.

married, unqualified women with little knowledge of the housing system, were more likely to be living in a direct access hostel at the point of losing accommodation. Thus the type of accommodation used may be a function of age, and the characteristics of homeless women will vary according to the accommodation provision sampled. Finally, a temporal system of classification may be helpful in tracing the pathway to homelessness.

Characteristics of homeless women

Reports indicate that single homeless women are younger and more socially stable than homeless men (Laidlaw, 1956; Digby, 1976; Drake *et al.*, 1982; Herzberg, 1987; Burt & Cohen, 1989). However, studies cannot be compared easily because of differences in definitions of age, sampling procedures and the location of samples (Table 5.1). Digby (1976) and Drake *et al.* (1982) reported their findings in terms of the proportion of the sample under 50 years and under 30 years, respectively. Fernandez (1984) and Herzberg (1987) carried out studies on similar populations of 'no fixed abode' admissions to psychiatric hospitals and reported similar results. Four British studies of homeless women in hostel accommodation in London sampled women from different age groups (Adams, 1991; James, 1991; Scott, 1991; Marshall & Reed, 1992). Adams (1991) found that 45% of his sample was under 44 years. The average age in James' (1991) selective sample of women referred to a visiting psychiatrist was 32.7

Table 5.2. *Age of homeless women compared with homeless men: American studies*

Study	Men:Women	Men	Women
Bassuk *et al.* (1984) *n* = 78	83%:17%	Median age 33.8	
Arce *et al.* (1983)	150:43	47% under 40	
Bassuk *et al.* (1986)	0:80	Median age 27	
Breakey *et al.* (1989)	298:239	39.7	32.9
Lipton *et al.* (1983) *n* = 100	75:25	63% aged 20–39	
Smith & North (1994)	0:300	29	

years. In Scott's (1991) study, 70% of the sample was under 40 years, whereas the mean age in Marshall & Reed's (1992) sample was 52.1 years.

Research from the USA corroborates the fact that homeless women are younger than homeless men (Table 5.2). The homeless women in Breakey *et al.*'s (1989) study were even younger than samples from Great Britain and Ireland and Lipton *et al.*'s (1983) hospital sample was also younger. Homeless mothers are the youngest group overall with a mean age in the late twenties (Bassuk *et al.*, 1986; Smith & North, 1994).

Homeless women are more likely than homeless men to have stayed on at school, to have obtained job training and to be employed (Digby, 1976; Drake *et al.*, 1982). They are also more likely to have maintained contact with their family, to have married and had children (Digby, 1976; Herzberg, 1987; Breakey *et al.*,1989). Homeless mothers (i.e. homeless women with dependent children), however, are seldom married, and have poor work histories (Bassuk *et al.*, 1986; Smith & North, 1994). Often there is a background of family violence and of abusive relationships with partners. Smith & North's (1994) study of 300 homeless women from shelters in St Louis found that 90% were mothers and that most were dependent on welfare.

In British studies the majority of homeless women have been white (Drake *et al.*, 1982), although more recently this profile has been changing. In James' (1991) study of 43 homeless women, 15 (35%) were black. In another study of 2308 pregnant women who booked into an antenatal clinic at a London teaching-hospital, over a 1 year period, 185 (8%) were found to be homeless (Paterson & Roderick, 1990). Compared to a housed group, the homeless group included a higher proportion of Indo-Pakistani women living in bed and breakfast accommodation. American studies of homeless women consistently report an over-representation of ethnic minorities on Skid Row (Garrett & Bahr, 1973; Blumberg *et al.*, 1978) and in urban areas (Breakey *et al.*, 1989). In Breakey *et al.*'s (1989) study of homeless men and women in missions, shelters and jails in Baltimore, 70.3% of the female sample was non-white, compared with 63.1% of the male sample. In Smith & North's (1994) sample of 300 homeless women, 76% were African-American.

Homeless women are less likely to have been in prison and institutions than homeless men (Digby, 1976; Drake *et al.*, 1982; Breakey *et al.*, 1989; Burt & Cohen, 1989; George *et al.*, 1991). Some surveys suggest that homeless women are more likely to be taken to psychiatric hospitals than homeless men. Herzberg (1987) found that homeless women were more likely than men to have been referred for admission on a Section 136 by the police. Perhaps the police, confronted by a woman behaving strangely are more likely to initiate admission to hospital, in circumstances where a man would be remanded to prison.

Mental illness in homeless women

Studies assessing mental illness in homeless women have largely used populations from hostels, shelters and no fixed abode admissions to hospital. Although the prevalence of self-reported mental illness has been as low as 8% (Drake *et al.*, 1982), the themes emerging are of high rates of serious mental illness (higher than in homeless men), with substantial co-morbidity (Table 5.3). While prevalence studies are not strictly comparable because of the different methods used in selecting the samples and in the assessment of psychiatric illness, they add further pieces to the jig-saw puzzle (James, 1991).

Digby (1976) interviewed one in ten residents in all common lodging houses and hostels. The 172 women interviewed (8.6% of the total sample of women) were a fairly settled group: 43% had been in the same hostel or lodging house for over 2 years and 55% of the women under 60 years were in employment. Over half had some record of an emotional or psychiatric problem, although only 10% had ever been an inpatient in a psychiatric hospital.

Brandon (1973) described a non-statutory project in London, run by social workers that catered for a disturbed population of destitute

Table 5.3. *Mental illness in homeless women: schizophrenia*

Studies	Men: Women	Men	Women
British hostel studies			
Adams (1991)	0:64		42% (27)
Scott (1991)	0:46		19% (9)
James (1991)	0:43		21% (9)
Marshall & Reed (1992)	0:70		64% (45)
Hospital studies			
Fernandez (1984)	115:28	33.3%	34.7%
Herzberg (1984)	62:48	25.8%	41.7%
American studies			
Bassuk et al. (1984)	65:13		85%
Breakey et al. (1989)	125:78	12.1%	17.1%
		42.0%[a]	48.7%[a]
Smith & North (1994)	0:300		1.0–12.5%[b]

[a] Major mental illness.
[b] Schizophrenia rates differed according to subgroup: non-mothers (6.5%); mothers with children (1.0%); mothers without children (10.0%); mothers with children over 16 years (12.5%).

women. A survey of residents on two separate days 4 months apart (46 and 48 women, respectively) found that residents were either young or old (under 20 or over 50 years) and that many had had psychiatric treatment. The women who used this project were more unstable than the women in hostels and common lodging houses.

Four more recent British studies of homeless women in London hostels reported different rates for schizophrenia: 42% (Adams, 1991); 21% (James, 1991); 19% (Scott, 1991); 64% (Marshall & Reed, 1992). This discrepancy can be explained on the basis of the age group studied. In the oldest sample only 16 of the 70 women (23%) interviewed were under 40 (Marshall & Reed, 1992), whereas 45% of the women in Adam's (1991) study were under 40 and the proportion was 70% in Scott's (1991) study. In three of these studies the older women were more likely to be schizophrenic (Adams, 1991; Scott, 1991; Marshall & Reed, 1992). James' (1991) sample was a selected one, made up of women referred by staff for a psychiatric opinion. He suggested that the lower prevalence of schizophrenia in his study could be due to the fact that the schizophrenic homeless in the hostel were less likely to present for treatment than other mentally ill groups and suspected that many of the women who did not present for assessment were suffering from schizophrenia.

In a retrospective study of 'no fixed abode' (NFA) admissions to a London psychiatric hospital, Herzberg (1987) reported that 41.7% of the homeless women were schizophrenic compared with 25.8% of men. Fernandez (1984) reported similarly high figures for psychosis in a Dublin sample of NFA admissions.

In Bassuk *et al.*'s (1984) study of a shelter in Massachusetts 65 men and 13 women were interviewed. Overall 40% had major mental illness, but the figure for the women was 85%. Breakey *et al.* (1989) interviewed a subsample of 125 homeless men and 78 homeless women and reported high levels of major mental illness, 42% in men and 48.7% in women. The figures for schizophrenia were 12% in men and 17% in women. Substantial co-morbidity was also found, 23% of men and 21.6% of women with major mental illness also having alcohol misuse. The figures for drug misuse co-morbidity were 9.1% and 9.5%, respectively.

In Bassuk *et al.*'s (1986) sample of 80 homeless mothers, 71% were given a DSM-III diagnosis of personality disorder. Smith & North (1994) divided their sample of 300 homeless women into non-mothers $(n=31)$, mothers with children present $(n=202)$, mothers without children present $(n=50)$ and mothers whose children were 16 years or over $(n=17)$. Mothers without children had the highest rates of DSM-III-R schizophrenia (10%), generalized anxiety disorder (16%) and alcohol abuse/dependence (33%), and 72% had a life-time psychiatric diagnosis.

Alcohol and drug problems in homeless women

Homeless women have a lower prevalence of alcohol and drugs problems compared with homeless men, but few good studies have been carried out (see Table 5.4). Although Digby (1976) reported that over half of the women living in hostel and common lodging house accommodation had some record of emotional or psychiatric problems, alcohol problems were not reported on separately. However, these women had a reasonably stable life-style in terms of retaining accommodation and employment and it is unlikely that women with serious drinking problems were found in these hostels and common lodging houses. They would have been more likely to have been sleeping rough or using the Reception Centres (Otto, 1980). This is borne out by a report from the Central London

Table 5.4. *Alcohol problems in homeless women*

Study	Men:Women	Men (%)	Women (%)
Adams (1991)[a]	0:64		8
James (1991)[b]	0:43		7
Marshall & Reed (1991)[c]	0:70		36
Herzberg (1984)	62:48	35.5	8.4
Fernandez (1984)	115:28	46.0	4.1
Breakey et al. (1989)[a]	125:78	56	16.5
Smith & North (1994)	0:300		Non-mothers: 19.4% Children present: 12.7% Children not present: 33.3% Children over 16: 12.5%

[a] Alcohol dependence.
[b] Alcohol seen as problem by staff.
[c] Drinking heavily.

Outreach Team (1984), which established contact with 399 people sleeping rough in London between April and December 1983. Their final sample of 318 included only 24 women, of whom 19 were identified as problem drinkers. These homeless women were considerably more withdrawn and isolated than the men and the team was unable to build up relationships with them. Female drunkenness was not as acceptable as male drunkenness on the 'sleeping rough scene', although their drinking was tolerated as part of their overall eccentricity. The women generally perceived their drinking as a problem, but only two were referred to the alcohol services for treatment.

Drake et al. (1982) reported that only 1% of 122 homeless women (compared with 3% of 398 homeless men) admitted to any problem with alcohol and drugs. The low prevalence may reflect the younger age group of the women in this sample (two thirds were under 30 and alcohol problems were commonest in the 35–44 age group), and the fact that self-report data is likely to be an underestimate. While similar proportions of men and women had taken at least one 'soft' drug (60% and 58%, respectively), women were more likely to have used barbiturates or tranquillizers, which they had obtained on prescription, and more men had used heroin. The most common age for having drug problems was the 20–24 age group followed by the 25–29 age group. This study was carried out in the late 1970s, and patterns of drug and alcohol misuse have changed since, thus the findings cannot be generalized to the present.

In Herzberg's (1987) retrospective study of no fixed abode admissions to a psychiatric hospital, 8.4% of women and 35.5% of men received a diagnosis of alcoholism. Fernandez (1984) reported similar figures, 4.1% for women and 46% for men. Breakey *et al.*'s (1989) Baltimore sample was assessed almost a decade later. Initially the Short Michigan Alcohol Screening Test (SMAST: Selzer *et al.*, 1975) was used to assess 298 homeless men and 230 homeless women in the missions, shelters and jails of Baltimore and 69% of men and 38% of women were found to be definite or probable alcoholics. When a subsample of 125 men and 78 women was interviewed, 56% of the men and 16.5% of the women fulfilled DSM-III criteria for the alcohol dependence syndrome (American Psychiatric Association, 1980).

Marshall & Reed (1992) reported that 25 (36%) of 70 women drank heavily and that 7 (10%) admitted to a current or serious drug problem. Seven (10%) had a history of opiate dependence and three were injecting at the time of the interview.

Physical illness in homeless women

Physical illness is common amongst the homeless (Drake *et al.*, 1982; Shanks, 1988; George *et al.*, 1991), particularly in those over 50 years (Drake *et al.*, 1982). Musculo-skeletal problems, respiratory, skin and gastro-intestinal disorders and alcohol-related problems have been reported as the most common problems in a sample sleeping rough in Central London (Ramsden *et al.*, 1989). Active tuberculosis has proved difficult to eradicate from the homeless of London and New York (Ramsden *et al.*, 1988). Unfortunately few studies have incorporated a physical examination in their design and the physical problems of homeless women are not always reported separately. Victor (1992) has investigated the health status of a temporarily homeless sample of 319 men and women in London. The sample was predominantly female (61%), young and belonging to an ethnic minority group. It included a large proportion of families with young children. Rates of both acute (10%) and long-standing (34%) illness were similar to those for regional residents, but the prevalence of mental morbidity was twice that for the region as a whole. The homeless population had higher utilization of general practitioner, accident and emergency departments and inpatient services.

Herzberg (1987) found no difference in the proportion of homeless men and women with physical illness in his sample of no fixed abode admissions, and in Fernandez' (1984) sample of a similar group 1.5% of the men and none of the women were reported as having 'mainly medical problems'.

Adams (1991) reported that 8 (12%) of 64 homeless women in a London hostel had some sort of physical illness, including asthma, hip pain, epilepsy and deafness. In Marshall & Reed's (1992) older sample, 19 (27%) of 70 women admitted to physical illness (epilepsy, 4; respiratory, 4; alcohol-related, 2; cardiovascular, 2; diabetes, 1; other, 6).

In the Baltimore study, Breakey et al. (1989) organized a comprehensive physical assessment of 120 homeless men and 75 homeless women, using a standardized protocol. This included a review of the past medical history, a physical examination and laboratory tests (an electrocardiogram, chest X-ray, blood count and liver function tests, urinalysis, tests for gonorrhoea and syphilis, tuberculin skin test and stool examination for parasites). Men had on average 8.3 problems and women 9.2, and each problem was considered sufficient for referral to primary care. Problems of the mouth and teeth (orodental) were the commonest in both sexes. Two thirds of women had gynaecological problems and some kind of arthritis was diagnosed in 32% of women and 26% of men. Anaemia was found in 35% of women and 18% of men.

Why do women become homeless?

While it is hard to generalize, women seem more likely than men to become homeless for social reasons, such as family break-up, marital and parental disputes (Drake et al., 1982). Social factors are intimately bound to economic factors such as the lack of affordable housing, due to a decrease in the supply over the past 30 years, and poverty. Younger homeless women often have a history of family break up and of being in care. Homelessness is not due to just one of these factors. Often a combination of factors occurring at a critical period precipitates homelessness or causes a further slide down the pathway.

Psychological factors are also important. There is evidence that women with psychiatric illness and substance abuse are likely to end up in hostels because they are unable to cope on their own, or to secure their own housing (Watson & Austerberry, 1986). De-institutionalization, together with the lack of provision of shelters for homeless women appear to have been factors in the USA (Bachrach, 1984).

Merves (1986) described three different pathways to homelessness for women – the skid or slide, periodical or cyclical homelessness and critical juncture. Skid or slide is the combination of several events, leading to a downward spiral. Periodical cyclical homelessness describes the situation where women are intermittently homeless. A critical juncture is a major change point where some women choose to leave home, perhaps in response to domestic violence, in order to take charge of their own lives. Periodical homelessness is more likely in younger women and the skid/slide process occurs particularly in older women.

Services for homeless women

The homeless mentally ill do not access psychiatric services, despite needing them (Padgett *et al.*, 1990). Homeless mentally ill women often avoid services or use them intermittently. This may be due to a variety of reasons, including negative experiences in the past, lack of insight, or a refusal to admit to mental illness because of the associated stigma. However, the literature suggests that they are resourceful in devising strategies to survive and are amenable to support services (Grella, 1994).

Few services have been designed specifically for homeless women but themes emerge from the studies that have evaluated such services. Homeless mentally ill women can engage in assertive clinical case management programmes while remaining residentially mobile (Harris & Bachrach, 1990; Goering *et al.*, 1992). They may benefit from periodic use of shelters as a respite from the streets and from daily support services provided by a day centre (Grella, 1994).

Harris & Bachrach (1990) described an assertive clinical case management programme for homeless women, based in the District of Columbia, USA. In the first 3 years of the programme, 25 homeless mentally ill women between the ages of 24 and 66 years were referred.

These women were a very disabled group and had histories of
multiple inpatient admissions; 16 had a diagnosis of schizophrenia
and 13 a history of alcohol or other substance abuse. Homelessness
had been a recurrent theme in their lives and they had frequently
moved in and out of the homeless population, many showing gross
geographical mobility. Despite these problems they engaged in an
assertive clinical case management programme and there was a
significant reduction in their use of psychiatric inpatient facilities.
Although the women continued to be residentially mobile this was
considered to be a restlessness rather than a rootlessness. Harris &
Bachrach (1990) hypothesized that the freedom to move about
among residential settings was instrumental in helping the women to
leave the streets and to become involved in a treatment programme.

Grella (1994) described a combined day centre and shelter
programme, based in Santa Monica, California, which aimed to help
homeless mentally ill women to achieve greater mental stability and
to obtain permanent housing. The role of the day centre was limited
to meeting the basic daily needs of the women, such as food, rest and a
place to wash. It also referred clients on to the shelter, which was more
structured, and operated a case management programme. Four
patterns of day centre and/or shelter use soon emerged. First, a small
proportion of women who could cope with the structure of the shelter,
had insight into their mental illness and agreed to treatment, were
able to move on to stable housing. The second pattern of use included
the majority of women who came to the shelter for periods of respite
and returned to the streets or to an unstable housing situation. These
women had more severe mental health problems for which they
refused help. They also refused to consider housing options associated
with mental illness e.g. group homes, preferring to maintain their
independence. The third pattern included women who used the day
centre but who were inappropriate for the shelter, either because of
overt psychosis and behavioural disturbance or because of alcohol/
drug misuse. Finally there was a group of women who used the day
centre but did not wish to move on to the shelter. These women were,
in many ways, like the women who made the transition, but they
were, in addition, independent and self-reliant loners. Although the
original goals were not fulfilled, the service was very effective in
taking on the role of primary service provider for these women.
Certainly a two-tiered system is one way of expanding the range of
service options available to this population in a climate of limited
resources and large demand.

Conclusions

Homeless women are a heterogenous group, largely younger and more socially stable than homeless men. Proportionally more have major mental illness than men. Older homeless women have high levels of schizophrenia while personality disorder and substance misuse are commoner in younger women. They are restless rather than rootless and can engage with appropriate services. Although the numbers of homeless women are rising, information is still sparse and more research on their problems and needs is required.

References

Adams, C. E. (1991). Homeless Women: a Prevalence Study of Homeless Women in London. Unpublished MSc. thesis. London School of Hygiene and Tropical Medicine.

American Psychiatric Association (1980). *Diagnostic and Statistical Manual of Mental Disorders*, 3rd edit. Washington DC: American Psychiatric Association.

Arce, A. A., Tadlock, M., Vergare, M. J. & Shapiro, S. H. (1983). A psychiatric profile of street people admitted to an emergency shelter. *Hospital and Community Psychiatry*, **34**, 812–17.

Bachrach, L. L. (1984). Deinstitutionalization and women. *American Psychologist*, **10**, 1171–7.

Bassuk, E. L., Rubin, L. & Lauriat, A. (1984). Is homelessness a mental health problem? *American Journal of Psychiatry*, **141**, 1546–9.

Bassuk, E. L., Rubin, L. & Lauriat, A. (1986). Characteristics of sheltered homeless families. *American Journal of Public Health*, **76**, 1097–101.

Blumberg, L. U., Shipley, T. E. & Barsky, S. F. (1978). *Liquor and Poverty: Skid Row as a Human Condition*. New Brunswick: Rutgers Centre of Alcohol Studies.

Brandon, D. (1973). Community for homeless women. *Social Work Today*, **4**, 167–70.

Breakey, W. R., Fischer, P. J., Kramer, M. *et al.* (1989). Health and mental health problems of homeless men and women in Baltimore. *Journal of the American Medical Association*, **262**, 1352–7.

Burt, M. R. & Cohen, B. E. (1989). *America's Homeless: Numbers, Characteristics and Programs that Serve Them*. Washington DC: Urban Institute.

Central London Outreach Team (1984). *Sleeping out in Central London*. London: Greater London Council.

Chesterton, C. (1926). *In Darkest London*. London: Stanley Paul and Co. Ltd.

Digby, P. W. (1976). *Hostels and Lodging Houses for Single People*. London: HMSO, Office of Censuses and Surveys.

Drake, M., O'Brien, M. & Biebuyck, T. (1982). *Single and Homeless*. London: HMSO, Department of the Environment Report.

Fernandez, J. (1984). In Dublin's fair city: the mentally ill of "no fixed abode". *Bulletin of the Royal College of Psychiatrists*, **8**, 187–90.

Fischer, P., Shapiro, S., Breakey, W. R., Anthony, J. C. & Kramer, M. (1986). Mental health and social characteristics of the homeless: a survey of mission users. *American Journal of Public Health*, **76**, 519–24.

Garrett, G. R. & Volk, D. H. (1970). *Homeless Women in New York City*. New York: Columbia University, Bureau of Applied Social Research.

Garrett, G. R. & Bahr, H. M. (1973). Women on skid row. *Quarterly Journal of Studies on Alcohol*, **34**, 1228–43.

George, S. L., Shanks, N. J. & Westlake, L. (1991). Census of single homeless people in Sheffield. *British Medical Journal*, **302**, 1387–9.

Goering, P., Wasylenki, D., St Onge, M., Paduchak, D. & Lancee, W. (1992). Gender differences among clients of a case management programme for the homeless. *Hospital and Community Psychiatry*, **43**, 160–5.

Grella, C. (1994). Contrasting a shelter and day centre for homeless mentally ill women: four patterns of service use. *Community Mental Health Journal*, **30**, 3–16.

Harris, M. & Bachrach, L. L. (1990). Perspectives on homeless women. *Hospital and Community Psychiatry*, **41**, 253–4.

Herzberg, J. (1987). No fixed abode. A comparison of men and women admitted to an East London psychiatric hospital. *British Journal of Psychiatry*, **150**, 621–7.

Higgs, M. & Hayward, E. (1910). *Where Shall She Live? The Homelessness of the Woman Worker*. London: P. S. King and Son.

James, A. (1991). Homeless women in London: the hostel perspective. *Health Trends*, **23**, 80–3.

Kroll, J., Carey, K., Hagedorn, D., Dog, P. F. & Benavides, E. (1986). A survey of homeless adults in urban emergency shelters. *Hospital and Community Psychiatry*, **37**, 283–6.

Laidlaw, S. I. A. (1956). *Glasgow Common Lodging-Houses and the People living in Them*. Glasgow: Corporation of Glasgow, Health and Welfare Department.

Lipton, F. R., Sabatini, A. & Katz, S. E. (1983). Down and out in the city: the homeless mentally ill. *Hospital and Community Psychiatry*, **34**, 817–21.

London County Council (1962). Southwark Reception Centre – Admission of Women with Histories of Mental Disorder. Report (19.9.62) by the Chief Officer of the Welfare Department.

McEwan, J. (1967). Preliminary Report of Visiting Medical Officer at Southwark Reception Centre. Unpublished report to the Ministry of Social Security.

Marshall, E. J. & Reed, J. L. (1992). Psychiatric morbidity in homeless women. *British Journal of Psychiatry*, **160**, 761–8.

Menzies, F. N. K. (1927). Common Lodging-houses and Kindred Institutions. London County Council Report No. 2489.

Merves, E. S. (1986). Conversations with Homeless Women: A Sociological Examination. PhD thesis. Ohio State University.

National Assistance Board (1966). *Homeless Single Persons*. London: HMSO.

Otto, S. (1980). Single homeless women and alcohol. In Camberwell Council on Alcoholism (eds.), *Women and Alcohol*, pp. 176–200. London and New York: Tavistock Publications.

Padgett, D., Struening, E. L. & Andrews, H. (1990). Factors affecting the use of medical, mental health, alcohol, and drug treatment services by homeless adults. *Medical Care*, **28**, 805–21.

Paterson, C. M. & Roderick, P. (1990). Obstetric outcome in homeless women. *British Medical Journal*, **301**, 263–6.

Ramsden, S. S., Baur, S. & El-Kabir, D. J. (1988). Tuberculosis among the central London single homeless. *Journal of the Royal College of Physicians of London*, **22**, 16–17.

Ramsden, S. S., Nyiri, P., Bridgewater, J. & El-Kabir, D. J. (1989). A mobile surgery for single homeless people in London. *British Medical Journal*, **298**, 372–4.

Ribton-Turner, C. J. (1887). *A History of Vagrants and Vagrancy and Beggars and Begging*. London: Chapman and Hall.

Scott, J. (1991). *Resettlement unit or asylum?* Paper presented at the Health Care Needs of the Homeless session of the Royal College of Psychiatrists Annual General Meeting, Brighton, 3 July 1991.

Scott, J. (1993). Homelessness and mental illness. *British Journal of Psychiatry*, **162**, 314–24.

Selzer, M. L., Vinokur, A. & van Rooijen, L. (1975). A self-administered Short Michigan Alcohol Screening Test (SMAST). *Journal of Studies on Alcohol*, **36**, 117–26.

Shanks, N. J. (1988). Medical morbidity of the homeless. *Journal of Epidemiology and Public Health*, **42**, 183–6.

Smith, E. M. & North, C. S. (1994). Not all homeless women are alike: effects of motherhood and the presence of children. *Community Mental Health Journal*, **6**, 601–10.

Tillard, M. A. & Booth, C. (1924). Homeless men. In Booth C. (ed.) *Life and Labour of the People in London*, vol. I, chapter IV, 2nd edit., London: Macmillan. (First published in 1891).

Victor, C. R. (1992). Health status of the temporarily homeless population and residents of North West Thames region. *British Medical Journal*, **305**, 387–91.

Watson, S. & Austerberry, H. (1986). *Housing and Homelessness: A Feminist Perspective*. London: Routledge and Kegan Paul.

6

Homelessness and criminality

PHILIP JOSEPH

Introduction

The relationship between homelessness, mental disorder and criminal behaviour is complex. Although many homeless people are not mentally disordered and have no criminal history, there is a strong association between homelessness and mental disorder on the one hand and homelessness and criminality on the other. The link between mental disorder and crime is more tenuous and is outside the scope of this chapter although a comprehensive review is provided by Wessely & Taylor (1991).

Theories of causation examining homelessness, mental disorder and crime vary according to ideological standpoint. Whilst criminological theories stress social and economic factors contributing to homelessness such as unemployment, lack of low cost housing and poverty, which in turn lead to mental disorder and crime, a psychological approach tends to focus on individual, intra-psychic factors, for example the onset of mental illness that precipitates homelessness and thence crime. Regardless of ideological perspective, homelessness provides the link between mental disorder and crime, and once an individual has become homeless, for whatever reason, the chances of being overlooked by mental health services or becoming ensnared in the criminal justice system are greatly increased.

This chapter will consider the plight of that most disadvantaged and chaotic group, namely those homeless people who are both mentally disordered and criminal. The historical review shows how homelessness has been criminalized since the Middle Ages as a means of social control. The review of studies of homelessness and criminality supports the strong links that exist with high rates of homelessness amongst prison and psychiatric hospital populations. Contemporary problems brought about by changes in mental health care policy over the last 30 years will be considered, particularly the increasing role of the policy as the main community response to disturbed behaviour. Finally some solutions will be offered, which in the light of the UK Reed Report (Department of Health and Home Office, 1992) will stress the early diversion of the mentally disordered from the criminal justice system as the first part of a package of measures in the community, such as access to primary care and a possible community treatment order, as a way of intervening in the cycle of disadvantage.

Historical background

The interaction between the law, social policy and public sentiment is clearly evident in society's response to the single homeless person. The fundamental quandary is whether the vagrant should be treated as a pauper or a criminal. Homelessness itself has been criminalized to varying degrees in the UK since the Middle Ages. Relief for the poor of the parish has always taken precedence over relief for poor people coming from outside the community. The poor, whether sick, frail, old or mentally ill relied on a dwindling proportion of the church tithes for their relief or on alms given indiscriminately by the wealthy. To leave the parish was considered a grave threat to society and attracted punitive legislation. The early statutes aimed to suppress vagrancy by punishment without any attempt at relieving the destitution that gave rise to it.

In the wake of the Napoleonic Wars, a combination of returning soldiers, the profound social changes set in motion by the beginnings of industrialization and the rapidly rising population, led to a dramatic increase in vagrancy. Workhouses, which had been set up sporadically during the eighteenth century were overcrowded and disease ridden. In 1821 it was estimated there were at least 60 000 people perpetually circulating up and down the country (Ribton-Turner, 1887, p. 232). The policy of returning them to their parish of origin under the Law and Settlement and Removal had become an expensive failure, open to abuse.

The Vagrancy Act 1824 entitled 'An Act for the Punishment of idle and disorderly Persons, and Rogues and Vagabonds...' abandoned the requirement that vagrants should be returned to their place of settlement and instead imposed a summary trial and imprisonment with hard labour. The two main offences under the Act were begging and sleeping out, which had thus clearly been made subject to the due criminal process of law. In 1830s the London Poor Law authorities regarded vagrants picked up by the police as a criminal concern, but the magistrates chose not to convict them but to use their powers under the New Poor Law of 1834 to send them to the workhouses.

As early as 1846 it was said that the Vagrancy Act was out of keeping with public sentiment. Nevertheless it remains in force today apart from an amendment of 1935, which abolished the simple offence of sleeping out. This amendment followed the tragic case of an ex-serviceman who was arrested and imprisoned for sleeping out whilst looking for work. He had never been imprisoned before and suffered a severe anxiety reaction in the prison leading to a fracas with prison officers that resulted in his death. A public outcry ensued and the feeling was summed up by Mr Spears MP in the House of Commons whose private member's bill led to the amendment. He said,

There never was a more blatant example of one law for the rich and another for the poor, for if you had money in your pocket and chose to sleep out as a health giving pursuit, the law would not touch you: but if you are so poor that you have not the price of a night's lodging in your pocket, you are a criminal and liable to be sent to jail.

(*Hansard*, 26 March 1935, col. 1743).

As well as the vagrancy legislation the life-style of the mentally disordered homeless was also regulated by the Poor Laws and later the mental health legislation. Initially there was little to distinguish between the treatment for acute mental illness and the punishment meted out to vagrants. The Vagrancy Act 1744 excluded pauper lunatics from punishment and empowered magistrates to order the confinement of those who were 'too furiously mad and dangerous to be permitted to go abroad'. This provision was entirely for the public's protection as few suitable places existed for their confinement and they usually ended up in gaols or bridewells.

Recorded convictions for begging and sleeping out, offences under the Vagrancy Act 1824, have varied greatly over the last century, with the main peak before the First World War. In 1910, the peak year in London, there were 7322 prosecutions for begging, a third of the total for England and Wales. The number prosecuted for sleeping out increased less dramatically, and tended to average one tenth of the begging prosecutions. During the 1920s and 30s, numbers were high and fairly constant, but never reached pre-war levels. A graphic account of homelessness between the wars has been provided by Orwell (1933; and see Chapter 2).

After the Second World War, prosecutions dropped markedly and the numbers of homeless sleeping out almost disappeared, partly due to the National Assistance Act of 1948. This led the then London County Council to suspend its annual homeless census. In the 1980s there has been a reversal of this trend, and although prosecutions for sleeping out have remained very low, probably due to a deliberate policy of not arresting those sleeping rough, the number of prosecutions for begging has begun to rise.

Of perhaps more importance is the propensity of the homeless single person to commit crimes outside the vagrancy statutes. Such crimes may themselves lead to the breaking of ties with society and the descent into an unsettled way of life, or they may be encouraged by this life-style and in either case may hinder escape from it. In earlier times the bands of 'sturdy rogues' roaming the country, causing havoc and spreading panic, were a real menace to society, but today's single homeless person is likely to be a recidivist petty offender.

Studies of homelessness and criminality

Studies of the criminal records of the homeless show high rates of criminality. The large single homeless persons survey of 1966 showed that 60% of reception centre residents admitted to a prison record, with 9.4% having been released from prison in the preceeding two months (National Assistance Board, 1966, p. 58). Edwards *et al.* (1968) found that a similar figure (59%) of their Camberwell Reception Centre sample had been imprisoned, but noted the longest sentence averaged 12.4 months with an average of 7.4 sentences, suggesting multiple petty offences were being committed. More recently, Marshall (1989) reported that 48% of hostel dwellers in Oxford had previously been imprisoned.

Tidmarsh (1977) analysed the criminal careers of his Camberwell Reception Centre residents according to psychiatric diagnosis. Those with no diagnosis had the lowest rate of previous convictions (38%).

The mentally ill were next with a rate of 55%, followed by those with personality disorder (69%), and finally the group with the highest rate of recorded criminality were the alcoholics at 76%. Tidmarsh also found that the more handicaps suffered by an individual, e.g. mental illness complicated by alcohol abuse, the higher the rate of criminality. The most common offences were theft, criminal damage and vagrancy; violence was much less likely, although higher than would be expected for the general population.

Tidmarsh then looked at the hospital careers of his homeless men. He showed that for those with a diagnosis of mental illness or alcoholism, a history of imprisonment was associated with previous psychiatric hospitalization. This finding is supported by a study of 529 homeless adults in Los Angeles, where those with a history of hospital treatment had higher rates of imprisonment and longer periods of homelessness than the non-hospitalized homeless (Gelberg et al., 1988).

Further evidence that confirms the close relationship between homelessness, mental disorder and criminality is provided by those studies of prison populations that show high rates of homelessness amongst prisoners prior to their incarceration, and studies of homelessness amongst psychiatric hospital admissions. Turning to the prison studies first; an early study of prisoners in the south-west of England found that of 174 sentenced men, 31% were homeless at the time of their arrest, and 42% expected to have no home to go to on their release. Those with no homes were older, more recidivist with higher rates of unemployment than the rest (South-West Regional Group Consultative Committee, 1969). A more extensive study covering London and south-east England showed higher rates of homelessness (Walmsley, 1972). He estimated that 7000 (58%) of the 12 000 prison releases annually were of men who were possibly homeless. They had either been sleeping rough or in common lodging houses for part of the year prior to their arrest. The homeless prisoners were older and serving shorter sentences, they were more likely to be single or separated and originate from Scotland or Ireland. In another survey of prisoners, Gibbens & Silverman (1970) showed that those who were alcoholic had three times the rate of homelessness than the other prisoners.

Turning to hospital admissions, Berry & Orwin (1966) retrospectively surveyed the admission of homeless patients to a Birmingham psychiatric hospital between 1961 and 1965. The percentage of male admissions who were homeless on admission rose from 8.3% to 13.6% during that period. The total sample consisted of 105 men and 40 women, of whom 49% were suffering from schizophrenia and 37% had a criminal record. Of the 107 patients (74%) who had a previous psychiatric admission, 60% had been discharged within the last year. Also, 69% of the schizophrenics had been admitted to hospital via the police or prison. A third of the sample remained in hospital less than 1 month, with little prospect of medical follow-up and rehabilitation. The authors concluded that 'the initial enthusiasm ... for the discharge of chronic psychotics into community care was premature, in view of the resources available, and has resulted in the overwhelming of community care' (Berry & Orwin, 1966, p. 1024).

The conclusions of the 1960s have a familiar ring to them and two studies in the 1980s showed that very little has changed in the disadvantaged world of the homeless mentally ill. First, Szmukler *et al.* (1981) reviewed all compulsory hospital admissions to a London borough and showed that the homeless were over-represented among those detained in hospital under both civil and criminal provisions of the Mental Health Act 1959, in force at that time. They tended to present management problems, have brief admissions and either abscond or be discharged prematurely. Secondly, Herzberg (1987) compared male and female homeless admissions to an East London psychiatric hospital over a 10 year period. He again painted a picture of social disadvantage, previous psychiatric admissions and previous episodes of imprisonment amongst his sample. Only just over a third were considered to have an improved mental state on discharge. Herzberg concluded 'It is sad to note the dearth of group home and small hostel accommodation during the 1970s ... Unfortunately this situation has not changed in the 1980s (Herzberg, 1987, p. 626).

In some cases hospitals may exacerbate homelessness by discharging patients to temporary hostel accommodation or even to the streets. Marshall's (1989) survey of Oxford hostel residents revealed that 48 (32%) showed persistent severe mental disability and 90% had previously been in a psychiatric hospital, many as long-term patients. Marshall concluded 'The two hostels, staffed by psychiatrically untrained workers and volunteers were effectively attempting to do the work equivalent to that in two long-stay psychiatric wards... We are witnessing the inadvertent creation of mini-institutions in hostels (Marshall, 1989, p. 708: for detailed discussion see Chapter 9).

Current problems

In England and Wales, a policy of community care has existed for over 30 years, during which there has been a decline in the mental hospital and mental handicap hospital population and a rise in the remand and sentenced prisoner population. From 1962 to 1990, the combined psychiatric inpatient population fell from 196 234 to 87 683, a 55% reduction; the combined prison population rose from 31 063 to 47 936, an increase of 54% (Home Office, 1962–1990; DHSS 1962–1990). The percentage changes are similar but the gross numbers differ widely, thus invalidating some of the wilder claims made about the wholesale transfer of the mentally ill from hospital to prison (Weller, 1989). However, when one narrows the focus on to the disadvantaged world of the homeless mentally ill, there is perhaps justified concern that many, who previously would have been admitted to psychiatric hospitals, are now becoming ensnared in the criminal justice system and ending up in prison.

The police are becoming increasingly recognized as an important community mental health resource, particularly as the focus of treatment for the mentally ill moves to the community. They are the only laymen in Great Britain who can act alone, without medical evidence, to detain a suspected mentally ill person in a place of safety. This power has existed in statutory form for over 100 years and the latest version is contained in section 136 of the Mental Health Act 1983, which states:

1. If a constable finds in a place to which the public have access a person who appears to him to be suffering from mental disorder and to be in need of care and control, the constable may, if he thinks it necessary to do so in the interests of that person or for the safety or protection of other persons, remove that person to a place of safety . . .
2. A person removed to a place of safety under this section may be detained there for a period not exceeding 72 hours for the purpose of enabling him to be examined by an Approved Social Worker and of making any necessary arrangements for his treatment and care.

This power coupled with the police's round-the-clock availability to intervene in emergencies, makes it hardly surprising that they become involved with the mentally ill, whether they see this as part of their job or not.

There is great variation across the country in the number of police referrals to psychiatric services. High rates are especially common in inner city areas and police in London are particularly likely to use their powers under section 136 Mental Health Act 1983, rather than rely on the attendance of approved social workers or other mental health professionals at the police station. In 1986, for example, 47% of all section 136 admissions in England took place in London. Rollin (1965) has attributed this excess in London to the city's role as a 'sump ... into which chronic psychotics from all over the United Kingdom ... are drained'.

The reasons that led the mentally ill to come to the attention of the police were identified by George (1972) in his study of police referrals to psychiatric services in west central London. Threatening or bizarre behaviour leading to public disturbance predominated, followed by suicide attempts or threats. George showed that those dealt with under section 136 differed from those admitted compulsorily under emergency civil provisions, i.e. section 29 of the then Mental Health Act 1959, which is now covered by section 4 of the 1983 Act. The police admissions had significantly more often shown aggressive behaviour before admission and presented more management problems during admission. They were more likely to be of no fixed abode and socially disorganized. Interestingly, those admitted compulsorily in the past tended to have been on the same section as the index admission.

Numerous studies have examined the characteristics of police referred psychiatric admissions in the UK and the USA and certain conclusions can be drawn. Police referrals have high rates of chronic serious mental illness, frequently requiring emergency compulsory psychiatric admission (Kelleher & Copeland, 1972). Diagnostically, the majority suffer from a psychotic illness, predominantly schizophrenia. For example, in George's (1972) sample of 856 section 136 admissions collected between 1967 and 1969, 57% had a diagnosis of schizophrenia. Very few referrals are considered to have no mental disorder, indeed Rollin (1965), suggested all 75 cases in his study had a psychiatric diagnosis. Other studies suggest a figure closer to 10% as having no mental disorder (Rogers & Faulkner, 1987; Fahy *et al.*, 1987). In the USA, Sheridan & Teplin (1981), have confirmed these diagnostic findings in their study of

838 police referrals to a Chicago community mental health centre.

In view of their serious mental illness, social disorganization and lack of psychiatric support, it is, perhaps, not surprising that police referrals do badly as a group following admission to hospital. They have a high rate of absconding or self-discharge from hospital, and they are less likely to attend follow-up appointments (Sims & Symonds, 1975; Szmukler *et al.*, 1981). They are a group to whom the term 'revolving door' (Rollin, 1969) has been applied to describe their frequent rotation between hospital, prison and the streets. Ways of breaking this cycle of disadvantage will now be considered.

Some solutions

Diversion from custody

When criminal proceedings are brought, the defendant who is mentally disordered has the same right as other defendants to be released on bail before trial unless one or more of the exceptions specified in the Bail Act 1976 apply. In practice the presumption in favour of bail is weakened for the mentally disordered defendant due to the clause allowing remand in custody for his own protection. This is compounded if the defendant is of no fixed abode, as 'lack of community ties' is cited as a reason for forming the belief that the defendant would fail to return to court. Thus, mentally disordered homeless defendants charged with minor offences are more likely to be remanded into custody than others charged with similar offences.

There has been mounting concern over the conditions endured by mentally disordered prisoners on remand (Herridge, 1989; HM Chief Inspector of Prisons, 1990). Suicide in prison is a matter of grave concern; between 1972 and 1989 there were 295 suicides in prisons in England and Wales with an increase in the yearly rate far in excess of the rise in the prison population (Dooley, 1990). In order to try and reduce the numbers of mentally ill prisoners the Home Office has issued guidelines to all courts regarding provision for mentally disordered defendants, which includes the statement: 'A mentally disordered person should never be remanded to prison simply to receive medical treatment or assessment' (Home Office, 1990).

It is not uncommon for there to be an inordinate delay following remand in custody whilst awaiting psychiatric assessment, with no guarantee of subsequent hospital admission (Bowden, 1978a,b). The process can be speeded up considerably by arranging for psychiatrists to conduct assessments at the magistrates' courts rather than in prison. A psychiatric assessment service based at two inner London courts was set up in 1989 to facilitate psychiatric assessment and diversion from custody (Joseph & Potter, 1993a,b). A total of 201 defendants were referred to the psychiatrist at court over an 18 month period. They were predominantly male, single, of no fixed abode and suffering from serious psychiatric disorder. The majority had received previous psychiatric treatment often as detained patients. They typically were recidivists charged with minor offences. Following initial assessment 25% were admitted directly to hospital and a further 50% were released. The time taken from arrest to hospital admission was 6 days, a considerable improvement on the figure of 50 days calculated by Dell *et al.* (1991) for comparable defendants remanded to Brixton Prison during the same period.

A follow-up was carried out on the 65 patients who were admitted to hospital. Fifty (77%) derived some or marked benefit from psychiatric treatment. Those who did badly were more likely to be homeless, with higher rates of criminality and previous compulsory admissions to hospital. Absconding was the largest management problem and 12 months after admission only one patient remained in hospital.

The population described bears many similarities to those patients taken to hospital by the police using their powers under section 136 of the Mental Health Act 1983 (Szmukler *et al.*, 1981). It also shares many features of those remanded into custody for medical reports (Bowden, 1978a,b; Coid, 1988a,b). The notion that these groups overlap is strengthened by the finding that approximately two thirds of this sample had previously been remanded in custody for medical reports or detained in hospital under civil or criminal provisions of the Mental Health Act or had been subject to section 136. Those with unsettled accommodation were particularly disadvantaged with higher rates of criminality and less contact with psychiatric services. The decision to charge these people with minor offences may be arbitrary yet once ensnared by the criminal process considerable delay many ensue, aggravated by the wait for psychiatric assessment, before diversion from custody can be achieved.

Psychiatric assessment at the Magistrates' Court places an extra burden on hospital resources both in terms of beds and staff, but creates savings in prison resources. However, the overall shift from prison to hospital is small due to the characteristics of the defendants seen, a group whose chronic mental illness, substance abuse, criminality and especially non-compliance with treatment makes admission to general acute unlocked psychiatric wards unsuitable in the majority of cases.

Early diversion from custody removes the last bastion of psychiatric treatment for many of this group, namely the hospital wing of the remand prison. In order to provide alternative psychiatric facilities there would need to be acute locked psychiatric wards providing psychiatric evaluations and reports on defendants remanded by the courts for such a purpose. The use of section 35 Mental Health Act 1983 would need to be substantially increased with treatment given compulsorily if required (Gunn & Joseph, 1993).

In addition, for those defendants currently remanded to prison who do not require compulsory hospital admission, their assessment could take place at specialist community based bail hostels, managed by the probation service with access to psychiatric consultation. Currently both these hospital and community based provisions either do not exist or are in short supply.

Access to primary care

The homeless mentally ill often suffer from multiple handicaps, yet there are administrative barriers that hinder their access to health care. Once homeless the mentally ill are at a serious disadvantage when they seek medical care. Their lack of accommodation makes it difficult for them to register with general practitioners and even when that has been accomplished, the slavish adherence by psychiatric services to catchment area boundaries may curtail further progress (see also Chapter 11).

This has been recognized to some extent by the Department of Health, which provided initial, direct funding for a primary care medical centre for homeless people in central London (El-Kabir, 1982) where a drop-in psychiatric clinic is attached (Joseph *et al.*, 1990). The clinic, Great Chapel Street Medical Centre, is a primary care health centre for the homeless set up in 1978 with direct government funding. The staff includes an administrator, general practitioners, district nurse and community psychiatric nurse, social worker, dentist, chiropodist and psychiatrists. There are close links with the local probation service and voluntary sector. Since its inception the number of patients attending has increased sharply; in 1992 there were approximately 7500 consultations of which 1500 were new patients. The majority of attendees are homeless and refer themselves, or are referred by the many voluntary hostels and day centres in the vicinity. Other referrals come from probation and social services.

Psychiatric consultations account for a quarter of referrals and form the largest single group attending the medical centre. Diagnostically four roughly equal groups are seen: first the chronic mentally ill, predominantly suffering from schizophrenia with previous hospital admissions; secondly, substance abusers, usually alcohol, as there is a facility for drug users nearby; thirdly, young people often labelled as personality disordered with a history of broken homes, periods in care and delinquency, who have gravitated to London, and are at risk of drug abuse and sexual exploitation. Finally a group of 'others', comprising situational and neurotic problems in people with inadequate coping reserves. Clearly these broad groups overlap, for example a schizophrenic patient with alcohol abuse and personality difficulties. Indeed it is a feature of the homeless mentally ill that there are often complicating factors that have led to them slipping through the net of conventional psychiatric care. Two important factors are non-compliance with medication and a criminal history, over one half of the psychiatric patients seen at the clinic over the last 10 years have a criminal record according to the Criminal Records Office data.

A residential care home, Wytham Hall is a sister organization to Great Chapel Street Medical Centre, providing 15 beds for homeless people suffering from a variety of physical and psychiatric conditions. It has 24 hour medical cover and can provide asylum for those psychiatric patients who are increasingly refused admission to overstretched inner city psychiatric units or who are discharged precipitously, once their acute symptoms have diminished.

A community treatment order?

Following well publicized cases of psychiatric patients who have harmed themselves or others following discharge from hospital,

attention has been focused on deficiencies in the government's policy
of care in the community, notably the lack of a community treatment
order to ensure compliance in those cases where compulsory admission to hospital, under existing provisions of the Mental Health Act
1983, is not considered appropriate.

Although community treatment orders are already in use in some
countries, notably Australia and part of the USA, they have been the
subject of little research, despite their widespread occurrence, estimated at 20% of all compulsory psychiatric treatment orders in the
USA (Miller, 1985). Even without a specific community treatment
order, mechanisms currently exist in the UK to ensure an element of
coercion in the community treatment of psychiatric patients.
Examples are a probation order with a condition of psychiatric
treatment or a guardianship order within the terms of the Mental
Health Act 1983. Both these provisions tend to be under-used and the
powers to ensure compliance are limited. However in Jersey, which
has its own Mental Health legislation, the powers of a guardian for
the purposes of a guardianship order are wider, allowing early
intervention to prevent a crisis (Moate *et al.*, 1993). Perhaps the most
effective mechanism to ensure compliance is the power exercised by
the Home Office regarding the supervision of section 41 (Mental
Health Act 1983) conditionally discharged restriction order patients,
but clearly this power is reserved for those who have committed
serious offences or who pose a serious threat to the community, and it
represents a severe infringement of personal liberty.

In England and Wales prior to 1983, the supervision of psychiatric
patients in the community following compulsory treatment in hospital was often ensured by granting the patient leave of absence under
section 39 of the then existing Mental Health Act 1959. This
provision created a 'liability to recall' to hospital for a period of 6
months following discharge, but the power could be renewed for a
further 6 months by simply re-admitting the patient to hospital for a
token 1 night. The arrangement was described by the Mental Health
Act Commission as the 'long leash' relationship and its legality was
challenged in 1985 when the absence of a clear provision in the 1983
Act similar to the previous legislation was noted and the practice
subsequently outlawed. In contrast in Scotland, under the Mental
Health (Scotland) Act 1984, the use of extended leave to ensure the
supervision of a patient in the community continues to be used.

Sensky *et al.* (1991a,b) used 'extended leave' patients as a starting
point to try and identify those patients who would be considered

suitable for a community treatment order if it existed. They followed up those patients who had been on extended leave prior to 1985 and found that its use had improved treatment compliance, reduced time spent in hospital and reduced levels of dangerousness. Psychiatrists who were asked to nominate patients under their care for a community treatment order, chose those, not surprisingly, who were less likely to comply with treatment and who had a history of recent dangerousness. It is uncertain how many patients will satisfy criteria for a proposed community treatment order but it is likely that the overwhelming majority of patients will suffer from a psychotic illness and for those suffering from personality disorder, particularly psychopathic disorder, there will continue to be a paucity of community based treatment facilities.

What has not been adequately addressed is the practical aspects of such an order and its applicability to homeless people. Although the Royal College of Psychiatrists support supervision in the community in their report of 1993, they comment on the undesirability of giving compulsory treatment in a community setting in the absence of consent. It is unclear what would happen to those patients who fail to comply but are not held to be detainable in hospital. The European Convention on Human Rights (Article 5.1) rules out compulsory treatment for those not suffering from mental disorder of a degree requiring detention. It is also unclear how such an order would ensure the homeless receive adequate support and what steps could be taken to maintain contact at a specified address. Whilst psychiatrists are generally enthusiastic about such a proposal there is less support from other mental health professionals, notably community psychiatric nurses and approved social workers (Burns *et al.*, 1993). There are others, for example Lucy Scott-Moncrieff, who are vociferous in their condemnation of such an order (Eastman, 1994) claiming that it will do nothing to stop further incidents of violence by the mentally ill and that the correct approach is to apply existing legislation properly and ensure adequate community resources to apply the principles of care in the community.

Conclusion

When homelessness is placed in its historical context it can be seen that its relationship with crime has always been close with the fate of the homeless person entwined with that of the criminal. For many years the vagrant, whether mentally disordered, criminal or both, could be swept off the streets into a large institution beyond the public gaze, but with the closure of long-stay psychiatric hospitals and other social changes, the homeless have become increasingly visible in society giving cause for public concern.

Public concern and sentiment is vital to ensure adequate provision for the homeless but it is fickle and changeable and what is worse, government policy seems to be overly influenced by changes in public attitudes. There is a cyclical pattern to the care of the disadvantaged in society with a tendency to re-invent the wheel (Allderidge, 1979). It is only to be expected that, as a liberal and humanizing approach is adopted, the clouds of a punitive backlash are already forming on the horizon. On the care side, the principles of early diversion from custody as set out in the UK Home Office (1990) Circular No. 66/90 and the recommendations of the Reed Report (Department of Health and Home Office, 1992), plus improvements to the prison system, the Criminal Justice Act 1991, prior to its hasty amendments, the policy of Care in the Community, rather than its implementation, have all helped to foster a caring, non-institutional approach to the homeless mentally disordered, whether or not they are offenders. The Royal Commission, set up in the wake of the much publicized miscarriages of justice, has examined the rights of suspects in criminal proceedings (Royal Commission, 1993).

However, the backlash is coming in the shape of disproportionate concerns about the dangerousness of recently discharged psychiatric patients, the public perception that people can do anything and not get sent to prison; or if they go to prison it is now a soft option, and the increasing emphasis on the infringement of the 'rights' of the victim rather than the alleged offender.

The direction of future policy will ultimately depend on public attitudes, which will determine, through government, the balance that is struck between care and custody, leading to the allocation of resources to this disadvantaged group. For example, without a recognition that diversion from custody requires increased funding of both community and hospital care, the schemes will crumble. As Rollin wipes the tears from his ageing eyes (Rollin, 1993), I am sure that he would agree that a return to institutional care is not the answer and that the only way forward is to resist the forced polarization between hospital and community, victim and perpetrator, bad or mad, treatment or punishment, which results in policy lurching from one extreme to the other, whilst the continual victim, the homeless, mentally disordered offender, is caught in a locked revolving door.

References

Allderidge, P. (1979). Hospitals, madhouses and asylums: cycles in the care of the insane. *British Journal of Psychiatry*, **134**, 321–4.

Berry, C. & Orwin, A. (1966). No fixed abode: a survey of mental hospital admissions. *British Journal of Psychiatry*, **112**, 1019–25.

Bowden, P. (1978a). Men remanded into custody for medical reports. I. The selection for treatment. *British Journal of Psychiatry*, **132**, 320–31.

Bowden, P. (1978b). Men remanded into custody for medical reports. II. The outcome of the treatment recommendation. *British Journal of Psychiatry*, **132**, 332–8.

Burns, T., Goddard, K. & Bale, R. (1993). Mental health professionals favour community supervision orders. *British Medical Journal*, **307**, 803.

Coid, J. (1988a). Mentally abnormal prisoners on remand. I. Rejected or accepted by the NHS. *British Medical Journal*, **296**, 1779–82.

Coid, J. (1988b). Mentally abnormal prisoners on remand. II. Comparison of services provided by Oxford and Wessex regions. *British Medical Journal*, **296**, 1783–4.

Dell, S., Grounds, A., James, K. & Robertson, G. (1991). Mentally Disordered Remanded prisoners. Unpublished report to the Home Office.

Department of Health and Home Office (1992). *Review of Health and Social Services for Mentally Disordered Offenders and Others Requiring Similar Services. (Reed Report)*. London: HMSO. (CM 2088).

DHSS (Department of Health and Social Security) (1962–1990). *Health and Personal Social Services Statistics for England (With Summary Tables for Great Britain). Annual Reports*. London: HMSO.

Dooley, E. (1990). Prison suicide in England and Wales, 1972–87. *British Journal of Psychiatry*, **156**, 40–5.

Eastman, N. (1994). Mental health law: civil liberties and the principle of reciprocity. *British Medical Journal*, **308**, 43–5.

Edwards, G., Williamson, V., Hawker, A., Hensman, C. & Postoyan, S. (1968). Census of a reception centre. *British Journal of Psychiatry*, **114**, 1031–9.

El-Kabir, D. (1982). Great Chapel Street medical centre. *British Medical Journal*, **284**, 480–1.

Fahy, T., Bermingham, D. & Dunn, J. (1987). Police admissions to psychiatric hospitals: a challenge to community psychiatry. *Medicine, Science and the Law*, **27**, 263–8.

Gelberg, L., Linn, L. & Leake, B. (1988). Mental health alcohol and drug use and criminal history among homeless adults. *American Journal of Psychiatry*, **145**, 191–6.

George, H. (1972). A study of police admissions to psychiatric hospitals. MD thesis. University of London.

Gibbens, T. & Silverman, M. (1970). Alcoholism among prisoners. *Psychological Medicine*, **1**, 73–8.

Gunn, J. & Joseph, P. (1993). Remands to hospital for psychiatric reports: a study of psychiatrists' attitudes to section 35 of the Mental Health Act 1983. *Psychiatric Bulletin*, **17**, 197–9.

Herridge, C. (1989). Treatment of psychotic patients in prison. *Psychiatric Bulletin*, **13**, 200–1.

Herzberg, J. (1987). No fixed abode. A comparison of men and women admitted to an east London psychiatric hospital. *British Journal of Psychiatry*, **150**, 621–7.

HM Chief Inspector of Prisons (1990). *Report*. London: HMSO.

Home Office (1962–1990). *Prison Statistics, England and Wales. Annual Reports*. London: HMSO.

Home Office (1990). Provision for Mentally Disordered Offenders. Home Office Circular no. 66/90.

Joseph, P. & Potter, M. (1993a). Diversion from custody. I. Psychiatric assessment at the Magistrates' court. *British Journal of Psychiatry*, **162**, 325–30.

Joseph, P. & Potter, M. (1993b). Diversion from custody. II. Effect on hospital and prison resources. *British Journal of Psychiatry*, **162**, 330–4.

Joseph, P., Bridgewater, J., Ramsden, S. & El-Kabir, D. (1990). A psychiatric clinic for the single homeless in a primary care setting in inner London. *Psychiatric Bulletin*, **14**, 270–1.

Kelleher, M. & Copeland, J. (1972). Compulsory psychiatric admissions by the police: a study of the use of section 136. *Medicine, Science and the Law*, **12**, 220–4.

Marshall, M. (1989). Collected and neglected: are Oxford hostels for the homeless filling up with disabled psychiatric patients? *British Medical Journal*, **299**, 706–9.

Miller, R. D. (1985). Commitment to outpatient treatment: a national survey. *Hospital and Community Psychiatry*, **36**, 265–7.

Moate, T., Ward, B. & Evans, G. (1993). A community treatment order in practice. *Psychiatric Bulletin*, **17**, 585–6.

National Assistance Board (1966). *Homeless Single Persons*. London: HMSO.

Orwell, G. (1933). *Down and Out in Paris and London*. Harmondsworth: Penguin.

Ribton Turner, C. (1887). *A History of Vagrants and Vagrancy and Beggars and Begging*. London: Chapman & Hall.

Rogers, A. & Faulkner, A. (1987). *A Place of Safety*. London: MIND.

Rollin, H. (1965). Unprosecuted mentally abnormal offenders. *British Medical Journal*, **1**, 831–5.

Rollin, H. (1969). *The Mentally Abnormal Offender and the Law*. Oxford: Pergamon Press.

Rollin, H. (1993). Community care: Italy's 'U' turn. *Psychiatric Bulletin*, **17**, 494–5.

Royal College of Psychiatrists (1993). *Community Supervision Orders*. London: RCP.

Royal Commission (1993). *The Royal Commission on Criminal Justice Report*. London: HMSO. (Cm 2263).

Sensky, T., Hughes, T. & Hirsch, S. (1991a). Compulsory psychiatric treatment in the community. I. A controlled study of compulsory community treatment with extended leave under the Mental Health Act: special characteristics of patients treated and impact of treatment. *British Journal of Psychiatry*, **158**, 792–98.

Sensky, T., Hughes, T. & Hirsch, S. (1991b). Compulsory psychiatric treatment in the community. II. A controlled study of patients whom psychiatrists would recommend for compulsory treatment in the community. *British Journal of Psychiatry*, **158**, 799–804.

Sheridan, E. & Teplin, L. (1981). Police-referred psychiatric emergencies: advantages of community treatment. *Journal of Community Psychology*, **9**, 140–7.

Sims, A. & Symonds, R. (1975). Psychiatric referrals from the police. *British Journal of Psychiatry*, **127**, 171–8.

South-West Regional Group Consultative Committee (1969). The Homeless Offender in the South-west of England. South-West Regional Group Consultative Committee for After-Care Hostels.

Szmukler, G., Bird, A. & Button, E. (1981). Compulsory admissions in a London borough. I. Social and clinical features and a follow-up. *Psychological Medicine*, **11**, 617–36.

Tidmarsh, D. (1977). Psychiatric Disorder in a Population of Homeless Destitute Men. MD thesis. University of Cambridge.

Walmsley, R. (1972). Steps from Prison. London: Inner London Probation and After-Care Services.

Weller, M. (1989). Mental illness – who cares? *Nature*, **339**, 249–52.

Wessely, S. & Taylor, P. (1991). Madness and crime: criminology versus psychiatry. *Criminal Behaviour and Mental Health*, **1**, 193–28.

PART II

SERVICES

7

Services for the mentally ill homeless

E. Jane Marshall and Dinesh Bhugra

Introduction

As for estimates of homeless populations in various countries (see Chapters 10, 12, 13 and 14) the estimates of various types of mental illness and other psychological morbidity in homeless populations vary. Most of the research so far has been in the 'captive' samples that are easy to approach and identify and findings from these populations cannot be generalized. We know from the existing literature that most homeless individuals do not receive help from any service agency and their distrust of statutory health services and the inflexibility of these services in return are important factors in continuing poor physical and mental conditions.

Between one third and one quarter of the homeless population suffers from serious mental illness (Tessler & Dennis, 1989; Dennis *et al.*, 1991; see Bhugra 1993, for a review). The relationship between homelessness and mental illness is complex and mental illness is only one of many interacting factors leading to and perpetuating homelessness. In addition, other factors include the reduction in availability of low cost housing, increasing unemployment, loss of the manufacturing base (in the UK) and closure of direct access hostels, which traditionally served as asylums for large numbers of the mentally ill (Craig & Timms, 1992; see Chapters 2 and 3). Cohen & Thompson (1992) argue that the distinction between the homeless mentally ill and the mentally ill homeless is not a semantic one but is vital in terms of addressing needs and in the development of services. They challenge the assumption that the fundamental problem of the homeless mentally ill is their mental illness and emphasize that the conceptual dichotomy between homeless persons with or without mental illness is purely illusory. 'Not mentally ill' homeless people are likely to have many mental health problems and the 'mentally ill' homeless may have non-psychiatric problems that arise from the socio-political elements affecting all homeless people. Their model views homelessness as the core element of the broader socio-economic and political context that in turn becomes intertwined with personal biography and illness.

Deinstitutionalization is often blamed for the increase in homelessness in the USA, but research data on this issue remain sparse (Fischer & Breakey, 1986; Dennis *et al.*, 1991; Cohen & Thompson, 1992). The British experience suggests that adequate follow-up and support for long-stay psychiatric patients discharged from hospital is critical in preventing homelessness (Dayson, 1992).

Most studies on the homeless mentally ill have been, until relatively recently, cross-sectional and lacking in methodological rigour. Longitudinal studies are needed to assess the extent to which individuals move in and out of homelessness and to evaluate the contributory impact of mental illness.

Homeless mentally ill and services

The homeless population is heterogeneous, disaffiliated from society and lacks trust in the statutory services. The homeless have complex and interrelated needs including food, housing, help for physical and psychological health problems and for substance misuse.

Studies sponsored by the National Institute of Mental Health (NIMH) in the USA between 1982 and 1986 highlighted the fact that although the mentally ill and non-mentally ill homeless populations were similar in terms of age, gender, ethnicity and the extent of substance abuse the former *were more likely* to have been ill for longer periods, to have less contact with family and friends, to be in poorer physical health, and to be in contact with the criminal justice system (Tessler & Dennis, 1989). The homeless mentally ill have great difficulty progressing beyond the homeless state and tend to accumulate in hostels, shelters and lodging houses (Leach & Wing, 1978). They may not be as geographically mobile as had previously been thought (Bachrach, 1987) and need an accepting non-judgemental environment with considerable support so that they can develop trusting relationships.

Services

The homeless mentally ill do not access psychiatric and substance abuse services, despite needing them (Padgett *et al.*, 1990). Breakey *et al.* (1989) reported that only 47% of 298 homeless men and 30% of 230 homeless women were able to name a usual source of health care. However, 20% overall had been hospitalized for a physical illness in the previous year and 23% of men and 33% of women had been psychiatric inpatients over the same period. Victor (1992) reported that 92% of 319 temporarily homeless people resident in bed and breakfast hotels in North West London were registered with a general practitioner. This sample was predominantly female (61%) and young (72% between the ages of 16 and 34 years). One tenth had had an acute health problem in the previous fortnight, 46% had been experiencing a health problem for 1 year or more and 34% had a health problem that had been limiting their daily activity for 1 year or more.

Factors related to service utilization amongst the homeless are poorly understood and little research has been carried out in this area. Higher rates of hospitalization have been reported among homeless women (Robertson, 1986; Grella, 1994; see Chapter 5). This may be due to the fact that homeless women are more likely to be admitted to hospital whereas homeless men in the same situation may be taken to prison (Herzberg, 1987).

The homeless and their use of mental health services

Some homeless mentally ill individuals do not come to the attention of services because they are withdrawn and isolated (Priest, 1976; Cohen *et al.*, 1984). Others may refuse services because they lack insight into their illness (Bassuk *et al.*, 1984), because of negative experience with the system (Cohen & Thompson, 1992), because they give higher priority to other basic needs such as food and shelter (Goering *et al.*, 1990), because of cognitive impairment (Herman *et al.*, 1993) or because they prefer to stay out of hospital.

Many homeless individuals are willing to accept help from the psychiatric services, but may find the services inflexible and inaccessible and unable to meet their multi-dimensional and complex needs. Many mentally ill homeless people are just too impaired to deal with the bureaucracy of the mental health services.

Traditionally, the mental health services have tended to 'medicalize' homelessness and have failed to recognize the broad range of needs of the mentally ill homeless, focusing on their 'psychiatric needs' and often engendering feelings of humiliation (Cohen & Thompson, 1992). Help has typically been in the form of inpatient treatment, often in crisis situations, with little concerted follow-up after discharge. Indeed, the tendency may be to discharge the homeless as fast as possible into temporary accommodation so that they do not 'clog' hospital beds. Follow-up often consists of outpatient appointments, which are low on the priority of the homeless person who needs shelter and food. Services have generally ignored the fact that even overtly psychotic patients may have adapted to life in hostels and/or the streets and are not in need of acute inpatient care.

Specific problems

Models of mental health care delivery

The emphasis on catchment areas and sectorization within catchment areas not only excludes individuals with no address but also those who are not interested in long-term follow-up. The geographical mobility of the homeless does not recognize catchment area boundaries and follow-up between catchment areas is often lacking.

Attitudes

Mental health professionals find it difficult to deal with the multiple complex problems of the homeless mentally ill. Many have been reluctant to work with the homeless, and the perceived dichotomy of the 'deserving' and the 'undeserving' poor has led to negative attitudes. Bachrach (1990) observed that the attitudes of the media towards the homeless do affect the services. In places where libraries and railway stations are used by the homeless, joint local planning has sometimes helped to improve services (Petroskey, 1988). Innovative and joint working between mental health workers and other organizations is also possible. Discrepancies between perceived needs by the homeless and by mental health professionals can create a dichotomy that leads to a rejection of the services (Herman *et al.*, 1993). Homeless women, despite having multiple mental and physical health problems, have been shown to express a strong preference for a normal independent living situation (Goering *et al.*, 1990). They also opposed being housed in settings with mentally ill persons, substance abusers and with those involved in criminal activities. Clearly the preferences and perceptions of the homeless must be taken into account when planning services. Voluntary organizations often deal more successfully with this than the statutory ones.

Mental illness: substance misuse, psychosis and dual diagnosis

Substance misuse and dual diagnosis

Homeless individuals with substance misuse problems are often seen as 'undeserving', and consequently have been poorly served by services. Although substance misuse was a prominent finding in Breakey *et al.*'s (1989) study, only one third of men and one tenth of women had recently obtained residential or ambulatory care for a substance misuse problem. Mavis *et al.* (1993) used residential mobility to identify 81 'homeless' out of a total of 938 subjects. Compared to housed clients, the homeless were more likely to be seeking admission to residential substance abuse programmes and a much larger proportion reported previous treatment for alcohol or drug problems.

Cognitive impairment is another important factor that is often unrecognized in the homeless mentally ill. In one study, nearly 40% of homeless men with a mean age of 55 years had severe or mild cognitive impairment and more than one in four showed severe cognitive impairment (Teesson & Buhrich, 1993). Of the group, 15% had alcohol related problems and 21% had a diagnosis of schizophrenia. The figures for dual diagnosis were not reported.

Rosenheck *et al.* (1993) reported that homeless persons with dual diagnosis appeared especially difficult to engage in treatment. In an earlier report Rosenheck & Leda (1991) observed that treatment programmes for homeless populations can be established within existing mental health institutions if supported with a clear mandate and appropriate resources. In that study compliant patients had a far higher chance of receiving services. Hartz *et al.* (1994) demonstrated that with decreasing housing stability, alcohol use increases and heroin use declines. Use of cocaine on the other hand was clearly linked with being unhoused rather than being homeless in the broader sense of lacking a permanent dwelling. African-Americans had higher rates of cocaine use even when housing status was controlled for. Wasylenki *et al.* (1993) reported that assertive care management for homeless mentally ill persons increased residential stability as well as reduced psychopathology. It is obviously important that the personnel who provide such care are well-trained and motivated. Specific models may prove to be more successful than generic ones. Grunberg & Eagle (1990) reported that a shelterization programme can be made more successful by helping the homeless person establish positive social networks and affiliation with social service and mental health providers. In Texas, Berman *et al.* (1993) have described a joint public–private and voluntary partnership that has succeeded in setting up 'work for pay' and substance abuse treatment programmes for the homeless.

Voluntary services

The vacuum left by the failure of mental health services to cater for anything other than the narrowly defined psychiatric needs of the homeless mentally ill has been filled by voluntary groups who provide shelter, food and support. However, the staff in these agencies, although qualified in other ways, may have had little training in mental health assessment or management. Lack of resources (Fischer & Breakey, 1986) and overwhelming demands (Marshall, 1989) have often put voluntary agencies under a tremendous strain. In addition, minimal liaison between various voluntary agencies and between voluntary and statutory groups has meant that a comprehensive mental health service for the homeless mentally ill cannot be delivered.

What is required?

Community mental health programmes must be adapted to meet the range of needs of the mentally ill homeless. The degree of disability of individuals, their personal strengths, vulnerabilities, preferences and limited social support networks must be recognized in planning any services (Breakey *et al.*, 1989). Special characteristics of the homeless population such as disaffiliation, co-morbidity and poor social networks should influence what is delivered. Any ideal community mental health service must be flexible, accessible, acceptable and widely available. These are also the essentials for the services targeting the homeless. Staff working on such programmes must have an understanding of the issues of homelessness and must be committed to the field. Special services for alcohol and drug misuse are needed. Services must be comprehensive and also provide long-term housing, support and psycho-social rehabilitation. The judicious use of resources can affect the housing and the take up rate of services (Dixon *et al.*, 1994).

Specific issues that need to be addressed in setting up services to meet the needs of the mentally ill homeless include outreach and engagement in non-traditional settings; long-term intensive case management, with smaller loads and increased frequency of contact; provision of services where needed; mental health and rehabilitation services; a wide range of housing options; supportive living programmes and links between services and housing (Hopper *et al.*, 1989; Dennis *et al.*, 1991).

Engagement and outreach

The first step in the provision of services to the homeless mentally ill is to ensure that they will engage. Engagement is a lengthy, labour-intensive process that may have little in common with the type of service envisaged. The regular provision of food at a drop-in service may be the first step in the process. The key to engagement is the building up of trust. Contact with homeless clients must, therefore, be non-threatening, flexible, repetitive and take place over long periods and be responsive to their needs (Rogg, 1988). Clinicians must be prepared to work in an unstructured way and to target individuals who would not otherwise use the services (Susser *et al.*, 1990). Newly set up outreach programmes were shown to increase the usage of outpatients as well as home assessments but did not affect the inpatient services (Rosenheck *et al.*, 1993).

Long-term intensive case management

Case management as originally described in the Social Services context has certain advantages but with a group that may be geographically mobile and residentially unstable, flexibility has to be maintained. In order to overcome catchment area problems a single consultant or team responsible for the whole of the district should be nominated to look after all the homeless mentally ill individuals. Members with outreach skills from within such a team can then attempt to make contact with homeless individuals and work as case managers. It must be emphasized that in order to achieve this a great deal of time needs to be spent with the individual in the initial stages. Homeless individuals should have one case manager who facilitates contact with community resources and often ongoing support. The case manager should have an understanding of homelessness and commitment and then intensive and long-term work should be reflected in a reduced caseload.

Provision of services where needed

The homeless mentally ill are willing to receive services that are flexible and accessible. In practice, this means that individuals need to be approached by outreach services and that service providers must be willing to do street assessments, clinics in hostels etc. (Slagg *et al.*, 1994). In the UK some innovative schemes are already operating (see Chapter 11). Whenever possible such services should offer multi-axial support and management.

Mental health and rehabilitation services

Community mental health programmes must be adapted to the needs of the homeless mentally ill. Essential components include flexibility in style of service delivery, time to establish rapport, patience and perseverance. Physical, psychiatric and substance misuse problems should be tackled together and not by different specialities.

A long-term view is needed in the planning of comprehensive services for the homeless, as is a willingness to work in non-traditional ways. Important pioneering programmes can serve as the models. For instance, the Skid Row Mental Health Service (1986) demonstrated how a statutory health service could offer regular consultation and case management, from a base in voluntary agencies.

Need for a wide range of housing options

Ongoing housing support is an essential part of any service package for the mentally ill homeless who may find it difficult to maintain residential stability when they are psychotic or depressed. This is a constant problem for many because of poor socialization and living skills. However, many mentally ill homeless individuals can remain in various types of housing with appropriate support for long periods of time.

Conclusion

The provision of comprehensive services for the mentally ill homeless is time-consuming and complex. However, it is also an opportunity to be innovative and flexible and may, in time, serve to inform the development of the standard mental health services.

References

Bachrach, L. L. (1987). Geographical mobility and the homeless mentally ill. *Hospital and Community Psychiatry*, **38**, 27–8.

Bachrach, L. L. (1990). The media and the homeless person. *Hospital and Community Psychiatry*, **41**, 963–4.

Bassuk, E. L., Rubin, L. & Lauriat, A. (1984). Is homelessness a mental health problem? *American Journal of Psychiatry*, **141**, 1546–50.

Berman, S., Barilich, J. E., Rosenheck, R. & Koerber, G. (1993). The VA's first comprehensive homeless centre: a catalyst for public and private partnership. *Hospital and Community Psychiatry*, **44**, 1183–4.

Bhugra, D. (1993). Unemployment, poverty and homelessness. In D. Bhugra & J. Leff (eds.), *Principles of Social Psychiatry*, pp. 355–84. Oxford: Blackwell Scientific Publications.

Breakey, W. R., Fischer, P. J., Kramer, M. J. *et al.* (1989). Health and mental health problems of homeless men and women in Baltimore. *Journal of the American Medical Association*, **262**, 1352–7.

Cohen, C. & Thompson, K. S. (1992). Homeless mentally ill or mentally ill homeless. *American Journal of Psychiatry*, **149**, 816–23.

Cohen, N. L., Putnam, J. F. & Sullivan, A. M. (1984). The mentally ill homeless. Isolation and adaption. *Hospital and Community Psychiatry*, **35**, 922–4.

Craig, T. J. & Timms, P. W. (1992). Out of the wards and onto the streets? Deinstitutionalisation and homelessness in Britain. *Journal of Mental Health*, **1**, 265–75.

Dayson, D. (1992). The TAPS Project. 12. Crime, vagrancy, death and readmissions of the long-term mentally ill during their first year of local reprovision. *British Journal of Psychiatry*, **162(supplement 19)**, 40–4.

Dennis, D. L., Buckner, J. C., Lipton, F. R. & Levine, I. R. (1991). A decade of research and services for homeless mentally ill persons. *American Psychologist*, **46**, 1129–38.

Dixon, L., Krauss, N., Myers, P. & Lehman, A. (1994). Clinical and treatment correlates of access to Section 8 certificate for homeless mentally ill persons. *Hospital and Community Psychiatry*, **45**, 1196–200.

Fischer, P. J. & Breakey, W. R. (1986). Homelessness and mental health: an overview. *International Journal of Mental Health*, **14**, 6–41.

Goering, P. Paduchak, D. & Durbin, J. (1990). Housing homeless women: a consumer preference study. *Hospital and Community Psychiatry*, **41**, 790–4.

Grella, C. (1994). Contrasting a shelter and day centre for homeless mentally ill women: four patterns of service use. *Community Mental Health Journal*, **30**, 3–16.

Grunberg, J. & Eagle, P. F. (1990). Shelterization: how the homeless adapt to shelter living. *Hospital and Community Psychiatry*, **41**, 521–5.

Hartz, D., Banys, P. & Hall, S. M. (1994). Correlates of homelessness among substance abuse patients at a VA medical centre. *Hospital and Community Psychiatry*, **45**, 491–3.

Herman, D. B., Struening, E. L. & Barrow, S. M. (1993). Self-assessed need for mental health services among homeless adults. *Hospital and Community Psychiatry*, **44**, 1181–3.

Herzberg, J. L. (1987). No fixed abode. A comparison of men and women admitted to an East London psychiatric hospital. *British Journal of Psychiatry*, **150**, 621–7.

Hopper, K., Much, D. & Morse, G. (1989). *The 1986–1987 NIMH-funded CSP Demonstration Projects to Seque Mentally Ill Homeless Persons: a preliminary assessment*. Rocksville, MD: NIMH.

Leach, J. & Wing, J. K. (1978). The effectiveness of a service for helping destitute men. *British Journal of Psychiatry*, **113**, 481–92.

Marshall, M. (1989). Collected and neglected: are Oxford hostels filling up with disabled psychiatric patients? *British Medical Journal*, **229**, 706 9.

Mavis, B. E., Humphreys, K. & Staffelmayr, B. E. (1993). Treatment needs and outcomes of two subtypes of homeless persons who abuse substances. *Hospital and Community Psychiatry*, **44**, 1185–7.

Padgett, D., Struening, E. L. & Andrews, H. (1990). Factors affecting the use of medical, mental health, alcohol and drug treatment services by homeless adults. *Medical Care*, **28**, 805–21.

Petroskey, D. (1988). Plan gives vagrants own library. *Indianapolis Star*, January 21, pp. B1, B8.

Priest, R. G. (1976). The homeless person and the psychiatric services: an Edinburgh study. *British Journal of Psychiatry*, **128**, 128–36.

Robertson, M. J. (1986). Mental disorder among homeless persons in the United States: an overview of recent empirical literature. *Administration in Mental Health*, **14**, 14–26.

Rogg, D. J. (1988). Engaging homeless persons with mental illness into treatment. Alexandria, VA; National Mental Health Association.

Rosenheck, R., Gallup, P. & Frisman, L. K. (1993). Health care utilization and costs after entry into an outreach programme for homeless mentally ill veterans. *Hospital and Community Psychiatry*, **44**, 1166–71.

Rosenheck, R. & Leda, C. (1991). Who is served by programmes for the homeless? Admission to a domiciliary care programme for homeless veterans. *Hospital and Community Psychiatry*, **42**, 176–81.

Skid Row Mental Health Service, Los Angeles County Department of Mental Health (1986). Gold Award: a network of services for the homeless chronically mentally ill. *Hospital and Community Psychiatry*, **37**, 1148–51.

Slagg, N. B., Lyons, J. S., Cook, J. A., Wasmer, D. J. & Ruth, A. (1994). A profile of clients served by a mobile outreach program for homeless mentally ill persons. *Hospital and Community Psychiatry*, **45**, 1139–41.

Susser, E., Golfinger, S. & White, A. (1990). Some clinical approaches to the homeless mentally ill. *Community Mental Health Journal*, **26**, 463–80.

Teesson, M. & Buhrich, N. (1993). Prevalence of cognitive impairment among homeless men in a shelter in Australia. *Hospital and Community Psychiatry*, **44**, 1187–90.

Tessler, R. C. & Dennis, D. L. (1989). *A Synthesis of NIMH-funded Research Concerning Persons who are Homeless and Mentally Ill.* Washington, DC: National Institute of Mental Health.

Victor, C. R. (1992). Health status of the temporarily homeless population and residents of North West Thames Region. *British Medical Journal, BMJ*, **305**, 387–91.

Wasylenki, D. A., Goering, P. N., Lemire, D., Lindsey, S. & Lancee, W. (1993). The Hostel Outreach Program: assertive case management for homeless mentally ill persons. *Hospital and Community Psychiatry*, **44**, 848–52.

8

Clinical work with homeless people in the USA

WILLIAM R. BREAKEY

Although psychiatric epidemiologists had demonstrated as early as the 1960s that the prevalence of psychiatric disorders was high among American homeless people, such as those who frequented the Bowery in New York (Spitzer *et al.*, 1969), it was not until the late 1970s that the issue was compellingly brought to the attention of American psychiatry (Reich & Siegel, 1978) and not until the 1980s that, stimulated by the National Institute of Mental Health, significant programmes of research and service development got under way (Tessler & Dennis, 1989).

In the past decade the problem of homelessness in the USA has, if anything, become more severe and there has been little improvement, overall, in the plight of the homeless mentally ill. After 10 years of research and programme development, however, the nature and extent of the problems are better documented and there has been progress in developing treatment, rehabilitation and resettlement approaches (Institute of Medicine, 1988; Burt & Cohen, 1989; Brickner *et al.*, 1990; Jahiel, 1992; Lamb *et al.*, 1992a; Robertson & Greenblatt, 1992).

Nevertheless, homelessness continues to be surrounded by debate and controversy, even as data on the problem accrue and the general public becomes increasingly resigned to the sight of homeless people in the streets and public places. The public perception continues to be that the homeless constitute a distinct class of individuals, alienated from the mainstream of society, often threatening to, or challenging, the general population of domiciled people. Among those who work with the homeless, however, the notion of an underclass has given way to a view of homelessness as a state into which people arrive for a wide variety of reasons. Not only are there many types of people in the homeless population, but in many respects they are not radically different from housed people. They are, however, the poorest of the poor, and often those who are the housed poor this week become the homeless poor next week, moving along a continuum of residential stability (Appleby & Desai, 1987; Breakey & Fischer, 1995). Solving the problem of homelessness will entail addressing the causes of poverty in the midst of affluence. People with mental illnesses tend to be poor (Cohen, 1993) and it is their poverty, along with their disabilities, that places them at enhanced risk of homelessness.

Debate continues, even among those who work with homeless people, regarding the rights of individuals who are mentally ill and homeless. On the one hand there are those who adopt a libertarian view, stressing the rights of individuals, including those who are mentally ill, to adopt life-styles that are eccentric, or even offensive to others. On the other hand there are those who stress the *parens* role of government and the helping professions and advocate for more authority to intervene where people are unwilling to accept psychiatric treatment. The issue of involuntary treatment for homeless mentally ill people has aroused considerable controversy in the USA. The issue was most hotly debated in New York City. Under New York statutes, people could only be compelled to accept involuntary treatment if they were considered to be dangerous to themselves or others. In the early 1980s, street outreach teams applied this criterion quite sparingly, so that only 3% of patients evaluated by the Project HELP teams in New York were involuntarily admitted to hospital (Cohen & Marcos, 1986). In 1985, the mayor of New York decreed that because of low temperatures, a 'cold weather emergency' existed, and street outreach teams were instructed to apply dangerousness criteria more liberally, conveying larger numbers of patients against their will to hospital emergency rooms for evaluation. Advocates for civil liberties were outraged and a series of court cases ensued. The issue was whether a mentally ill person's right to independence and self-determination should be respected even where his or her behaviour is endangering his or her own health and is offensive to other citizens. Most psychiatrists and others involved in caring for homeless people believe that existing laws and policies are adequate to permit action to be taken where a person's life or health is seriously at risk. Another view is sometimes expressed, however, that restrictions on involuntary admission should be relaxed, so that seriously ill people could be more easily hospitalized, that this respects their right to treatment, even when they are unable to consent to it, and that admitting a person to a substandard facility is the lesser of two evils, when compared to having that person stay on the streets (Lamb *et al.*, 1992b). However, the majority of those who work in the field are of the opinion that the great majority of mentally ill people can be treated or sheltered without resorting to involuntary treatment procedures, and that, instead of looking to institutional models of care, policy makers' attention should be focused upon the great poverty of many mentally ill people, the lack of suitable housing and the need for better community support systems, which might prevent their homelessness. What is more, Appelbaum (1992) points out that the literature on involuntary hospitalization provides little evidence that creating more draconian commitment laws would have the effect of reducing homelessness among the mentally ill.

The consumer movement has also had considerable impact on thinking about services for homeless people in recent years, as it has in other areas of public life and in community mental health. Organizations of homeless and formerly homeless people have had important roles, through advocacy and confrontation, in sensitizing the public and those in power to the dilemmas homeless people face. Consumer-run programmes have been able to reach out to homeless people in ways that may be more effective than conventional professional approaches (Van Tosh, 1993).

The American homeless population

Within the diversity of homeless people, certain subgroups can be defined, with their own profiles of needs (Fischer & Breakey, 1986). These include the *street people*, eccentric and bizarre individuals who have made the streets their home; *chronic alcoholics*, whose activities centre around satisfying the craving for alcohol; *situationally homeless* people, whose homelessness has resulted from a change in circumstances, such as unemployment, spousal abuse or urban redevelopment; and the *chronically mentally ill*, whose mental illness interferes with their capacity to solve problems, settle in stable housing and function socially. Among the mentally ill, the most difficult to treat are those with co-morbid substance use disorders, often dubbed the *dually diagnosed*. Other subgroups are *homeless families*, now estimated to comprise perhaps 20% of the homeless population; *homeless children and adolescents*, 'runaways' and 'throwaways', living on the streets of major cities; and people with *HIV infection*, many of whom are also substance abusers. These groups are not mutually exclusive. Within groups, people vary in their educational levels, their personal strengths and vulnerabilities and the helping resources available to them, so that the patients of a clinician working with homeless people are likely to be as varied as any others.

Homeless people frequently suffer from a relative lack of networks of personal support. Linkages to family, to friends, to neighbours, or to other occupational or social groupings are lacking or fragmentary. Disaffiliation and isolation make it more difficult for a person to cope with life's hardships. In therapy with homeless patients, the lack of family or other support networks deprives them of a source of support that is ordinarily available in the treatment and rehabilitation of other psychiatric patients. What is more, those personal attributes that impair a person's ability to develop and maintain social networks also impair the capacity to establish effective therapeutic relationships. Homeless people frequently distrust authority and are suspicious of psychiatrists and other mental health professionals. They may have had unpleasant experiences with hospitals or doctors, which lead them to be wary of further involvement. Some former patients who have experienced unpleasant medication side-effects choose to stay away from psychiatrists to avoid being pressured into another course of treatment.

Homeless people, more than most, present to the service provider a multiplicity of needs. There are very few simple or uncomplicated cases. Apart from assistance with obtaining shelter, clothing, food, financial support and other basic needs, their physical health is often very poor. They not only suffer from the same disorders that affect others, but also from health problems that are especially common because of their peculiar life-style. Infectious diseases, parasitic diseases, respiratory diseases, skin and joint problems are common, in addition to the results of trauma and the complications of substance abuse (Wright & Weber, 1987; Breakey *et al.*, 1989; Gelberg & Linn, 1989).

Substance abuse disorders are ubiquitous (Fischer, 1990). Any treatment programme for the homeless must expect that 40–60% of patients, including those whose primary diagnosis is schizophrenia or major affective disorder, will have substance abuse or dependence and should plan accordingly.

The high prevalence of psychiatric disorders in homeless people, relative to the general population, is well documented (Fischer & Breakey, 1991; Fischer *et al.*, 1992). The reasons for the high levels of psychiatric morbidity are several. First, there are the difficult circumstances of homeless people – poverty and homelessness are extremely stressful. The streets are dangerous; homeless people are especially prone to be victims of assault and robbery; some have become homeless as a result of unbearable relationships or abuse; others have suffered the indignities of redundancy, unemployment and eviction. Secondly, many homeless people have become vulnerable, and thus ultimately homeless, because they were already disabled by mental illness or dependence on alcohol or other drugs. Although psychiatrically disabled persons are eligible for Social Security and other income supports, the level of these payments is insufficient to raise the person out of poverty, and of limited benefit to a person whose money management skills may be compromised by illness or cognitive impairment.

Prevalence rates of specific psychiatric disorders vary in different subgroups, and from place to place, but a broad consensus is emerging from a series of research studies over the past decade. Of homeless people residing in shelters, about one third have significant psychiatric problems. This estimate can be derived from reports that about one third have been admitted to a psychiatric inpatient facility at some time, but is documented more precisely by epidemiological surveys of homeless people using standardized diagnostic methods (Koegel *et al.*, 1988; Breakey *et al.*, 1989; Susser *et al.*, 1989; Smith *et al.*, 1992, 1993). Data from the Baltimore Homeless Study are typical (Table 8.1). Approximately 35% of men and 48% of women were found to have a major mental illness: schizophrenia was diagnosed in 9% of men and 16% of women, and major affective disorders in 17% of men and 24% of women. Note that these mentally ill people vary in their degree of disability, as do mentally ill people in general. If criteria of extensive histories of in-patient admissions and significant functional impairment are applied to those patients with major mental illnesses, the number who are severely mentally ill is many fewer. It is this group, 17% of men and 24% of women in the Baltimore sample, who present the greatest needs for treatment and rehabilitation.

Alcohol and other drug dependence have traditionally been the major disorders of homeless people. With attention focused recently

Table 8.1. *The Baltimore Homeless Study: prevalence (%) of DSM-III psychiatric disorders*

	Men	Women
Major mental illnesses		
Schizophrenia		
Total	9.0	16.3
SMI	7.3	10.3
Bipolar disorder		
Total	4.7	9.7
SMI	1.3	9.3
Major depression		
Total	12.6	13.8
SMI	6.3	2.3
Other major mental illnesses[a]		
Total	8.3	8.3
SMI	2.0	1.8
Substance use disorders		
Alcohol abuse or dependence	67.0	26.2
Other drug use disorder	28.8	11.1
Dual diagnosis		
(major mental illness + substance use disorder)	24.7	24.3
Other DSM-III Axis I disorders	30.0	46.2
Personality (DSM-III *Axis II*) disorders	46.5	45.3

SMI, severely mentally ill: mental illness diagnosis, with history of extensive hospitalization and/or severe functional impairment.
[a] Includes paranoid disorder, atypical psychosis, organic hallucinosis, etc.

on mental illness, less public prominence has been accorded to homeless addicts. Again, data from Baltimore are typical of data from other American cities in showing that alcoholism and drug use are extremely prevalent, occurring in two thirds of men and one third of women – more prevalent than major mental illness.

The third major group of psychiatric disorders is the personality disorders. These conditions are more difficult to document in a systematic way, based on a single interview in an epidemiological survey. The Baltimore Homeless Study data, however, suggest that approximately 40% of men and of women suffer from personality disorders.

Co-morbidity is the rule, rather than the exception. Apart from the many physical health problems, many people have more than one psychiatric disorder. Substance use disorders occur in mentally ill people with the same frequency as in those who are free of mental illness. This 'dual diagnosis' of mental illness and substance dependence, which was found in one quarter of the Baltimore sample, creates major problems for treatment and rehabilitation.

These data were obtained from men and women surveyed in the general shelter system and the city jail in Baltimore. Other subgroups of homeless people may have different profiles of disorders. For example, a survey of mothers in shelters for families in Massachusetts revealed a different profile in these young women. Personality disorders were more frequently diagnosed, major mental illnesses less frequently (Bassuk *et al.*, 1986). Several studies of women have found high prevalence rates of post-traumatic stress disorder (Smith *et al.*, 1993). Prevalence rates may also vary over time. A recent survey of homeless women in Baltimore has shown a massive increase in cocaine abuse between the mid-1980s and the early 1990s, in keeping with trends in the general population.

Providing services for the homeless mentally ill

Experience in providing psychiatric services for homeless people has shown that there are four principal stages: engagement, basic service provision, transition and integration. *Engagement*, gaining a person's confidence to the point where he or she will enter treatment, is often a major issue because of the reluctance of many homeless mentally ill people to accept help, their fear of being forced into hospital or into accepting treatment they do not want, or their lack of insight into the fact that they are ill. It is not sufficient to establish a clinical service programme and expect homeless people to come in for services. Thus, health programmes for homeless people are often located in areas where homeless people already congregate – such as shelters, Skid Rows, or in mobile units or temporary buildings that can be strategically placed for maximum accessibility. One of the first psychiatrists to take seriously the need for special services for the homeless was Rodger Farr who established a clinical programme on Skid Row in Los Angeles (Farr, 1986; Lomas, 1992). It was clear that homeless mentally ill people were not going to come to a conventional clinic, so he went to where they were. Others have confirmed that the only way to be accessible to homeless people is to take the services to those places where homeless people normally congregate. Valencia and Susser and their colleagues (Susser *et al.*, 1992) work within a massive shelter in New York, and the health care programme for homeless people in Baltimore began its operations within two daytime walk-in shelters. There are many other examples. Still, it is necessary to reach out beyond the walls of the clinic or shelter. Many programmes employ outreach workers who go to the streets and alleys, parks and railroad terminals. Several, such as that in Milwaukee (Blackwell *et al.*, 1990) have developed multi-disciplinary outreach teams. Outreach is an ideal role for formerly homeless people, whose knowledge of the territory and ability to establish rapport with homeless people is frequently superior to that of most professionals. An outreach worker or outreach team's role is, first, to establish contact with a person in need, then gain his or her confidence, which may take many contacts over a long period of time, and then to persuade the individual to accept help. Ovrebo (1992) notes that professional help may be seen by some mentally ill people as a direct path to institutionalization, which means loss of autonomy and self-respect. This is, of course, quite contrary to reality. Lomas (1992) notes that individuals cared for in the Los Angeles Skid Row mental health programme are likely to experience less institutional care than in the period prior to their entry to the programme.

Not all homeless people require long periods of persuasion and familiarization before they are willing to accept psychiatric help. Many, who have benefited from previous treatment, are grateful that services are made available to them. Diagnostic and treatment services may be brought to a person on the street, or the person may be persuaded to go to a clinic or service centre, where help is available. Whichever is the case, a range of *basic services* will be needed to assist the individual. Shelter is a first requirement for those who have been living rough. Income support, clothing and general health care will be needed in most cases, in addition to whatever psychiatric treatments may be indicated.

Homeless people themselves are clear about the existence of a hierarchy of needs. Ball & Havassy (1984), for example, listed the needs expressed by homeless mentally ill people in San Francisco. Mental health treatment was far down the list. Herman *et al.* (1993) found in a survey of shelter users in New York, that while the interviewers considered that mental health services were needed by 41% of those surveyed, only 17% of the homeless people themselves thought that they needed mental health services. First priority in their minds went to housing, food, clothing and money. It is unrealistic to expect homeless people to participate in treatment programmes until their basic needs have been met. Psychiatric treatment providers, therefore, must work closely in concert with providers of basic subsistence needs.

Co-ordinating the various social and health agencies is a major problem. In some cases this may be facilitated by setting up multi-disciplinary teams of social workers, nurses, psychiatrists and advocates; basing mental health clinics in centres that provide a number of services under one roof is helpful; but case management has come to be the major strategy employed. A case manager's primary role is to ensure that the variety of services needed by a particular person are made available. The role involves evaluation of the individual's particular set of needs, co-ordination of the several service systems, support of the client and advocacy, where barriers to service have to be overcome (Billig & Levinson, 1987; Morse & Calsyn, 1992; Swayze, 1992).

Clinical services needed by homeless people cover the full range of clinical and support services generally provided by a community mental health centre. Diagnosis and evaluation, pharmacological and psychotherapeutic treatments and co-ordination with general health care providers are first provided at outpatient level. Inpatient admissions are needed in some cases, and for this, good relations with psychiatric hospitals or inpatient units are essential. In the American context, where capacity to pay is very important for gaining admission to hospitals, and where the patients concerned are not only very poor, but often considered to be unattractive 'problem' patients, and where arranging post-hospital disposition is likely to be very difficult, admission offices may do all they can to avoid such an admission. The homeless service provider must thus develop good working professional relations with the hospital staff, so that when an admission is needed, it can be arranged with a minimum of obstruction.

The tension between libertarian and paternalistic views of the rights of homeless people is often apparent when an involuntary admission is needed. Non-medical colleagues who are generally allies of the psychiatrist in bringing help to homeless people may become adversaries when involuntary treatment is proposed. The solution to this problem often lies in the doctor's role as teacher. Many individuals who work with homeless people have limited professional training, or have backgrounds in social sciences, with little appreciation of the realities of mental illness. Working together over a period of time, and helping them to understand concepts of disease in psychiatry will reduce misunderstanding and disagreement.

Services must be provided to address some of the peculiar problems facing homeless people. For example, a mailing address is generally necessary to receive a Social Security cheque. A homeless service centre can provide such an address. Purchasing medications, and storing them safely, can be a major difficulty for a person living on the street. Providing facilities for storing medicines can be extremely helpful (Lomas, 1992).

The third stage is that of *transition*. A programme for the homeless can not, by definition, provide indefinite care for people. Once they have been engaged, and their basic needs met, they must be moved into the mainstream mental health service system. This may take time, however. The very reason for their being in a special programme for homeless people may have been their reluctance to enter the mainstream service system (Surber *et al.*, 1988). The therapist will therefore need to engage the patient, establish trust, and then use this trusting relationship to enable the transition to another treatment provider. For a while the patient will become a regular client of the homeless programme. When the idea of moving the patient to another setting is broached, it is likely to be perceived by the patient as yet another in a series of rejections that may have been life-long. For the therapist, transferring a patient with whom he or she is working effectively is also a loss, and may be consciously or unconsciously resisted. Nevertheless, mental health programmes for homeless people are generally limited in their resources and unable to care for very large numbers of people. Patients can generally be helped to understand this and to accept the need to move on to a mainstream clinical setting.

The fourth stage and ultimate goal in providing care for homeless mentally ill people is that of *integration*. The person moves out of settings and programmes designed for homeless people, into the general community, with regular housing and other supports. This is an area that has been relatively poorly documented. To what extent can homeless people lose their identity of homeless or formerly homeless, and what will facilitate this? The success of this final step depends on the ability of the mainstream mental health service system to accept and retain patients who may be reluctant participants. Case managers and clinicians may need to make special efforts to ensure that the person integrates effectively into the culture of the programme and the community, recognizing that formerly homeless people are more vulnerable than others to slip back into homelessness.

Clinical considerations

What are the practical implications for the clinician? What special understanding or techniques are needed to work with homeless people? As the words 'homeless mentally ill' indicate, there are two broad strategic objectives: to treat the illness and to end the homelessness. At each stage, both objectives need to be kept in mind. Without treating the illness, the person is unlikely to be able to obtain or retain housing; without addressing the housing problem, attempts at treatment of the mental illness will be futile.

Often a clinician must exercise great patience to establish trust. Simply offering a friendly word, or some food or clothing, may be all that is possible at first. Over time, as trust develops, more active interventions become possible. Susser (1992) took many months to gain the confidence of both staff and residents of the residence in which he was trying to provide service. The role he identified as one that would permit him to move into the hotel and be accepted initially was that of organizer of a weekly Bingo game. This role was sufficiently unthreatening to the women in the hotel for him to gradually gain their confidence enough to move into other areas. Social workers with Project Outreach at the Goddard Riverside Community Center in New York were the first to adopt a trust-building technique that has since been adopted widely. Each day they would make trips out into their community with a store of sandwiches to distribute and to exchange a greeting or engage in a brief conversation with the men and women they encountered. They took months on occasion to establish contact with some of the most timid of the street people; many contacts were often needed before the individual gained sufficient confidence in the workers to establish some sort of tenuous relationship.

In many cases, homeless patients are among the most severely and chronically ill that a therapist is likely to encounter. They are 'treatment resistant' and have minimal resources in material terms as well as in terms of their social environment. To avoid disillusionment, it is wise to keep in mind that the prognosis in many cases is poor. Some homeless people may be reluctant to contemplate change in their life-style, or may not believe that a better way of life is feasible for them. For some it seems as if the street offers a haven of anonymity, an environment to which they have made a bizarre adjustment, but one that satisfies their needs. Some have developed a routine whereby their needs are met, albeit at marginal subsistence level, and for them adjusting to a new, domiciled life-style would be too much to contemplate. They have achieved a level of competence in coping with a dangerous, even hostile environment, and to leave that environment for another, in which their incompetence would be all too apparent is not an attractive prospect. So when we offer help along conventional lines, homeless people may reject it (Drake & Adler, 1984). This should not be a cause for despair, rather a stimulus to develop more creative or effective approaches. The striking success that can be achieved with some patients enables us not to be discouraged in spite of what often seem to be overwhelming odds.

Consultation with shelter providers and others involved with homeless people is an important function for psychiatrists or other mental health professionals. Often it is the staff or helpers in shelters and soup kitchen, police officers or others who are first in line to provide help for a person with a mental illness or substance use disorder. Often these people are not well-informed about mental illness, fearful of the mentally ill, and unskilled in handling the situations that may develop, often at night, or at other times when help is not easily available. Time devoted to education and skill-building with such people is time well-spent. The increase in sophistication of these service providers will be repaid in smoother handling of emergencies and an increasingly collaborative relationship with the mental health team (Susser, 1992).

A consideration of the many tasks and skills involved in providing services to homeless people indicates the necessity of team work. A psychiatrist, psychologist, nurse or social worker working alone can certainly be of assistance to many people, but to provide an adequate service requires the efforts of a team of specialists who combine their several special skills.

Programmes, models and service systems

Increasing accessibility

Special programmes are needed for homeless people because of accessibility problems with conventional services. One set of problems is within the person: a distaste for conventional clinical settings, an exaggerated fear of how they will be treated, or a level of disorganization that makes it difficult for the person to get to the treatment facility. A second set of factors relates to the service programmes themselves. There may be reluctance on the part of providers to deal with dirty or bizarre individuals, or a concern that such clients might scare away others. A clinic or agency may be located in a neighbourhood that is off the beaten track for homeless people or the cost or the complexity of its intake and registration procedures may serve as a deterrent (Stark, 1992). A classic example of the latter occurred during the 1980s, when the application procedures for Supplemental Security Income (SSI) were made so complex that most mentally ill people could not complete them without considerable assistance. The situation has now changed. Not only has the procedure been simplified, but a special cadre of staff from the Social Security Administration now goes out in the streets of some cities to assist homeless people in making applications for SSI.

Programmes should be situated in areas frequented by homeless people. Public transport should be available. Buildings should not be intimidating, as many hospitals are. Facilities should be comfortable and attractive, as an inducement to enter, and as an indication that homeless people are respected and that their dignity and comfort are of concern to the programme providers. There should be signs to assist people to find the programme, but sufficiently discrete to avoid stigmatization. The availability of services should be publicized through all the available media. In particular, other agencies serving homeless people should be fully aware of the location and hours of availability of mental health services.

Linkage and collaboration

An individual programme generally is only able to provide a partial response to the treatment needs of homeless people. This is reasonable in the light of the slender resources generally available. However, in the light of the wide range of services needed by many homeless people, clinicians must take advantage of community service systems that are already in place. It often requires a lot of diplomacy and hard work to establish linkages with other treatment or rehabilitation programmes in the area so that, through active liaison, the combined resources can be mobilized when needed. Considerable effort often needs to go into advocacy and obtaining support from state or local health service administrators.

Even then, the scope of services is likely to be severely limited, because probably no state has yet provided adequate funds to cope with the development of community services for deinstitutionalized psychiatric patients or for the long-term treatment or rehabilitation of chronic alcoholics or drug abusers. Clinicians must join forces with advocates, political activists, rehabilitation experts and others to form coalitions that will bring pressure on policy-makers to develop service systems adequate for the needs of the nation's most disadvantaged citizens.

Dual diagnosis

The treatment of people with both mental illness and substance abuse or dependence (Drake & Wallach, 1989) perplexes service providers in community psychiatry programmes generally (Minkoff & Drake, 1991), but especially in those working with homeless people, where the rates of co-morbidity are so high (Table 8.1). The problems encountered in attempting to treat dually diagnosed persons are both clinical and organizational.

The clinical problems arise from the difficulty of dealing with two types of disorder. The psychiatric treatment of schizophrenia, for example, will lead to a diminution or elimination of many of the symptoms of the disease. Rehabilitation of the person, however, requires a concerted effort on the part of the patient and the professionals to move him or her in the direction of independence and self-sufficiency. Substance abuse greatly impedes this process. Conversely, remaining drug and alcohol free is, for an addict, a considerable feat, requiring volition, persistence, resilience and a supportive milieu, all of which may be lacking for a mentally ill person, especially one who is homeless. Each condition undermines the treatment of the other. The organizational problems arise because of the traditional separation of substance abuse and mental illness treatment services. This separation is reflected at the federal, state and local levels, where separate bureaucracies deal with these problems. Planning and implementing services to bring together treatment for mental illness and substance abuse is often complex and requires a great deal of work to overcome organizational, philosophical and professional differences.

Traditional service systems therefore often provide separate services for substance abuse and mental illness treatment, and efforts may be made to enroll a patient in both. Most often these plans do not succeed, and it has been found that integrated treatment programmes are most effective, where treatment for mental illness and treatment for substance abuse are provided in a co-ordinated fashion, in the same setting, by the same staff (Ridgely, 1991).

The problems are compounded when the person is homeless (Minkoff & Drake, 1992). Alcohol has traditionally had an important place in the lives of homeless people (Hopper, 1989) and, for example, insisting on abstinence from alcohol or drugs as a prerequisite for participation in treatment may be counter-productive. Treatment programmes for homeless dually diagnosed individuals, therefore, may have abstinence as a goal to be attained, but accept individuals who are still drinking or using drugs (Minkoff & Drake, 1992).

Federal programmes for the homeless mentally ill

Since the early 1980s, the Federal government has played an important role in stimulating research and programme development for homeless mentally ill people, specifically through the National Institute for Mental Health, and the Center for Mental Health Services since its establishment in 1993. The Center supports the development of mental health services for homeless people through a system of PATH (Program for Assistance in Transition for the Homeless) grants to states. These grants support a range of services for homeless mentally ill people in cities across the country, provided by a variety of non-profit or local government groups.

In 1991 the federal government appointed a Task Force on Homelessness and Severe Mental Illness, which brought together senior representatives of the several federal agencies who have roles to play in combating homelessness, particularly among the mentally ill, including the Department of Housing and Urban Development (HUD), the Department of Health and Human Services, the Department of Veterans' Affairs (VA), the Department of Labor, the Social Security Administration, the Department of Justice, etc. The Task Force produced a report in 1992, containing a series of 58 recommendations for steps the several agencies could take under their existing mandates to ease the plight of people who are mentally ill and homeless (Federal Task Force on Homelessness and Severe Mental Illness, 1992).

One specific problem identified in that report is the fractionation of the service systems and the numerous agencies whose activities need to be integrated in order to provide homeless people with what they need. The Task Force report recommended the development of ACCESS (Access to Community Care and Effective Services and Supports), an initiative to promote service integration. A series of demonstration projects have been funded in nine states to test new models, which include innovations such as inter-agency joint management teams, to co-ordinate the work of the various social agencies; peer engagement teams, which employ former homeless people for outreach, support and linkage; multi-service centres, where various agencies provide co-ordinated services; and the use of advanced data systems integration, so that consumers do not have to register repeatedly with different agencies to obtain services.

The Federal Task Force also introduced the concept of Safe Havens, based on the experience of many workers in the field, that many homeless people desire, and will accept, little more than a safe and sanitary place to obtain shelter from the elements and the dangers of the streets.

Innovative programmes at the local level

Activity at the national level has been matched by creativity at the local level. A wide variety of programmes have been developed, many with federal grant support, but also relying heavily on support from states, local communities and private philanthropy (Center for Mental Health Services, 1994).

Community Connections in Washington, DC provides clinical case management to severely mentally ill men and women, many of whom have been homeless, many of whom are dually diagnosed and virtually all of whom are at risk of homelessness. A particular set of interventions is aimed at addressing the deficiencies in the social networks of many homeless people, believed to be a factor in precipitating or prolonging homelessness. Their Social Network Treatment model includes a number of innovative techniques to assist people in developing and maintaining networks of supportive relationships (Bebout et al., 1993).

In Baltimore, a joint project of the University of Maryland and the city's mental health administration, Baltimore Mental Health Systems, Inc., has adapted the Assertive Community Treatment (ACT) approach of Stein & Test (1985). The mobile ACT Team consists of psychiatrists, nurses, social workers and counsellors who provide services, wherever they are needed, for a group of patients who were homeless at the time of entry to the programme. A particularly interesting aspect of this programme is the inclusion of 'consumer advocates', people who have experience as psychiatric patients and in some cases also of homelessness. Their own past histories provide them with skills and authenticity that professionals may lack in gaining the trust of the homeless individuals they are trying to help (Dixon et al., 1994).

A group at Columbia University in New York has developed the concept of Critical Time Intervention (CTI). They believe that the time at which a person makes the transition from a homeless shelter to more permanent housing is critical, and that a person is especially vulnerable to relapse or default at this period in time. A CTI team, based in a men's shelter, provides case management, treatment and social skills training to assist individuals who are moving out of the shelter. The team has identified four major functional areas that are the focus of the intervention: medication adherence, money management, substance use management and crisis management. For a 9 month period they support and provide continuity of care as the men settle in their new surroundings and move towards integration in the community (Susser et al., 1992). Preliminary data on the effectiveness of the programme in reducing the probability of return to homelessness are encouraging.

The need for an intermediate level of care for people who are too ill to care for themselves on the streets or in the shelter system, but not ill enough to be admitted to hospital, has been recognized in a number of places. Christ House, in Washington, DC, provides an excellent example (Goetcheus et al., 1990). While not focusing specifically on mentally ill people, but rather those with other health problems, psychiatric care and treatment for substance abuse disorders is provided to the many residents who need such help. People stay at Christ House for up to a month as they regain their health and strength.

Another approach to providing a supportive environment for mentally ill people has been developed in Baltimore. The city's Mental Health Agency has developed a list of room and board providers, who are given some basic training in dealing with mentally ill people, and whose homes are inspected for health and fire safety. Mentally ill people can rent rooms in these houses, with case management and other support and treatment services provided by local community mental health programmes or by homeless health care teams (S. Diehl, personal communication).

In the area of housing, an approach currently being developed and evaluated by Stephen Goldfinger and his colleagues in Boston, sets up 'evolving consumer households' for homeless mentally ill individuals. This concept provides housing for a group of homeless people, with staff support at the outset, as they establish their household. As the group becomes more skilled in establishing their own house rules and managing their own affairs, staff gradually withdraw until the group is functioning independently. An evaluation, currently in progress, will determine to what extent mentally ill people can establish independent households in this way, and what the longer-term outlook for such households may be (Center for Mental Health Services, 1994).

The future

Those who engage in providing services for homeless people do so in the hope that their services will soon no longer be needed, because homelessness will cease to be a major problem in American society. However this hope seems increasingly naive. As the years pass, the numbers of homeless people seeking help from service agencies only increases. The enormous deficiency in the supply of housing in America may take decades to remedy. Public opinion is not support- ive of significant increases in assistance to the poor. Education for the masses of young Americans is not fitting them well for employment in an increasingly technological employment market.

America is struggling to reform its health care system. In spite of the efforts of the Clinton administration, federal health care reform remains a distant hope. At state levels, reforms are taking place piecemeal, but the emphasis is on controlling cost rather than on guaranteeing health care for all the citizens. Many states, for example, are radically changing their Medicaid plans to introduce the methods of managed care. Poor people in some cases are forced into health maintenance organizations that are not equipped to provide the types of services needed by the mentally ill or by homeless people. Health care programmes for homeless people, up to now supported by a mixture of funds from Medicaid, special federal or state grant programmes and local philanthropy, view their future with grave misgivings.

Prevention

Mental health service providers must focus their energies, therefore, not only on providing appropriate services for those who are mentally ill and homeless, but also on prevention. Prevention of mental illness is still beyond our capabilities, but prevention of homelessness should be more feasible. As research continues to provide more and more information about homeless people, it is becoming possible to identify risk factors for homelessness. Co-morbid substance dependence has been shown to be a risk factor (Drake & Wallach, 1989). Histories of problems in childhood, such as foster care placement or running away from home, are also associated with homelessness in mentally ill men (Susser *et al.*, 1991). Risk factors such as these could be used to identify individuals at special risk of homelessness, who could be provided with additional preventive interventions. Simply improving the quality and extent of community mental health services would be of significant help. Many major cities' service systems are very inadequate to meet the needs of their mentally ill citizens for treatment, rehabilitation and support. With the knowledge base already existing, a great deal more could be done not only to improve the safety net that should protect mentally ill people from becoming homeless, but to greatly increase the quality of their lives.

Whether there is progress along these lines will depend upon there being sufficient political will to make it possible. For this reason, psychiatrists and others who are concerned about these issues see it as important that they involve themselves in political advocacy and public education, in concert with other groups who are active in this field.

References

Appleby, L. & Desai, P. (1987). Residential stability: a perspective on system imbalance. *American Journal of Orthopsychiatry*, **57**, 515–24.

Appelbaum, P. S. (1992). Legal aspects of clinical care for severely mentally ill, homeless persons. *Bulletin of the American Academy of Psychiatry and the Law*, **20**, 455–73.

Ball, F. L. J. & Havassy, B. E. (1984). A survey of the problems and needs of homeless consumers of acute psychiatric services. *Hospital and Community Psychiatry*, **35**, 97–9.

Bassuk, E. L., Rubin, L. & Lauriat, A. S. (1986). Characteristics of homeless sheltered families. *American Journal of Public Health*, **76**, 1097–101.

Bebout, R. R., Harris, M., Swayze, F. V. *et al.* (1993). *The Community Connections Social Support Network Intervention Model*. Washington DC: Community Connections, Inc.

Billig, N. & Levinson, C. (1987). Homelessness and case management in Montgomery County, Maryland: a focus on chronic mental illness. *Psychosocial Rehabilitation Journal*, **11**, 59–66.

Blackwell, B., Breakey, W. R., Hammersley, D., Hammond, R., McMurray-Avila, M. & Seagar, C. (1990). Psychiatric and mental health services. In P. W. Brickner, L. K. Sharer, B. A. Conanan, M. Savarese & B. Scanlan (eds.), *Under the Safety Net: the Health and Social Welfare of the Homeless in the United States*, pp. 184–203. New York: Norton.

Breakey, W. R. & Fischer, P. J. (1995). Mental illness and the continuum of residential stability, *Social Psychiatry and Psychiatric Epidemiology*, **30**, 147–51.

Breakey, W. R., Fischer, P. J., Kramer, M. *et al.* (1989). Health and mental health problems of homeless men and women in Baltimore. *Journal of the American Medical Association*, **262**, 1352–7.

Brickner, P. W., Sharer, L. K., Conanan, B. A., Savarese, M. & Scanlan, B. (eds.) (1990). *Under the Safety Net: The Health and Social Welfare of the Homeless in the United States*. New York: Norton.

Burt, M. R. & Cohen, B. E. (1989). *America's Homeless*. Washington, DC: The Urban Institute.

Center for Mental Health Services (1994). *Making a Difference: Interim Status Report of the McKinney Demonstration Program for Homeless Adults with Serious Mental Illness*. Washington, DC: US Department of Health and Human Services.

Cohen, C. I. (1993). Poverty and the course of schizophrenia: implications for research and policy. *Hospital and Community Psychiatry*, **44**, 951–8.

Cohen, N. L. & Marcos, L. R. (1986). Psychiatric care of the homeless mentally ill. *Psychiatric Annals*, **16**, 729–32.

Dixon, L., Kraus, N. & Lehman, A. (1994). Consumers as providers: the promise and the challenge, *Community Mental Health Journal*, **30**, 615–25.

130   W. R. BREAKEY

Drake, R. E. & Adler, D. A. (1984). Shelter is not enough: clinical work
    with the homeless mentally ill. In H. R. Lamb (ed.), *The Homeless
    Mentally Ill*, pp. 141–52. Washington, DC: American Psychiatric
    Association.
Drake, R. E. & Wallach, M. A. (1989). Substance abuse among the
    chronically mentally ill. *Hospital and Community Psychiatry*, **40**,
    1041–5.
Farr, R. K. (1986). A mental health treatment program for the
    homeless mentally ill in the Los Angeles Skid Row area. In B. E.
    Jones (ed.), *Treating the Homeless: Urban Psychiatry's Challenge*,
    pp. 65–92. Washington, DC: American Psychiatric Press, Inc.
Federal Task Force on Homelessness and Severe Mental Illness (1992).
    Outcasts on Main Street. Washington, DC: National Institute of
    Mental Health.
Fischer, P. J. (1990). Estimating prevalence of alcohol, drug and mental
    health problems in the contemporary homeless population: A
    review of the literature. *Contemporary Drug Problems*, **16**, 333–90.
Fischer, P. J. & Breakey, W. R. (1986). Homelessness and mental
    health: an overview. *International Journal of Mental Health*, **14**, 6–41.
Fischer, P. J. & Breakey, W. R. (1991). The epidemiology of alcohol,
    drug and mental disorders in the homeless. *American Psychologist*, **46**,
    1115–28.
Fischer, P. J., Drake, R. E. & Breakey, W. R. (1992). Mental health
    problems among homeless persons: A review of epidemiological
    research from 1980–1990. In H. R. Lamb, L. L. Bachrach & F. I.
    Kass (eds.), *Treating the Homeless Mentally Ill*, Washington, DC:
    American Psychiatric Association.
Gelberg, L. & Linn, L. S. (1989). Assessing the physical health status of
    homeless adults. *Journal of the American Medical Association*, **262**,
    1973–9.
Goetcheus, J., Gleason, M. A., Sarson, D., Bennett, T. & Wolfe, P. B.
    (1990). Convalescence: for those without a home – developing
    respite services in protected environments. In P. W. Brickner, L. K.
    Sharer, B. A. Conanan, M. Savarese & B. Scanlan (eds.), *Under the
    Safety Net: the Health and Social Welfare of the Homeless in the United
    States*. New York: Norton.
Herman, D. B., Struening, E. L. & Barrow, S. M. (1993). Self-assessed
    need for mental health services among homeless adults. *Hospital and
    Community Psychiatry*, **44**, 1181–3.
Hopper, K. (1989). Deviance and dwelling space: notes on the
    resettlement of homeless persons with alcohol and drug problems.
    Contemporary Drug Problems, **16**, 391–414.
Institute of Medicine (1988). *Homelessness, Health and Human Needs*.
    Washington, DC: National Academy Press.
Jahiel, R. I. (ed.) (1992). *Homelessness: A Prevention-oriented Approach*.
    Baltimore, MD: Johns Hopkins University Press.
Koegel, P., Burnam, A. & Farr, R. K. (1988). The prevalence of

specific psychiatric disorders among homeless individuals in the inner city of Los Angeles. *Archives of General Psychiatry*, **45**, 1085–92.

Lamb, H. R., Bachrach, L. L. & Kass, F. I. (eds.) (1992a). *Treating the Homeless Mentally Ill.* Washington, DC: American Psychiatric Association.

Lamb, H. R., Bachrach, L. L., Goldfinger, S. M. & Kass, F. I. (1992b). Summary and Recommendations. In H. R. Lamb, L. L. Bachrach & F. I. Kass (eds.), *Treating the Homeless Mentally Ill*, pp. 1–10. Washington, DC: American Psychiatric Association.

Lomas, E. (1992). Skid-row based services for people who are homeless and mentally ill. In R. I. Jahiel (ed.), *Homelessness: A Prevention-oriented Approach*, pp. 193–206. Baltimore, MD: Johns Hopkins University Press.

Minkoff, K. & Drake, R. E. (eds.) (1991). *Dual Diagnosis of Major Mental Illness and Substance Disorder.* San Francisco: Jossey-Bass.

Minkoff, K. & Drake, R. E. (1992). Homeless and dual diagnosis. In H. R. Lamb, L. L. Bachrach & F. I. Kass (eds.), *Treating the Homeless Mentally Ill*, pp. 221–48. Washington, DC: American Psychiatric Association.

Morse, G. A. & Calsyn, R. J. (1992). Mental health and other human service needs of homeless people. In M. J. Robertson & M. Greenblatt (eds.), *Homelessness: A National Perspective*, pp. 117–32. New York: Plenum Press.

Ovrebo, B. (1992). Understanding the needs of homeless and near-homeless people. In R. I. Jahiel (ed.), *Homelessness: A Prevention-oriented Approach*, pp. 139–50. Baltimore, MD: Johns Hopkins University Press.

Reich, R. & Siegel, L. (1978). The emergence of the Bowery as a psychiatric dumping ground. *Psychiatric Quarterly*, **50**, 191–201.

Ridgely, M. S. (1991). Creating integrated programs for severely mentally ill persons with substance disorders. In K. Minkoff & R. E. Drake (eds.), *Dual Diagnosis of Major Mental Illness and Substance Disorder*, pp. 29–41. San Francisco: Jossey-Bass.

Robertson, M. J. & Greenblatt, M. (eds.) (1992). *Homelessness: A National Perspective.* New York: Plenum Press.

Smith, E. M., North, C. S. & Spitznagel, E. L. (1992). A systematic study of mental illness, substance abuse and treatment in 600 homeless men. *Annals of Clinical Psychiatry*, **4**, 111–20.

Smith, E. M., North, C. S. & Spitznagel, E. L. (1993). Alcohol, drugs and psychiatric comorbidity among homeless women: an epidemiological study. *Journal of Clinical Psychiatry*, **54**, 82–7.

Spitzer, R. L., Cohen, G., Miller, J. D. & Endicott, J. (1969). The psychiatric status of 100 men in Skid Row. *International Journal of Social Psychiatry*, **15**, 230–4.

Stark, L. (1992). Barriers to health care for homeless people. In R. I. Jahiel (ed.), *Homelessness: A Prevention-oriented Approach*, pp. 151–64. Baltimore, MD: Johns Hopkins University Press.

Stein, L. & Test, M. A. (eds.) (1985). *The Training in Community Living Model: A Decade of Experience*. San Francisco: Jossey-Bass.

Surber, R. W., Dwyer, E., Ryan, K. J., Goldfinger, S. M. & Kelly, J. T. (1988). Medical and psychiatric needs of the homeless. *Social Work*, **33**, 116–19.

Susser, E. (1992). Working with people who are mentally ill and homeless: the role of a psychiatrist. In R. Jahiel (ed.), *Homelessness: A Prevention-oriented approach*, pp. 207–17. Baltimore, MD: Johns Hopkins University Press.

Susser, E., Struening, E. L. & Conover, S. (1989). Psychiatric problems in homeless men. *Archives of General Psychiatry*, **46**, 845–50.

Susser, E., Valencia, E. & Goldfinger, S. M. (1992). Clinical care of homeless mentally ill individuals: strategies and adaptations. In H. R. Lamb, L. L. Bachrach & F. I. Kass (eds.), *Treating the Homeless Mentally Ill*, pp. 127–40. Washington, DC: American Psychiatric Association.

Susser, E., Lin, S. P., Conover, S. A. & Struening, E. L. (1991). Childhood antecedents of homelessness in psychiatric patients. *American Journal of Psychiatry*, **148**, 1026–30.

Swayze, F. V. (1992). Clinical case management with the homeless mentally ill. In H. R. Lamb, L. L. Bachrach & F. I. Kass (eds.), *Treating the Homeless Mentally Ill*, pp. 203–20. Washington, DC: American Psychiatric Association.

Tessler, R. C. & Dennis, D. L. (1989). *A Synthesis of NIMH-funded Research Concerning Persons who are Homeless and Mentally Ill*. Rockville, MD: National Institute of Mental Health.

Van Tosh, L. (1993). *Working for a Change: Employment of Consumers/Survivors in the Design and Provision of Services for Persons who are Homeless and Mentally Disabled*. Rockville, MD: Center for Mental Health Services.

Wright, J. D. & Weber, E. (1987). *Homelessness and Health*. Washington, DC: McGraw-Hill.

9

The severely mentally ill in hostels for the homeless

Max Marshall

Introduction

The terms 'shelter', 'hostel' and 'lodging house' have been used interchangeably by most UK commentators on homelessness. Unfortunately the imprecise use of these terms has obscured important differences between two distinct types of accommodation that have traditionally been provided for the single homeless in the UK. In this chapter these two types of accommodation will be referred to as shelter accommodation and hostel accommodation. If we are to make sense of the UK studies of homeless people with mental disorder it is necessary to reassert the distinction between shelter and hostel accommodation. Consequently this chapter will begin by defining hostel and shelter accommodation. Studies of homeless people in the UK will then be classified into hostel or shelter populations. The findings revealed by this reclassification will then be discussed. Finally, on the basis of these findings, the size of the mentally ill hostel population, and the characteristics of its members, will be discussed. The effectiveness of hostels for the homeless in caring for people with severe psychiatric disorder is discussed in Chapter 16.

Shelters and hostels

Definition of shelter and hostel accommodation

Shelters will be defined as buildings offering emergency overnight accommodation to single homeless people. Hostels will be defined as buildings (other than cheap bedsits) offering board and lodgings to

133

single homeless people. Because of their different functions, shelter and hostel accommodation tend to cater for different populations. Shelter accommodation caters for a transient population consisting of whoever happens to turn up on a particular night, whereas hostel accommodation caters for a relatively 'permanent' group of 'residents', who will live in the hostel by day and occupy the same bed, or room, at night. Sometimes both hostel and shelter accommodation may be provided within the same building, as, for example, in the now defunct Camberwell Reception Centre (Wood, 1976).

Origins of shelter and hostel accommodation

The origins of shelter accommodation may be traced to the pre-war casual wards, subsequently reorganized in the post-war period as 'reception centres', under the surveillance of the National Assistance Board. Although these reception centres ostensibly had a rehabilitative function, contemporary research indicated that for the majority of occupants they largely provided emergency accommodation, particularly for 'wanderers' and 'vagrants' (Wade, 1963). The widespread closure of reception centres in the 1950s appears to have been followed by the creation of shelter accommodation staffed by voluntary organizations. Many of these shelters were permanent; others were opened only during cold weather emergencies or at Christmas (Weller et al., 1989). Such shelters served not only as emergency accommodation, but also as 'contact points' where suitable clients for hostel accommodation could be identified and assessed (Leach & Wing, 1978).

The origins of hostels may be traced to the squalid privately run lodging houses of the Victorian era. Concern over conditions in these establishments led to increasing regulation, and in many cases closure or rebuilding by local authorities (Laidlaw, 1956). With the introduction of the welfare state the demand for lodging house accommodation dropped. The remaining lodging houses were increasingly run as hostels, either by local corporations or by religious charities such as the Salvation Army and Church Army. Many of the residents of such hostels were 'permanent' and were allocated their own beds, cubicles, or (if lucky) rooms. Conditions in these hostels were basic, but meals, cheap provisions and laundry facilities were provided. In the 1950s about 50% of hostel residents were working men.

The latter part of the century saw further developments in hostel accommodation, against a background of further decreases in the numbers of lodging house beds. First, there was a general attempt by religious charities to improve the quality of their hostel accommodation by building new hostels in which shared or private rooms replaced dormitory accommodation. However, despite these efforts much old-style dormitory accommodation remained, particularly in London. Secondly, new charitable bodies such as the Simon Community and the St Mungo's community began to set up a network of smaller scale hostels run as therapeutic communities, where staff and residents lived together on an equal footing. These new hostels attracted increasing numbers of mentally ill residents. Under the pressure of caring for the mentally ill, these organizations tended to become increasingly bureaucratized, so that by the late 1970s the distinction between the 'new hostels' and those run by religious bodies was often blurred (Leach, 1979).

Separating hostel studies from shelter studies

Table 9.1 summarizes the findings of UK studies of mental disorder amongst the homeless. At first sight the findings of these studies vary widely, for example Priest (1971) in an Edinburgh study found a much higher level of schizophrenia amongst the homeless than was found in a study in London by LCSS (1960).

There is a temptation to consider the findings of these UK studies as practically worthless, given the wide variations in study design and sample selection. This temptation is reinforced by the tendency of some authors to make incredible extrapolations from the findings of these studies. For example, in a recent review Scott (1993) estimated that there were 1–2 million homeless people in the UK, 30–50% of whom were suffering from mental disorder, predominantly 'functional psychosis'. According to these figures, the minimum estimate for the number of homeless people with 'functional psychoses' in the UK is 300 000; considerably larger than a generous estimate of the total yearly prevalence of schizophrenia (approximately 291 000; calculated by taking the maximum estimate of the yearly prevalence in the UK, 5.3/1000 and multiplying by an estimated adult population of 55 000 000).

However, despite such flights of fancy, it is unnecessarily nihilistic to accept that no coherent picture can be extracted from the available

Table 9.1. *Summary of UK studies of the prevalence of schizophrenia in homeless populations*

Study	City	Date	Prevalence of schizophrenia (%)
Laidlaw (1956)	Glasgow	1954	3
LCSS (1960)	London	1955	5
Priest (1971)	Edinburgh	1965	32
Crossley & Denmark (1969)	Bolton	1969	24
Lodge Patch (1971)	London	1970	15
Tidmarsh & Wood (1972)	London	1971	16
Leopoldt & Lynch (1981)	Oxford	1979	17
Timms & Fry (1989)	London	1987	31
Marshall (M) (1989)	Oxford	1988	27
Marshall (J) & Reed (1992)	London	1988	64
Reed et al. (1992)	London	1988	13
Stark et al. (1989)	Various centres	1989	18–25
Adams et al. (1996)	London	1990	50
Geddes et al. (1994a)	Edinburgh	1992	9
Newton et al. (1994)	Edinburgh	1992	3
Weller et al. (1989)	Various centres	1985	22[a]

Note: the date column in the table records the year when the study was begun, not the year of publication.

[a] No estimate for schizophrenia was given in this study, but 22% had 'active psychotic symptoms'.

data. When the findings of existing UK studies are considered in the light of the distinction between hostel and shelter accommodation, a more coherent picture emerges. To demonstrate this coherence we must first reclassify the studies along these lines.

Shelter studies

Two of the studies listed in Table 9.1 are unequivocally studies of shelter populations: a study of users of an emergency cold-weather shelter in London (Reed et al., 1992); and a study of users of a Cyrenian shelter in Oxford, located in an abandoned air raid shelter (Leopoldt & Lynch, 1981). The study by Lodge Patch (1971), although conducted on two Salvation Army hostels, is also a study of a shelter population. In this study the hostels are described as 'large dormitories', where 'there was no privacy and no room for personal possessions' (Lodge Patch, 1971). Furthermore, the 'men used the hostel for little more than a clean bed . . . most of the occupants moved their beds within the hostel, were transient, or spent periods elsewhere'.

Hostel studies

Eight of the studies listed in Table 9.1 are unequivocally studies of hostel populations: a study of Glasgow Common Lodging houses (Laidlaw, 1956); a study of London Common Lodging Houses (LCSS, 1960); a study of Edinburgh Common Lodging houses (Priest, 1971); and three recent studies: one of hostels in Oxford (Marshall, 1989), and the other two of women's hostels in London (Marshall & Reed, 1992; Adams *et al.*, 1996). In addition, the study by Crossley & Denmark (1969) of a Salvation Army hostel, unlike the study of Lodge Patch (1971), is considered to be a true hostel survey, because the hostel was 'a full board hostel . . . the population being mainly long-stay'.

Mixed studies

In addition there are three studies that have reported the prevalence of mental disorder in accommodation that was functioning as a shelter for some persons and as a hostel for others. The first of these studies reported the rates of mental disorder amongst casual users and recognized residents of the Camberwell Reception Centre (Tidmarsh & Wood, 1972). Recognized residents were said to differ from the casual users in that residents: had agreed to stay for a period of time; worked in the Centre (cleaning or preparing food, or working in the workshops); ate separately from the 'casuals'; and could stay in the Centre during the day and have a midday meal. The second of these studies compared the rate of mental disorder amongst new admissions to a Salvation Army Hostel with that amongst long-term residents (Timms & Fry, 1989). The third study was a random sample of residents of nine Edinburgh hostels (Geddes *et al.*, 1994a), in which approximately 10% of the beds were short-term 'shelter accommodation' (J. Geddes, personal communication). In view of the small number of shelter beds in this study it will be classified as a hostel study.

Table 9.2. *Summary of UK studies of the prevalence of schizophrenia in homeless populations, grouped by whether 'hostel', 'shelter', or 'roofless' population*

Location of subjects	Study	Date begun	Sample size	Percentage with schizophrenia
Hostel	Laidlaw (1956)	1954	800	3
Hostel	LCSS (1960)	1955	?	5
Hostel	Priest (1971)	1965	79	32
Hostel	Crossley & Denmark (1969)	1969	55	24
Hostel	Tidmarsh & Wood (1972)	1971	63[a]	29
Hostel	Timms & Fry (1989)	1987	58	38
Hostel	Marshall (M) (1989)	1988	146	27
Hostel	Marshall (J) & Reed (1992)[b]	1988	70	64
Hostel	Adams et al. (1966)[b]	1990	64	50
Hostel	Geddes et al. (1994a)	1992	136	9
Shelter	Lodge Patch (1971)	1970	123	15
Shelter	Tidmarsh & Wood (1972)	1971	?	16
Shelter	Leopoldt & Lynch (1981)	1979	76	17
Shelter	Timms & Fry (1989)	1987	65	25
Shelter	Reed et al. (1992)	1988	96	13
Roofless	Newton et al. (1994)	1992	65	3

[a] There is some ambiguity about the sample size in the original paper, this figure may be inaccurate.
[b] Study carried out in women-only hostels. In other studies subjects were predominantly or entirely male.

Unclassified studies

Three of the studies listed in Table 9.1 cannot be classified as studies of shelter or hostel accommodation. In one study this is because data collected over several years from shelter and hostel populations have been combined (Weller et al., 1989). This study is therefore omitted from the subsequent analysis. In another study, of the users of reception centres (Stark et al., 1989), subjects were selected on the grounds of being 'hard to place', therefore the study does not provide a representative sample of the users of the centres. This study will also be omitted from the following analysis. The final study (Newton et al., 1994) is the only UK prevalence study of mental disorder amongst rough sleepers. This study cannot be classified as a shelter study, but its findings are of interest and will be shown alongside the shelter and hostel data for comparative purposes.

Trends in the prevalence of mental disorder amongst users of shelter and hostel accommodation

The discussion that follows will focus on the prevalence of schizophrenia because it is more narrowly defined than severe mental disorder and is also by far the most common severe mental disorder amongst the homeless (see below). Table 9.2 shows the findings of UK studies of the prevalence of schizophrenia amongst homeless people, when these studies are regrouped into studies of hostel populations and shelter populations.

From this table two findings emerge:

1. With the exception of the study by Geddes *et al.* (1994a), since the 1960s the levels of schizophrenia found in hostels are consistently higher than those found in shelters.
2. Overall (with the exception of Geddes *et al.*, 1994a) the levels of schizophrenia in hostel accommodation appear to have increased markedly, whilst the levels in shelter accommodation have remained stable.

These two findings will be analysed below.

The higher prevalence of schizophrenia in hostels

The first finding (that the levels of schizophrenia in hostels are consistently higher than those in shelters) refutes the commonly held belief that 'the lower the standard of accommodation from lodging house, to hostel, to reception centre, to the street, the greater is the proportion of . . . mentally disabled people found' (Herzberg, 1987). In fact people suffering from severe psychiatric disorder are much more common in better quality hostel accommodation. This can be seen clearly from Table 9.3 in which a weighted prevalence is computed for each decade from 1950 onwards (calculated by taking all relevant studies in each 10 year period, multiplying each study prevalence by the number of subjects in the study, dividing by the total number of subjects in all the studies in the period, and then adding together these weighted prevalences). The table shows that the weighted prevalence of schizophrenia in shelters remained stable

Table 9.3. *Estimated mean percentage of hostel, shelter and roofless subjects with schizophrenia over the past four decades*

	1951–60	1961–70	1971–80	1981–90	1991–
Hostel (%)	3–5	28.7	29	41(30.1)[a]	9
Shelter (%)	?	15	16–17	17.6	?
Roofless (%)	?	?	?	?	3

[a] Mean percentage when data from women-only hostels are excluded.

at about 17%, whilst in the 1960s, 1970s and 1980s the prevalence in hostels was about twice this figure. These findings, the exact opposite of accepted wisdom (Scott, 1993), are further reinforced by the findings of Newton *et al.* (1994) who (using the same methodology of Geddes *et al.*, 1994a) found a prevalence of only 3% schizophrenia in their survey of Edinburgh rough sleepers.

There are four possible explanations of the higher prevalence of schizophrenia in hostels:

1. Hostels offer care that is attractive to persons with severe mental disorder. Since hostels cater for semi-permanent residents they tend to have higher staff ratios and better facilities than shelters. Thus hostels are better placed to provide support to people suffering from schizophrenia. Such support could include: getting meals, assisting with personal hygiene and domestic chores, and obtaining benefits and managing money.
2. Admission procedures to hostels select people with severe mental disorders. There is a tradition of using shelter accommodation as a contact service from which those suitable for hostel accommodation are selected. When this occurs those selected are often suffering from severe mental disorder. For example, a programme of action research in the St Mungo's hostels found that homeless men coming from the street tended to remain in hostels for only short periods of time. To overcome this problem the researchers suggested that a 'contact service' should be set up to make contact with, and to assess, potential residents, before a place was offered. This new approach was highly successful in increasing length of stay, but an unforeseen consequence was that amongst those who settled 'psychiatric disabilities were particularly prominent' (Leach, 1979). Many hostels are associated with shelters that act

as a contact service in the way described by the St Mungo's researchers.

3. People with severe mental disorder find hostel environments congenial. This suggestion was first mooted in a study of Edinburgh Common Lodging Houses (Priest, 1976). The author stated that 'many (people with schizophrenia) ... prefer the anonymous sanctum of their "eight-by-four two bit room"'. Other researchers have noted that hostels 'exhibit two features strikingly reminiscent of the old mental hospitals: (a) the wide range of bizarre behaviours tolerated; (b) the general non-intrusiveness of other residents and staff' (Timms & Fry, 1989). The same authors have suggested that hostels provide 'low expressed emotion' environments where persons with severe psychiatric disorder are less likely to relapse. It is not yet clear how far these impressions are correct. Moreover high rates of re-admission to hospital of hostel residents (Marshall & Gath, 1992) would tend not to support the suggestion that hostels are low expressed emotion environments.

4. Once resident in hostels, people with severe mental disorder are difficult to resettle elsewhere.

Mentally disordered hostel residents have limited access to suitable accommodation in the public or private sector housing. Thus a follow-up of mentally disordered hostel residents in Oxford found that only 10 of the 48 residents were rehoused in an 18 month period. Those residents who were rehoused went either: back to their families, to private bedsits, or to accommodation provided by the hostels. No residents obtained accommodation supported by health, social services or housing associations (Marshall & Gath, 1992). This 'log-jam' phenomenon (Wood, 1976) may make a considerable contribution to the high prevalence of severe mental disorder in hostels.

The apparent rise in the level of schizophrenia in hostels

The second finding from the reclassified studies was that levels of schizophrenia in hostels appear to have increased markedly, whilst the levels in shelter accommodation have remained relatively constant. Before discussing this finding in more detail it is first necessary to discuss the study by Geddes *et al.* (1994a), because the findings of this study are at variance with all other recent hostel studies. This study is by far the most methodologically rigorous of all UK prevalence studies. The study was based on a random sample of 198 residents of nine Edinburgh hostels. Subjects were assessed by trained interviewers using standardized diagnostic instruments. The findings of the study were compared with the earlier study of Priest (1976) after suitable adjustment of confounding factors. The conclusion of the study was not only that the prevalence of schizophrenia in Edinburgh hostels was much lower than expected (9%), but also that it had actually fallen since the time of Priest's study which began in 1965.

The study has been criticized by some authors (see Connolly & Crown, 1994; Connelly & Williams, 1994) who have questioned the validity of the comparison with Priest's earlier study on two grounds. First, that different standardized instruments were used in the two studies. Secondly, that only 36% of the population in the later study (carried out in 1992) came from the hostels surveyed by Priest in 1965.

Both criticisms, whilst not entirely groundless, miss the most important point of Geddes et al.'s study, namely that a very well conducted survey has established that the true prevalence of schizophrenia in Edinburgh hostels in 1992 was much lower than anyone (including the researchers) expected. Moreover, whilst it is true that the comparison with Priest's work has some methodological limitations, the fact remains that two well conducted surveys in the same hostels 27 years apart appear to show a large fall in the numbers of residents with schizophrenia (Geddes et al., 1994b).

If, as seems likely, the findings of Geddes et al. are correct, how can they be reconciled with recent prevalence studies such as those by Marshall & Reed (1992) and Adams et al. (1996)? A re-examination of these two studies suggests an explanation – both are studies of hostels for homeless women. Women make up only a small proportion of residents of hostels for the homeless, but it is well established that they are more likely to suffer from schizophrenia than male residents (Virgona et al., 1993). If these two studies are excluded from the weighted prevalence in Table 9.3 (see figure in brackets in column 5 (1981–90)) an interesting and unexpected trend emerges – namely that the prevalence of schizophrenia in hostels for the homeless has been stable from the mid-1960s to the late 1980s, with a major increase occurring in the 1950s to early 1960s and perhaps a major fall occurring in the 1990s.

These findings lead us to question why was there such a steep rise in the prevalence of mental disorder in hostels between the 1950s and mid-1960s? There are two possible answers to this question. The first answer is that the increase was related to the reduction in the number of beds in psychiatric hospitals that began in the mid-1950s. The rise in the percentage of hostel residents with schizophrenia, from 5% in the mid 1950s to around 25% by the mid-1960s is contemporaneous with a fall in psychiatric inpatients from 3.5/1000 in 1954, to 3/1000 in 1961, to 2.1/1000 in 1970 (Gunn, 1974). However, if this explanation is correct, it is difficult to explain why the continuing fall in bed numbers was not reflected in further increases in the prevalence of mental illness in the hostels in the 1970s and 1980s.

The second answer is that the same period saw an important change in the nature of hostels, as they moved away from being residences for poor single working men to becoming places of last resort for those with disabilities. As the availability of cheap council housing increased, working men moved away from hostels, leaving behind the mentally ill and socially disabled. The effect of this movement, would have been to increase the prevalence of psychiatric disorder in the remaining hostels without there being any absolute increase in the numbers of mentally ill homeless people.

In summary, an analysis of prevalence data in terms of hostel and shelter studies appears to overturn a number of widespread beliefs about the homeless mentally ill in the UK. First, in UK studies at least, the proportion of people with schizophrenia or 'functional psychoses' is considerably lower than the 30–50% generally cited. Secondly, there is no evidence that the proportion of hostel residents with schizophrenia has increased since the mid-1960s. Thirdly, the proportion of people with schizophrenia increases from street to shelter to hostel – the opposite direction to that widely cited in the literature.

The numbers and characteristics of hostel residents with severe mental disorders

Estimating the numbers of people with schizophrenia in hostels

This author's most recent estimate is that there are between 2400 and 8100 persons with schizophrenia living in hostels for the homeless in the UK. This estimate is arrived at as follows. First, it is estimated that

Table 9.2. *Characteristics of hostel residents*

	Hostel males (*mainly*)			Hostel females	Shelter males
Study	Timms & Fry (1989)	*Marshall (1989)*	Geddes ea (1994a)	Marshall & Reed (1992)	Reed ea (1992)
Age	59.2	*48.1*	50.7	52.1	40
Ethnic	12	*2*	—	—	—
Imprisoned	—	*48*	42	30	52
Organic disorder (%)	2	*3*	—	4	—
Length of stay	—	*44% > 3yrs*	—	*50% > 2yrs*	—
Ever admitted (%)	—	*90*	20	64	18
Ever married (%)	—	*12*	47	42	29
Last contact with relatives	—	*42% > 1yr*	—	*66% > 1yr*	—
Unemployed (%)	94	*100*	95	100	—
Admitted from hospital (%)	—	*46*	—	11	—

Data in italics were derived from a sample of mentally ill residents. Data in normal font were derived from a sample of all residents.
ea, *et al.*

there are 27 000 hostel beds in hostels for the homeless in the UK (based on doubling the accepted figure for London of 13 500 (Balazs, 1993)). Secondly, it is estimated that from 9–30% of the occupants of these beds are suffering from schizophrenia. The lower 9% figure is derived from the recent work of Geddes *et al.* (1994a), whilst the higher figure is derived from the weighted prevalence figure for the 1980s (see Table 9.3). Until further data become available it is difficult to determine which of these figures is most accurate. From the prevalence data discussed below, we may assume that about 80% of hostel residents with severe psychiatric disorders are suffering from schizophrenia, hence the figures for all severe psychiatric disorder are in the region of 2880–9720.

Social and psychiatric characteristics of hostel residents

Some of the characteristics of hostel residents are summarized in Table 9.4 below. The contents of the table are derived from recent hostel studies only, as it is not clear how far data from studies conducted in the 1960s can be applied to the hostel populations of today. For purposes of comparison the findings of a recent study of shelter users, based on a representative sample, are included (Reed *et al.*, 1992).

Social characteristics

Hostel residents (including those with mental disorder) tend to be in late middle age. They have limited social networks in that: nearly all are unemployed, and only a minority have ever been married. Rates of imprisonment amongst hostel residents are high, usually for minor offences. Probably about one in five hostel residents have been in psychiatric hospitals, with this figure rising to about 90% amongst those residents who are known to be mentally ill. Mentally ill hostel residents tend to have lost contact with their relatives, but it is not clear how far this is true for non-mentally ill residents.

The data from Table 9.4 indicate some differences between hostel residents (both male and female) and shelters users. Hostel residents tend to be older than shelter users and are more likely to have been admitted to psychiatric hospitals. Female hostel residents differ from male residents in that they are more likely to have been married.

Otherwise the social situations of male and female hostel residents are fairly similar.

There are insufficient data to reach firm conclusions about the ethnic composition of modern hostel populations. It appears that people of Scottish and Irish origin are over-represented. There are also indications that, in London at least, people of West Indian origin are over-represented. Little recent data is available concerning the original social class of hostel users. It is of interest however that Marshall & Reed (1992) found that the fathers of 32 out of 53 women in two women's hostels were members of social classes 1, 2 or 3.

There are indications that the health of mentally disordered hostel residents is poor. Several authors have reported physical problems to be common amongst residents with mental disorder (Stark *et al.*, 1989; Marshall & Reed, 1992). High mortality rates amongst mentally disordered hostel residents were suggested in the Oxford follow-up study described above (Marshall & Gath, 1992).

Psychiatric characteristics

There is general agreement amongst hostel studies that schizophrenia is by far the most common diagnosis amongst mentally ill hostel residents. Thus, for example, a study of Oxford hostels found that 40 out of 48 severely disabled residents were suffering from schizophrenia (Marshall & Gath, 1992), whilst in a London hostel 22 out of 31 mentally disordered residents were given a diagnosis of schizophrenia (Timms & Fry, 1989). Organic brain disease would also appear to be relatively common. A study of women's hostels in London (Marshall & Reed, 1992) found that 3 out of 45 women with schizophrenia also suffered from epilepsy (in two cases the epilepsy was due to head injury and in one due to a previous leucotomy). The same study reported that, of 63 women with mental disorder, 6 had organic mental disorder. Similarly in the London hostel study referred to above (Timms & Fry, 1989), 3 out of 27 mentally disordered residents were suffering from organic brain disease (dementia, amnesic syndrome and mental retardation). There is insufficient evidence to estimate the prevalence of other causes of severe psychiatric disorder, such as bipolar disorder or severe depression, in hostel residents. It seems likely however that people with these disorders make up less than 5% of the hostel population.

A further characteristic of mentally disordered hostel residents is the extent of the social disability caused by their disorder. In a survey of two large Oxford hostels for the homeless, standardized rating scales were used to measure psychiatric symptoms and social disability. Forty-eight residents were found to have chronic disabling mental disorders (one third of the total residents). Half of these 48 residents, according to national norms, were as severely socially disabled as the most disabled long-stay patients in psychiatric hospitals (Marshall, 1989). The same study also showed that mentally disordered hostel residents showed high levels of socially unacceptable behaviour, including violence, self-harm, incontinence and sexually offensive behaviour.

In conclusion, the findings from UK studies of the homeless show a remarkable degree of consistency once reclassified into studies of shelters and studies of hostels. Viewed in this light, the findings contradict two commonplace beliefs: (a) that there is evidence for a recent increase in the numbers of homeless mentally ill, and (b) that the proportion of people with mental disorder is greatest in the least supportive environments, i.e. shelters or the street. The evidence consistently shows that people with severe mental disorders are most common where the highest degree of support is offered – in hostels. The effectiveness of hostels in caring for the severely mentally ill will be discussed in Chapter 16.

References

Adams, C. E., Duke, P. J., Pantelis, C. & Barnes, T. R. E. (1996). Homeless women: A prevalence study. *British Journal of Psychiatry*, (in press).

Balazs, J. (1993). Health care for the single homeless. In K. Fisher (ed.), *Homelessness, Health Care and Welfare Provision*, pp. 51–93. London: Routledge.

Connolly, J. & Crown, J. (eds.) (1994). *Homelessness and Ill Health. A report of a working party of the Royal College of Physicians*. London: RCP.

Connelly, J. & Williams, R. (1994). Schizophrenia among residents of hostels for homeless people. *British Medical Journal*, **308**, 1572 (letter).

Crossley, B. & Denmark, J. C. (1969). Community care – a study of the psychiatric morbidity of a Salvation Army hostel. *British Journal of Sociology*, **20**, 443–9.

Geddes, J., Newton, R., Bailey, S., Young, G., Freeman, C. & Priest, R. (1994a). Comparison of prevalence of schizophrenia among residents of hostels for homeless people in 1966 and 1992. *British Medical Journal*, **308**, 816–19.

Geddes, J., Bailey, S., Young, G., Freeman, C., Newton, R. & Priest, R. (1994b). Schizophrenia among residents of hostels for homeless people. *British Medical Journal*, **309**, 195 (letter).

Gunn, J. (1974). Prisons, shelters and homeless men. *Psychiatric Quarterly*, **48**, 505–12.

Herzberg, J. (1987). No fixed abode: a comparison of men and women admitted to an East London psychiatric hospital. *British Journal of Psychiatry*, **150**, 621–7.

Laidlaw, S. I. (1956). *Glasgow Common Lodging-houses and the People Living in Them*. Glasgow: Glasgow Corporation.

LCSS (London Council of Social Services) (1960). *Forgotten Men*. London: NCCS.

Leach, J. (1979). Providing for the destitute. In J. K. Wing & R. Olsen (eds.), *Community Care for the Mentally Disabled*, pp. 90–105. Oxford: Oxford University Press.

Leach, J. & Wing, J. K. (1978). The effectiveness of a service for helping destitute men. *British Journal of Psychiatry*, **113**, 481–92.

Leopoldt, H. & Lynch, B. (1981). Homeless men in Oxford. *Nursing Times*, **77**, 53–6.

Lodge Patch, I. C. (1971). Homeless men in London. 1. Demographic findings in a lodging house sample. *British Journal of Psychiatry*, **118**, 313–17.

Marshall, E. J. & Reed, J. L. (1992). Psychiatric morbidity in homeless women. *British Journal of Psychiatry*, **160**, 761–9.

Marshall, M. (1989). Collected and neglected: are Oxford hostels for the homeless filling up with disabled psychiatric patients? *British Medical Journal*, **299**, 706–9.

Marshall, M. & Gath, D. G. (1992). What happens to homeless mentally ill people? Follow up of residents of Oxford hostels for the homeless. *British Medical Journal*, **304**, 79–80.

Newton, J. R., Geddes, J. R., Bailey, S., Freeman, C. P., McAleavy, A. & Young, G. C. (1994). The mental health problems of the Edinburgh "roofless". *British Journal of Psychiatry*, **165**, 537–40.

Priest, R. G. (1971). The Edinburgh homeless. *American Journal of Psychotherapy*, **25**, 194–213.

Priest, R. G. (1976). The homeless person and the psychiatric services: an Edinburgh study. *British Journal of Psychiatry*, **10**, 233–5.

Reed, R., Ramsden, S., Marshall, J. *et al.* (1992). Psychiatric morbidity and substance abuse among residents of a cold weather shelter. *British Medical Journal*, **304**, 1028–9.

Scott, J. (1993). Homelessness and mental illness. *British Journal of Psychiatry*, **162**, 314–25.

Stark, C., Scott, J. & Hill, M. (1989). *A Survey of the Long-stay Uses of DSS Resettlement Units: A Research Report*. London: Department of Social Security.

Tidmarsh, D. & Wood, S. (1972). Psychiatric aspects of destitution. In
   J. K. Wing & A. M. Haley (eds.) *Evaluating a Community Psychiatry
   Service. The Camberwell Register, 1964–71*, pp. 328–40. Oxford: Oxford
   University Press.
Timms, P. W. & Fry, A. H. (1989). Homelessness and mental illness.
   Health Trends, **21**, 70–1.
Virgona, A., Buhrich, N. & Teesson, M. (1993). Prevalence of
   schizophrenia among women in refuges for the homeless. *Australian
   and New Zealand Journal of Psychiatry*, **27**, 405–10.
Wade, C. C. (1963). Survey of inmates of a common lodging house. *The
   Medical Officer*, **109**, 171–3.
Weller, M., Tobiansky, R. I., Hollander, D. & Ibrahimi, S. (1989).
   Psychosis and destitution at Christmas 1985–8. *Lancet*, **ii**, 1509–11.
Wood, S. M. (1976). Camberwell Reception Centre: a consideration of
   the need for health and social services of homeless single men.
   Journal of Social Policy, **5**, 389–99.

10

Old and homeless in London and New York City: a cross-national comparison

Carl I. Cohen and Maureen Crane

Introduction

Persons aged 50 and over are estimated to comprise about one fifth of the homeless in New York City (NYC) and nearly one third of the homeless in London (Weeden & Hall, 1985; Kelling, 1991). The proportion of those aged 50 and over living in substandard single-room occupancy (SRO) hotels or hostels may be even higher (Keigher, 1991). However, older homeless have been an unwanted stepchild of both the fields of homelessness and geriatrics. In contrast to the scholarly literature on younger homeless that has mushroomed in recent years, there have been relatively few papers written about ageing homeless (Cohen, 1996). On a service level, most senior citizen centres have shown little interest in this group, and public shelters have been typically avoided by older homeless persons because of fear of aggression by younger homeless, insensitive staff and accommodations that are not suitable for their physical disabilities (Coalition for the Homeless, 1984). Finally, governmental policy has failed to recognize the special needs of this ageing group, and even when statutory entitlements exist, many older homeless have not obtained such benefits (Kelling, 1991; Crane, 1993).

Although the absolute numbers of homeless persons in London are lower than in NYC, the former has the highest number of homeless persons among Western European cities (Adams, 1986; Toro & Rojansky, 1990; Schmidt, 1992). This commonality of large-scale homelessness in both cities creates an opportunity to undertake cross-national comparisons of ageing homeless. Such comparisons can provide answers to: (a) the proportionate contribution to the causes of homelessness of individual pathology and behaviour versus socio-political (structural) forces; (b) the effect of political, economic and cultural differences on creating policies for the solution of homelessness; (c) the ability of innovative, model programmes to successfully address the problems of the homeless, and the effect of broader structural forces on such programmes.

Definitions

What is 'old' among homeless persons?

For the most part, there has been a consensus in the literature that studies of 'older' homeless should include persons aged 50 and over (Gelberg *et al.*, 1990). This is because many of these persons at age 50 look and act like persons 10–20 years older in the general community. However, there are important differences between the 'younger' homeless (i.e. ages 50 to 60 or 65) and the 'older' homeless (i.e. ages 65 and over). The latter, especially in the USA, are entitled to considerably more social and health benefits, and this may have important implications for their well-being.

What is homelessness?

The definition of homelessness in Britain and the USA has represented a compromise between social justice and social expediency (Hopper, 1991). Until about 1980, homelessness in the USA included persons living in marginal housing such as SRO hotels and low-cost boarding houses (Bogue, 1963; Wallace, 1968). With the dramatic expansion of homelessness that occurred after 1980, homelessness became more narrowly defined, sometimes to include only street persons but usually encompassing those persons living in public or private shelters (Federal Task Force on Homelessness and Severe Mental Illness, 1992). In Britain, a broader definition of homelessness is generally used that comprises persons in hostels, bed and breakfast hotels, squats and on the streets ('sleeping rough') (Gay, 1989; Gay & Greener, 1990). However, economic constraints have increasingly led many local councils in Britain to exclude all the above categories except street living from the definition of homelessness (Gay, 1989).

Because of some of these problems with definitions, precise comparisons of the number of homeless in London and NYC are difficult.

The number of homeless in NYC of all ages living on the streets or in public or private shelters is estimated to be 70 000–90 000 (New York State Coalition for the Homeless, 1989). Similarly, the number of homeless in London of all ages living in unfit housing stock, squats, bed and breakfast hotels, hostels and the streets is estimated to be 75 000 (Greve, 1991). O'Flaherty (1991) suggested that if we viewed shelters, hostels, hotels and squats all as measures that were defences against street living, then the number of persons living on the street is one point of comparability. It is estimated that there are 10 000 to 35 000 street persons in NYC and 1000 to 3000 street persons in London (New York State Coalition for the Homeless, 1989; Greve, 1991; Havesi, 1991). Therefore, based on estimates that 20% and 33% of homeless persons in NYC and London are aged 50 and over, respectively, then the absolute number of persons aged 50 and over living on the streets of NYC are roughly 2–21 times that of London.

Theoretical approach

A cross-national comparison provides an excellent laboratory for testing a general model of homelessness proposed by Susser *et al.* (1993), and its adaptations for use with older homeless populations (Cohen, 1996). This model theorizes that various background factors (e.g. gender, race, parental socio-economic status), disruptive events in youth and adulthood experiences (e.g. occupational history, physical and psychiatric status, deviant behaviour, social supports) may predispose persons to homelessness. These predisposing factors interact with structural forces such as housing and economic conditions. Finally, there may be immediate precipitating events that tip a person into homelessness. On becoming homeless, a person may quickly find housing, remain chronically homeless, or alternate between homelessness and domiciled status. A combination of individual and structural forces affect the ability of an individual to become successfully re-domiciled.

Methods for comparison

The paucity of data on older homeless persons in the USA and the UK makes comparisons difficult. Fortunately, there have been a few reasonably well-constructed studies of older persons in both cities that allowed for at least some provisional analyses. In NYC, three studies provided the data base. Two were studies by Cohen and colleagues: a study of 281 homeless men aged 50 and over living on the streets or in the flophouses of New York's Skid Row, 'The Bowery' (Cohen & Sokolovsky, 1989) and a study of 237 homeless women aged 50 and over living in shelters or on the streets (Cohen, 1996). For clarity, data from these two samples have been merged, except when gender differences warranted separation. The third NYC study was by Ladner (1992) and comprised 353 persons aged 60 or older living in 14 public shelters.

Data on London's homeless were derived from five investigators: a study of 130 men and women aged 60 and over living on the streets in London (Crane, 1993, 1994); a series of one-night surveys of 319 homeless persons, nearly all men, living in direct access hostels or on the streets who had a mean age of 49 years (Weller *et al.*, 1989); a study of 70 women with a mean age of 52 years living in two direct access hostels in inner London; a subsample of 58 male residents with a mean age of 59 years living in a direct access hostel near Waterloo Station; a subgroup of 55 men with a median age of 70 years living in a direct access hostel in the London Borough of Camden (Wake, 1991).

In addition, review articles of older homeless persons in the USA and the UK by Cohen (1996) and Kelling (1991), respectively, were used to supplement the data from the specific studies described above.

Comparison of individual characteristics of older New York City and London homeless populations

Demographics

Among younger homeless samples in both NYC and London, the proportion of women has been estimated at 10–25% (Bachrach, 1987; Scott, 1993). This proportion is probably similar among the older homeless in both cities, although in Crane's (1993) study of London's street homeless and in Ladner's (1992) study of public shelter clients the proportion of women was nearly one third.

There are dramatic differences in the racial composition of older homeless persons in NYC and London. In NYC, roughly half the ageing street and shelter homeless were non-white (Ladner, 1992; Cohen, 1996), whereas in London only about 1% of the ageing street homeless are non-white (Kelling, 1991; Crane, 1993). Minorities may be more prevalent in hostels; for example, Timms & Fry (1989) reported 12% of their sample were black. Most vulnerable older minorities double-up with friends or relatives, although some may be hidden amongst the shop doorways or clubs in the black community (Kelling, 1991). In London, the Irish were disproportionately represented among the older street homeless, comprising one quarter of the sample (Crane, 1993). In some London hostels, more than one third of older residents are Irish (Wake, 1991).

The percentage having never married was 36% in Cohen's (1996) studies in NYC and between 42 and 67% among London's older homeless (Timms & Fry, 1989; Marshall & Reed, 1992; Crane, 1993). In both cities, women had married more frequently than had men. Conversely, rates of divorce and separation were higher among NYC homeless persons (about one half in NYC versus one third in London); roughly one fifth to one quarter of the homeless in both cities were widows. By contrast, all groups differed from the general elderly population in NYC and London, among whom 7–11% never married, 3–5% were divorced or separated, 39–41% were widowed and 46–47% were currently married (Gurland et al., 1983).

Kelling's (1991) survey indicated that most older British homeless have a life-time history of low income. Marshall & Reed (1992) found that among London women in direct access hostels, 70% had held unskilled jobs as domestics or factory workers. About one sixth held white collar jobs (mostly clerical). Very similar occupational histories were found among older homeless in NYC (Martin, 1982; Cohen, 1996). Approximately three fifths had skilled or semi-skilled jobs, one fifth had unskilled jobs, and one fifth had white collar jobs (mostly women who were in clerical or sales jobs). Occupational histories among the homeless in both cities reflected the relatively lower educational levels found among the homeless (Cohen, 1996).

Disruptive experiences in youth

A number of investigators (Susser et al., 1993) have identified disruptive experiences in childhood and adolescence as predisposing to homelessness. Among NYC homeless (Ladner, 1992; Cohen, 1996), roughly 1 in 5 or 6 experienced disruptive events such as foster care or institutional living in their youth, and about two thirds were raised by both parents. Although there are no data regarding foster or institutional care among London's ageing homeless, Marshall & Reed (1992) reported that nearly one fifth of their sample had experienced significant separations from one or both parents and 16% reported an alcoholic parent.

Deviant behaviour

It is difficult to gauge the meaning of criminal arrests among ageing homeless persons because many were arrested for loitering, vagrancy, public intoxication and the like. There were considerable similarities in history of incarceration between the two cities. In NYC, history of arrests were 49% and 15% for men and women, respectively (Cohen, 1996). In London, arrest rates were 52% for men in Weller *et al.*'s (1989) one-night surveys between 1985 and 1988 and 30% for women in direct access hostels (Marshall & Reed, 1992).

Alcohol abuse was a common problem among the homeless in both cities, with rates among older men being considerably higher than among older women. Currently, about two fifths of the men in Cohen's study in NYC and Crane's (1993) study in London were problem drinkers. A survey of older residents at Arlington House (Wake, 1991), a large direct access hostel for men, found one third were heavily 'dependent' on alcohol. However, Timms & Fry (1989) found only 3% of older direct access hostel residents to be clinically diagnosable as alcohol-dependent. Among homeless women the prevalence rate was 8% in NYC (Cohen, 1996) and 0–16% in various London sites (Marshall & Reed, 1992; Crane, 1993). However, in both cities, as many as one third of women may have life-time histories of alcoholism (Marshall & Reed, 1992; Cohen, 1996). History of substance abuse was less than 5% in both cities (Ladner, 1992; Marshall & Reed, 1992; Cohen, 1996).

Mental health

Mental illness has been identified as a major contributory factor to homelessness in both the USA and Britain. Between 20% and 70% of London's older homeless have been found to have active psychotic symptoms, 'thought disturbances', a diagnosis of schizophrenia, or prior psychiatric history (Timms & Fry, 1989; Weller *et al.*, 1989;

Marshall & Reed, 1992; Crane, 1994). Rates for women were about twice that of men. These figures were remarkably similar to those of NYC's ageing homeless. For example, Cohen (1996) found 54% of women and 23% of men exhibited psychiatric symptoms or had prior psychiatric hospitalization; and among shelter residents aged 50 and over, Crystal (1984) found 27% of women and 12% of men had prior psychiatric hospitalization.

Prevalence of depression was also very high in both cities. Two fifths of London's elderly street homeless and one third of NYC's older street and shelter homeless reported substantial levels of depressive symptoms (Crane, 1994; Cohen, 1996). This widespread despair was illustrated by the fact that 30% of NYC's older homeless agreed that 'life was not worth living'. Whether these symptoms correspond to actual clinical diagnosis is unclear. For example, the prevalence of diagnosable affective disorders was less than 2% among London's older hostel dwellers (Timms & Fry, 1989; Marshall & Reed, 1992).

Levels of cognitive deficits differed between the two cities. Moderate or severe cognitive disturbance was found in 39% of London's street homeless (Crane, 1994), approximately half of whom were judged to have severe problems. However, fewer than 4% of older hostel dwellers had clinical diagnoses of organicity and dementia (Timms & Fry, 1989; Marshall & Reed, 1992). In NYC, 9% of street, shelter, or flophouse dwellers had moderate or severe deficits, and one third of these were judged to be severe (Cohen, 1996).

Physical health

In both cities, the ageing homeless were thought to have impaired physical health. Many suffered from the so-called 'Skid Row Syndrome' of respiratory disease, gastro-intestinal disease, hypertension, seizures and physical trauma (Feldman *et al.*, 1974; Ashley *et al.*, 1976; Timms & Fry, 1989). Among London's street homeless (Crane, 1993), 17% of the sample had mobility problems whereas 30% of the NYC street and shelter sample (Cohen, 1996) had ambulatory difficulties. Weller *et al.* (1989) reported that two fifths of London's homeless persons required medical treatment. Many London hostels housed very impaired older persons. For example, one hostel reported (Wake, 1991) that one fifth of its tenants were unable to walk three to four steps without help or were dependent on a wheelchair, and two fifths had difficulty with stairs.

NYC homeless had twice the prevalence of somatic symptoms as a community sample of elderly (Gurland *et al.*, 1983; Cohen, 1996). Ladner (1992) reported that nearly three fifths of older shelter residents had current medical problems. Interestingly, ability to perform daily activities was only slightly worse among the NYC older homeless versus an elderly community sample (Gurland *et al.*, 1983), and actually substantially better than a sample of elderly living in SRO hotels (Cohen *et al.*, 1988).

Although by law persons cannot be rejected by general practitioners (GPs) in Britain because they are homeless, surveys have found that one fifth of older homeless persons reported such rejections (Kelling, 1991), and Weller *et al.* (1989) found half of the ageing homeless did not have a GP. Consequently, some older persons have been compelled to seek medical care at emergency rooms and hospitals, where discharge plans are often poorly arranged. This resembles findings in NYC, in which most homeless use public clinics and emergency rooms. Despite these problems, 83% of NYC older homeless persons had seen a physician in the past year, and half of these persons had seen a physician in the past month; rates of hospitalization were very high, with 32% reporting at least one hospitalization in the past year (Cohen & Sokolovsky, 1989). In the mid-1960s, Scott *et al.* (1966) reported that London's Skid Row men were 'high consumers of hospital outpatient services'. This pattern of health care utilization seemingly has persisted in both London and NYC to the present day.

Social networks

There were marked differences between Londoners and New Yorkers in the percentage of persons having and seeing children and other relatives. Of the older London street homeless, 34% had children but none had contact with them; 31% had living siblings or other relatives, but only 3% of the sample were in contact with them (Crane, 1993). Weller *et al.* (1989) found that roughly half of their homeless sample reported no friends, and Marshall & Reed (1992) found that only 14% of their hostel-dwelling women were in regular contact with friends or family. Two thirds had no social contacts other than with hostel staff. By contrast, 55% of the NYC homeless had children and 81% had living siblings; three fifths of the NYC homeless sample had contact with at least one child or relative

(Cohen, 1996). Moreover, older NYC homeless men and women had mean social networks of 8.5 and 11.4 persons, respectively.

Patterns and pathways of homelessness

There was little evidence in either NYC or London that older homeless persons were largely dischargees from institutions. Fewer than 12% had been in institutions prior to becoming homeless (Marshall & Reed, 1992; Crane, 1993; Cohen, 1996). Among those in shelters or streets in NYC and London (Crane, 1993; Cohen, 1996) about two thirds had reported living in apartments or houses and about one quarter had been living in SRO hotels, hostels, or boarding homes prior to becoming homeless. In NYC, half reported living independently and two fifths said they had been living with family or friends (Ladner, 1992; Cohen, 1996).

Although many persons stated that they had drifted into homelessness, in some instances the first episode of homelessness was triggered by a specific event. The factors identified by self-report as more immediate causes of homelessness were similar in NYC and London (Ladner, 1992; Crane, 1993; Cohen, 1996): (a) financial, e.g. loss of welfare support when children or grandchildren moved, rent raised, loss of work; (b) breakdown of relationships due to death of spouse or kin, conflict, or abuse; (c) eviction, sale of property, fire, or unsafe conditions; (d) dissatisfaction with residence. Observations by researchers in both cities suggested that alcoholism and mental health problems such as paranoid ideation also appeared to contribute to creating homelessness (Marshall & Reed, 1992; Crane, 1993, 1994; Cohen, 1996). On the basis of a variety of factors such as life-style, family support and availability of public welfare, women are much less apt to become homeless (Marin, 1991). Moreover, in NYC, (Cohen, 1996), there was approximately a 10 year gap in the age that women first became homeless (early fifties) versus men (early forties).

Those older persons in both cities who lived in the lowest level of accommodations such as hostels or flophouses were able to develop a greater level of stability than those in shelters or streets. For example, the median length of time in flophouses or hostels was 2 years whereas women in NYC shelters had a median length of stay of 4 months (Marshall & Reed, 1992; Cohen, 1996). Among the older women in NYC shelters, three common patterns were discerned: (a) prolonged homelessness of 2 or more years (37%); (b) usually domiciled except for a recent relatively brief episode (30%); (c) alternating between homelessness and being domiciled (32%).

A 2 year follow-up study (Cohen, 1996) of these women indicated that of 13 variables examined only 2 – psychoses and a prior history of homelessness of 1 or more years – were significant predictors of remaining homeless. On follow-up, only 40% of women were re-domiciled. The data pointed to the inadequate level of low-cost housing options for older homeless women, especially for those with severe mental illness.

Structural factors and homelessness among older persons

In turning to social (i.e. structural) factors, we find that despite re-trenchment over the past decade, the British system provides indigent persons over 60 and those with disabilities levels of income that exceed the official poverty level of £57 (note: £1 = $1.50) per week for a single person (Piachaud, 1992). The poverty level is calculated as half the average national income after housing costs. The basic weekly income benefits are £42.45 and £59.15 for indigent persons aged 59 and under and 60 and over, respectively (Camden Welfare Rights Unit, 1992), which is equivalent to monthly benefits of £183.95 ($275.93) and £256.22 ($384.48), respectively. Additional benefits are available for physical or mental disabilities that can bring weekly benefits to over £100. Importantly, housing benefits are also provided on a sliding scale to all persons with savings of less than £16 000, who are in rented accommodation where the rent has been set at a fair market rate.

By contrast, levels of support for indigent Americans are much lower. In NYC, which provides some of the most generous levels of support in the country, indigent persons under 65 receive $358 per month (approx. £239) for housing and general support, plus $111 (£74) in food stamps. For those persons 65 and over or for those with serious mental or physical disabilities, the level of income support is $520 (£347) per month plus $111 (£74) in food stamps. The poverty level for a single person is $580 (£387) per month (Tiadail, 1992), meaning that most needy New Yorkers receive supports below the poverty level.

A second structural factor that may reduce the absolute number of homeless in London is the greater availability of extremely low-cost housing in London versus NYC. While there has been a loss of roughly 8000 direct access (emergency) hostel bed spaces between 1983 and 1987 (Crane, 1990), there has also been an increase in smaller and special needs hostels, that have offset many of the losses (Gay & Greener, 1990). There are now 18 000 hostel spaces in London (Gay & Greener, 1990). Moreover, London continues to have approximately 25 000 spaces in bed and breakfast hotels, of which one quarter are occupied by single persons (Gay & Greener, 1990). By contrast, in NYC the number of SRO hotel units decreased from 127 000 to 14 000 between 1970 and 1985 (Interagency Council on the Homeless, 1991).

Both cities have experienced a decline in low-cost housing stock generated by conversions of rentals to private ownership, the absence of government support for public rental housing, and the competition for living space in the central city as these sections were transformed from manufacturing to service centres (Adams, 1986; Hopper, 1988; Greve, 1991). However, despite these common trends, London has a much greater supply of public (council) housing than does NYC, although both cities now have substantial waiting lists. NYC has 190 000 units in public housing and a waiting list of 200 000 applicants (Marcuse, 1990). London has 742 000 council units and a waiting list of 306 000 applicants (Department of Environment, 1993; Greve, 1991). About two thirds of all new council lettings in London now go to homeless applicants. While there are differences between council housing in London and public housing in NYC – the former is often used by the middle class whereas the latter is exclusively for the poor – London does have more opportunities for affordable low-cost housing. Importantly, in Britain, the Housing Act of 1985 stipulates that certain groups, including the elderly and those with mental or physical disabilities, have priority for permanent accommodation (Gay, 1989). By contrast, there are no statutory provisions for permanent housing in NYC, and local authorities have been under judicial decree to provide emergency shelter.

Because the safety net is stronger in Britain for individuals as well as their families, there is a tendency for families to provide shelter through doubling-up and the like. In NYC, families often have less public support, and when coupled with drug problems and other family strains, older persons, particularly minorities, may not be housed by children or other relatives. However, older NYC women generally remain in contact with the family, even if they are living in a shelter. In Britain, on the other hand, because separation from the family is rare, when it occurs, it usually reflects a severe rift, sometimes triggered by an older person's psychopathology. Consequently, the older homeless in London report few contacts with kin and many years of isolation.

There are several structural factors that affected older British and American homeless alike (Hopper, 1988; Greve, 1991). Both Britain and the USA experienced economic downturns in the early 1980s. Accompanying this recession was the permanent loss of manufacturing jobs as London and NYC shifted increasingly to service economies. Many persons, especially those who were older and blue collar workers, were unable to re-enter the workforce during the economic recovery that ensued.

Secondly, both Britain and the USA have undergone large-scale release of patients from psychiatric hospitals, although the pace in Britain has lagged behind that of the USA. Thus, there was an 80% drop of psychiatric inpatients in the USA between 1955 and 1990, whereas the British experienced a 60% decrease over the same time period (Murphy, 1991). In both countries many older inpatients were 'trans-institutionalized' into nursing homes, although this practice has been curtailed in both countries. In Britain, for example, more older inpatients are being discharged to residential care programmes (Murphy, 1991). Nevertheless in both countries, there is an inadequate array and supply of residential treatment programmes that cater to older adults (Lipmann, 1995).

A third important structural factor concerns access to benefits, health care and housing. Thus, whereas all Britons aged 60 and over are legally entitled to sufficient income to live above the poverty level, to health and psychiatric care under the National Health Service and to priority placement for permanent housing, there is evidence that the poorest segments of the elderly population do not always receive these benefits. For example, with respect to housing, local authorities had varying interpretations of age vulnerability; they often considered any 'reasonable' offer of permanent housing to fulfill their obligations; interpretations of homelessness differed with only 30–40% of authorities considering persons in bed and breakfast hotels or hostels as homeless; and many authorities were often insensitive to older persons and perceived them as 'lost causes' (Gay, 1989; Kelling, 1991). Weller *et al.*'s (1989) survey found that one fifth of ageing London homeless persons were receiving no benefits at all.

Similarly, with respect to health care, homeless persons may be discouraged from registering with a GP because they are incorrectly told that they need a permanent address (Primary Care for Homeless Team, 1991). As GPs are now assuming management of their budgets, they may be even more reluctant to register persons with complex needs. Not registering with the GP means that homeless persons are denied access to medical specialty service, district nursing, psychiatric care, health visiting services and other community services (Kelling, 1991, 1992). Advocates for the homeless have contended that many of the increased health problems found among homeless persons and families such as high levels of tuberculosis, gastro-intestinal disturbances and low immunization levels – conditions that resemble those found among the homeless in the USA – are related to the shortcomings of primary care (Access to Health, n.d.). Finally, access to benefits are often impeded by local authorities or by the central government. For example, persons with mental illness frequently have difficulty obtaining additional disability payments, allowances to establish independent housing, or crisis loans. Many persons, especially the elderly, are unaware of their statutory rights (Crane, 1993).

Homeless persons in NYC have fewer statutory entitlements than those in London, and what is potentially available is often not obtained. Although virtually all older homeless persons in NYC are entitled to Medicaid, nearly three fifths were not receiving this benefit. Similarly, despite eligibility, fewer than one third were receiving food stamps, and between 40 and 50% were not receiving supplemental social security or public assistance (Ladner, 1992; Cohen, 1996). Thus, for example, a recent survey found that fewer than half of single shelter residents have any form of public assistance or social security disability despite virtually all being eligible (New York City Commission on the Homeless, 1992). What is evident in both countries is that in times of shortage and economic retrenchment, there is little incentive to encourage applications for entitlements. Thus, bureaucratic conspiracy or indifference coupled with ignorance about benefits have worked to exclude certain segments of the population from benefits.

Towards a causal model of ageing and homelessness

When the cross-national comparison of ageing homeless persons presented here is tested within the theoretical model outlined at the beginning of the chapter, our comparison validates the model's assumption that certain individual factors are associated with homelessness. As summarized in Table 10.1, in contrast to older persons in the general population, older homeless persons in both countries have considerably higher levels of social, psychiatric and physical problems. To what extent these factors predispose to homelessness and/or are risk factors for remaining homeless is unclear. Also, some of these factors (e.g. depression, diminished social contacts) may be by-products of being homeless. It is evident from our analysis that older homeless persons in both cities are remarkably similar. Nevertheless, the prevalence of homelessness among the ageing is substantially lower in London. Thus, we believe that the differences in prevalence can be best explained by the structural forces, particularly the housing and economic variables, described in the second half of this chapter. Moreover, the cross-national comparison suggests that systemic forces are much more potent than individual factors in determining the extent of homelessness, although individual factors may have more of a role in shaping qualitative features (i.e. patterns) of the ageing homeless population. However, the latter still represents an interplay between systemic and individual elements.

Solutions

On a broader societal level, there are important differences in how the British and Americans must approach the problem of ageing homeless. In Britain, in theory there are a variety of statutory social programmes that should provide adequate income support, health care and housing. There are less firm supports for psychiatric aftercare, but this has begun to be addressed under the new legislation (Murphy, 1991). In the USA, considerably less statutory support is available to older persons – especially for those between the ages of 50 and 64 – and what is available may not be easily accessed. Thus, we

Table 10.1. *Older homeless and community samples in New York City and London: individual characteristics*

	London homeless	New York City homeless	New York City and London community[a]
Physical disorders	+ + +	+ + +	+
Activity limitations	NA	+ +	+ +
Psychosis/prior psychiatric hospitalization[b]	+ + +	+ + +	+
Depression	+ + +	+ + +	+
Cognitive deficits (moderate/severe)	+ / + + +[d]	+	+
Low social contacts	+ + +	+ +	+
Marital status			
Never married	+ + +	+ +	+
Divorced/Separated	+ +	+ + +	+
Widowed	+	+	+ + +
Never had children	+ + +	+ +	+
Alcohol use[c]	+ +	+ + +	+
Poor grooming/ hygiene[c]	+ + +	+ + +	+
Low skilled occupations	+ + +	+ + +	+
Racial minorities	+	+ + +	+ +
Disruptive youth	+ +	+ +	+
History of imprisonment	+ + +	+ + +	+

Note: For each variable, the lowest score is given a value of (+) and the other scores are approximate multiples of this baseline score.
[a] Gurland *et al.* (1983).
[b] Women > men.
[c] Men > women.
[d] Street homeless.

find in the USA, those between 50 and 64 years of age have prevalence rates of homelessness that are proportional to their representation in the general population (12%), whereas those over 65 have disproportionately low rates of homelessness, i.e. 3% homeless versus 12% in the general population (Cohen, 1996). Therefore, in Britain, a significant component of the solution must entail linking older homeless persons with organizations who can advocate on their behalf. In the USA, while case advocacy is likewise necessary, efforts must be directed to obtaining more statutory benefits and supports for older persons, especially for those between the ages of 50 and 64.

In Britain, there seems to be substantially fewer emergency shelters and drop-in centres for older persons than in the USA, especially those that cater for women (Kelling, 1991; Crane, 1993). A number of such drop-in/social centres have arisen in NYC and other large American cities. While there is a general consensus that these centres should be age-segregated, there is less consensus about whether there should be separate programmes for the mentally ill. Our data from a service programme for seniors in NYC indicate that a generic, age-segregated programme can be successful in attracting those persons with serious mental illness (Cohen *et al.*, 1993). This programme, which revolves around a senior lunch programme, is open to all persons aged 60 and over. Situated one block from the Bowery, it attracts many indigent elderly, about one third of whom have serious mental illness. Once engaged in the programme, those with mental illness are sometimes willing to seek additional treatment. However, even among those who do not want specialized services, their quality of life and well-being have been enhanced by the regular meals, free clothing, assistance with entitlements and housing, and by the socialization that they have received.

Although one must be mindful of respecting civil rights, mobile units of the type used by Project Help in NYC (Cohen & Sullivan, 1990) to involuntarily hospitalize persons may be useful for certain segments of London's older homeless population, such as persons with moderate or severe organic mental syndromes. These persons' cognitive deficits usually render them incapable of making informed decisions about their well-being, and placement in a more supportive environment is warranted.

Finally, we have no evidence that most older homeless persons whether mentally ill or not, prefer to live on the streets rather than in safe accommodation. A range of housing options are needed in both countries. Some of those with mental illness are fearful of being segregated with other psychiatric cases. Nearly half of London's elderly street persons had lived in hostels, but they had found them too noisy, too restrictive, too violent and lacking in privacy (Crane, 1993). However, nearly two fifths of London's elderly street homeless expressed a desire to have a room in a home with others, and one third wanted an independent flat or room. For older women already living in hostels, Marshall & Reed (1992) found that among those expressing residential preferences, nearly half wanted their 'own place' and about one third would be content to remain in the hostel if they could have more privacy. These desires were not dissimilar to those of NYC's homeless (Cohen & Sokolovsky, 1989; Cohen, 1996). For example, among older homeless women offered placement from a shelter, fear of new neighbours or residents, financial concerns and distance from familiar neighbourhoods were cited as the principal reasons for not accepting the placement. Likewise, older Skid Row men were willing to accept apartment programmes that were relatively close to their former neighbourhoods, convenient to shopping and that afforded independence and security.

Summary

A comparison of older homeless in London and NYC indicated the following:

1. Although personal biography and traits contribute to individual homelessness, structural forces largely determine the extent of homelessness and, to a lesser degree, the patterns of homelessness.
2. Statutory regulations are necessary but not sufficient to provide housing and income support to older persons. In difficult economic periods, governments may discourage persons from seeking assistance, and strong advocacy is required to secure entitlements.
3. Most older homeless persons in both cities do not prefer to live on streets or in shelters. However, any housing scheme must recognize the desire for independence expressed by many older homeless persons as well as the high levels of physical and mental illness – both psychoses and cognitive disorders – that may necessitate more intensive supervision and care. Thus, any solution must entail a suitable mix of age-segregated, safe and supportive housing programmes.

Acknowledgements

The authors greatly appreciate the assistance of Heather Petch, Mary Carter, Jay Sokolovsky, John Mason, Kim Hopper, Frank Lipton, Diane Sonde, Ellen Baxter, Eric Roth, Eugene Feigelson and Carole Lefkowitz. This work was supported in part by NIMH Center for Mental Disorders Branch grant no. RO1-MH45780.

References

Access to Health (n.d.) *Health Problems of Homeless People*. London: Access to Health.

Adams, C. A. (1986). Homelessness in the postindustrial city. *Urban Affairs Quarterly*, **21**, 527–49.

Ashley, M. J., Olin, J. S., le Riche, W. H., Kornaczewski, A., Schmidt, W. & Rankin, J. G. (1976). Skid row alcoholism: a distinct sociomedical entity. *Archives of Internal Medicine*, **136**, 272–8.

Bachrach, L. (1987). Homeless women: a context for health planning. *The Milbank Quarterly*, **65**, 371–96.

Bogue, D. J. (1963). *Skid Row in American Cities*. Chicago: University of Chicago Press.

Camden Welfare Rights Unit (1992). *Report on the Benefits and Mental Health Project*. London: Corporate Services.

Coalition for the Homeless (1984). *Crowded Out: Homelessness and the Elderly Poor*. New York: Coalition for the Homeless.

Cohen, C. I. (1996). The elderly homeless: a conceptual model. In P. Szwabo & G. T. Grossberg (eds.), *Psychosocial Needs of Special Populations of the Elderly*, (in press).

Cohen, C. I. & Sokolovsky, J. (1989). *Old Men of the Bowery*. New York: Guilford.

Cohen, N. L. & Sullivan, A. M. (1990). Strategies of intervention and service coordination by mobile outreach teams. In N. L. Cohen (ed.), *Psychiatry Takes to the Streets*, pp. 63–79. New York: Guilford Press.

Cohen, C. I., Onserud, H. & Monaco, C. (1993). Outcomes for the mentally ill in a program for older homeless persons. *Hospital and Community Psychiatry*, **44**, 650–6.

Cohen, C. I., Sokolovsky, J., Teresi, J. & Holmes, D. (1988). Gender, networks, and adaptation among an inner-city population. *Journal of Aging Studies*, **2**, 45–56.

Crane, M. (1990). *Elderly Homeless People in Central London*. London: Age Concern England and Age Concern Greater London.

Crane, M. (1993). *Elderly Homeless People Sleeping on the Streets in Inner London: An Exploratory Study*. London: Age Concern Institute of Gerontology.

Crane, M. (1994). The mental health problems of elderly people living on London's streets. *International Journal of Geriatric Psychiatry*, **9**, 87–95.

Crystal, S. (1984). Homeless men and homeless women: the gender gap. *Urban Social Change Review*, **17**, 2–6.

Department of Environment (1993). *Quarterly Statistics*. December, 1993. London: HMSO.

Federal Task Force on Homelessness and Severe Mental Illness (1992). *Outcasts on Main Street*. Washington, DC: Interagency Council on the Homeless.

168   C. I. COHEN AND M. CRANE

Feldman, J., Su, W. H., Kaley, M. & Kissin, B. (1974). Skid row
and inner-city alcoholics. A comparison of drinking patterns
and medical problems. *Quarterly Journal of Studies on Alcohol*, **35**,
565–76.

Gay, O. (1989). *Homeless*. Background Paper No. 229. London: House of
Commons Library Research Division, 4 July 1989.

Gay, O. & Greener, K. (1990). *The young single homeless*. Background
Paper No. 242. London: House of Commons Library Research
Division, 9 March 1990.

Gelberg, L., Linn, L. S. & Mayer-Oakes, S. A. (1990). Differences in
health status between older and younger homeless adults. *Journal of
the American Geriatrics Society*, **38**, 1220–9.

Greve, J. (1991). *Homelessness in Britain*. York: Joseph Rowentree
Foundation.

Gurland, B., Copeland, J., Kuriansky, J., Kelleher, M., Sharpe, L. &
Dean, L. L. (1983). *The Mind and Mood of Aging*. New York:
Haworth Press.

Havesi, D. (1991). Census count of homeless is disputed. *New York
Times*, 13 April, p. 26.

Hopper, K. (1988). More than passing strange: homelessness and mental
illness in New York City. *American Ethnologist*, **15**, 155–67.

Hopper, K. (1991). Homelessness old and new: the matter of definition.
Housing Policy Debate, **2**, 757–813.

Interagency Council on the Homeless (1991). *Executive Summary. The 1990
Annual Report*. Washington, DC: Interagency Council on the
Homeless.

Keigher, S. M. (ed.) (1991). *Housing Risks and Homelessness Among the
Urban Elderly*. New York: Haworth Press.

Kelling, K. (1991). *Older Homeless People in London*. London: Age
Concern.

Kelling, K. (1992). Meeting the health needs of older homeless people.
Health Visitor, **10**, 346–7.

Ladner, S. (1992). The elderly homeless. In M. J. Robertson & M.
Greenblatt (eds), *Homelessness: A National Perspective*, pp. 221–6. New
York: Plenum Press.

Lipmann, B. (1995). *The Elderly Homeless*. Williamstown, Australia:
Wintringham Hostels.

Marcuse, P. (1990). Homelessness and housing policy. In C. L. M.
Caton (ed.), *Homeless in America*, pp. 138–59. New York: Oxford
University Press.

Marin, P. (1991). Why are the homeless mainly single men. *The Nation*,
253, 46–51.

Marshall, E. J. & Reed, J. T. (1992). Psychiatric morbidity in homeless
women. *British Journal of Psychiatry*, **160**, 761–8.

Martin, M. A. (1982). Strategies of Adaptation: Coping Patterns of the
Urban Transient Female. PhD thesis, Columbia University, NY.

Murphy, E. (1991). *After the Asylums*. London: Faber and Faber.

New York City Commission on the Homeless (1992). *The Way Home. A New Direction in Social Policy*. New York: Office of the Mayor.

New York State Coalition for the Homeless (1989). *One Hundred Thousand, and counting ... Homelessness in New York State*. Albany, NY: New York State Coalition for the Homeless.

O'Flaherty, B. (1991). What's homelessness? Comparing New York and London. Paper presented at the 13th Annual Conference of the Association for Public Policy Analysis and Management, Bethesda, MD, 24–26 October.

Piachaud, D. (1992). Hopes that turned to dust. *The Guardian*, 30 September, p. 21.

Primary Care for Homeless People Team (1991). *Annual Report 1991*. London: Camden & Islington Family Health Services Authority.

Schmidt, W. E. (1992). Across Europe, face of homeless become more visible and vexing. *New York Times*, 5 January, pp. 1, 8.

Scott, J. (1993). Homelessness and mental illness. *British Journal of Psychiatry*, **162**, 314–24.

Scott, R., Gaskell, P. G. & Morrell, D. C. (1966). Patients who reside in common lodging houses. *British Medical Journal*, **2**, 1561–4.

Susser, E., Moore, R. & Link, B. (1993). Risk factors for homelessness. *American Journal of Epidemiology*, **15**, 546–56.

Tiadail, S. (1992). U.S. poor get poorer. *The Guardian*, 5 September, p. 9.

Timms, P. W. & Fry, A. H. (1989). Homelessness and mental illness. *Health Trends*, **21**, 70–1.

Toro, P. & Rojansky, A. (1990). Homelessness: some thoughts from an international perspective. *Community Psychologist*, **24**, 8–11.

Wallace, S. E. (1968). The road to skid row. *Social Problems*, **16**, 92–105.

Wake, M. (ed.) (1991). *Housing and Care Needs of Older Homeless People*. London: Arlington House.

Weeden, J. & Hall, C. (1985). *The Homeless Mentally Ill Elderly*. University of California, S.E.: Institute for Health and Aging.

Weller, M., Tobiansky, R., Hollander, D. & Ibrahami, S. (1989). Psychosis and destitution at Christmas 1985–88. *Lancet*, **ii**, 1509–11.

11

Primary health care of the single homeless

DAVID EL-KABIR AND SIMON RAMSDEN

To write about the primary care of the single homeless suggests that there are particular factors in that population that are in some way different to the general population, and that these influence care. It is important to understand these factors if we are to look at primary care in this setting. To start with, who exactly do we mean and can we define the population? This is far from straightforward but definitions should include inadequate accommodation and some degree of disaffiliation from society. 'Single' homeless usually means those who are unmarried or divorced and without close supportive relationships, but occasionally married couples are seen within groups considered to be single homeless. In this chapter, we will look at the care of a wide and disparate population, living on the streets, in hostels, night shelters and bed and breakfast accommodation, as well as those in more permanent accommodation but who have previously had more tenuous accommodation.

A morbidity profile

A number of studies have described the physical and psychiatric morbidity of a variety of single homeless populations. In terms of physical health, frequent infectious, respiratory and skin diseases and infestations are usually described, along with trauma (Hewetson, 1975; Powell, 1987; Shanks, 1988). Within this perhaps obvious pattern are more serious diseases, less prevalent in the general population. Tuberculosis is the best known (Patel, 1985) although others such as epilepsy are found more frequently than expected. Over 50% of hostel populations are usually found to suffer from a

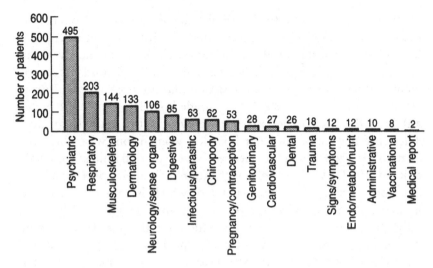

Figure 11.1. Presenting problems of new patients. Note that 40% of new patients presented with psychiatric problems.

chronic disease (Scott *et al.*, 1966). Studies of psychiatric disorders show wide variations, schizophrenia is common and its prevalence has been estimated in one study as over 40% (Weller *et al.*, 1989). Personality disorder, a term not usually defined precisely, has been described at up to 50% in some studies (Lodge Patch, 1971). Major affective disorders are often found to be more common than expected. Alcoholism is common, as is drug abuse, and often co-exists with severe psychiatric or physical illness. Figure 11.1 shows the morbidity pattern of presenting patients at our medical centre in 1992–1993, and is typical of that recorded amongst homeless populations.

The variation in morbidity patterns reported in various studies is wide, and in large part reflects the different settings in which the studies were conducted. This has important implications as the single homeless are often erroneously thought to be an essentially homogeneous group by politicians and health planners. The studies showing a high prevalence of schizophrenia, usually with much lower levels of alcohol abuse, have generally been conducted in hostels or in ill-defined groups such as those attending the Crisis at Christmas emergency shelter. Street dwellers are more difficult to assess, but in our study of those staying at a cold weather shelter in London at a time of deep snow, the pattern was predominantly that of alcohol abuse (over 60%) and only 9% were defined as definitely or probably psychotic (Reed *et al.*, 1992). Whilst the shelter stayed open, the number of alcoholics fell rapidly due to aggressive and disruptive behaviour, whilst the number of schizophrenics rose as they were far easier to cope with. Studies of young homeless people find less severe mental illness but high levels of anxiety, family problems and drug abuse. Overall, around 80–90% of single homeless people are male, although the sex balance is far more even in the younger groups. There are few studies of older homeless women, but what data are available suggest a high prevalence of severe mental illness (Marshall & Reed, 1992). A number of classifications of homelessness have been described, perhaps the most useful of which is that of Fischer & Breakey (1986). They recognized four groups: the chronically mentally ill, alcohol abusers, the situationally distressed and street dwellers. These groups vary in terms of morbidity, age structure and life-styles. The young (age < 20 years) are more likely to suffer situational distress, the chronically mentally ill are more likely to reside in hostels as described, and alcohol abusers on the streets, and both of these groups tend to be older. One way to look at the morbidity patterns is to distinguish between those illnesses that are a consequence of homelessness, and those which may result in homelessness. Surprisingly, the pathways of social, psychological and medical problems underlying homelessness have received little attention as yet. There is some evidence that schizophrenia precedes the onset of homelessness, and that the mental, family and social deterioration that the illness causes underlies the subsequent homelessness (Tidmarsh & Woods, 1972). Similar evidence is available for homeless people who abuse alcohol (Myerson & Mayer, 1966), and recently it has been suggested that the social and psychiatric problems that are more common in children with epilepsy predisposes to subsequent homelessness, explaining to an extent the excess of this condition seen among the homeless (Ramsden, 1994). It has been considered that many of those who previously were in long-stay psychiatric hospitals would subsequently become homeless although in contrast to the USA, there is little evidence as yet that this is the case (Geddes *et al.*, 1994). Tuberculosis in this context is a result of homelessness: one hostel study from the USA showed that the likelihood of a positive tuberculin test increased with the duration of stay at the hostel (McAdam *et al.*, 1985).

A demographic and psycho-social profile

Reference has already been made to the diversity of the population, and to some extent the demographic and psycho-social profile reflects this. However, there are common strands. As mentioned most are male. The age distribution is wide. In terms of place of origin, there is a preponderance of people from the north of England, Scotland and Ireland. Most are white, though increasingly people from ethnic minorities are being seen. In particular, among the younger homeless, many come from institutional care and many from broken homes. Educational achievement is usually low and many have not sustained prolonged periods of employment. Many have prison records, although often for petty or drink-related offences. Few have close relationships and many describe intense social isolation. The picture that emerges is of individuals who have multiple medical and social handicaps, often beginning early in life, and who are isolated and disaffiliated from society.

Factors underlying presentation to medical services

The decision to consult a doctor is for most people a complex decision based on an assessment of symptoms, their perceived significance and the likely effect of consultation, as well as family and peer advice and pressure. Similar factors affect the decision to seek medical advice amongst homeless people, although other pressures, such as the need to find shelter, food and, for some, alcohol may take priority. We often see people who have ignored illnesses until they are advanced, for example severe leg ulceration, cellulitis or tuberculosis. Some have argued that the principal barrier is that doctors discourage the homeless and discriminate against them. However, in practices that are freely available and perceived as such, patients often still delay seeking advice. Projects that have tried to ensure that the patients are registered on general practitioners' lists find, contrary to received dogma, that the patients often fail to consult or follow-up, and that little difference has been made to those the project aimed to help (Editorial, 1989; Williams & Allen, 1989). The reasons underlying this are that whilst some of the external barriers to consultation have been addressed, the internal barriers particularly emotional ones are ignored. Many patients express guilt at their circumstances and life-style, and others an expectation that they will be unwell. Some find sitting in waiting rooms with patients who are not homeless threatening and humiliating. Nonetheless illness is frequent and may necessitate consulting a doctor. 'Flu' or leg ulcers or injuries may make coping with the demands of homelessness difficult, and other symptoms such as cough or abdominal pain may be understood as evidence of a life-threatening disease, that the individual feels is the result and perhaps desserts of social failure and homelessness.

Aspects of the consultation

This emotional baggage is necessarily evident when homeless people consult with doctors. In many ways the consultation is the doctor's moment of truth where his authenticity, humanity, understanding, knowledge and intentions are put to the test. Much has been written about various aspects of it, particularly by Balint (1964) and Pendleton et al. (1982), but the particular needs of homeless patients necessitate a very much broader view of its nature, dynamics and possibilities. In conventional circumstances, the role of the doctor and the patient are fairly well defined, and subject to the norms of conduct that are, generally, accepted within social contexts common to them both (El-Kabir, 1993). Even in these circumstances grey areas are encountered, from time to time, where both the doctor and the patient are ill-equipped – disability, misfortune and infirmity, degeneration and death for example, or even stresses and disaffections of daily life. The best that can be expected (and it is good) is summed up by the old aphorism '*guérir quelquefois, soulager souvent, consoler toujours*' (cure sometimes, relieve often, console always). This, alas, is not quite good enough for the vulnerable people we describe in this chapter. Their deprivation firmly puts the onus of what can be done for them in the lap of the carer.

The consultation cannot therefore be understood in isolation of the social context and the mores in which it takes place. It represents the meeting point of two pasts and two presents, and the only way in which it can have a sustained continuity in the future (and that is surely a potent index of effectual care) depends on what can be created by mutual trust.

The first point of contact is the most crucial one, and its model applies to all subsequent encounters. The role of the receptionist is therefore, in this respect, crucial in setting the ambience of the consultation. The aim is the same for all the care workers: to make manifest one's intentionality, the basic motive behind one's choice of action. One's perception of another's situation leads to a number of different options, to which the doctor may not be sensitive, owing to his own past, or other circumstances of which he may not be entirely aware. To do that implies a degree of self-awareness that requires training and development. One has to put across one's humanity rather than one's sympathy, and also one's desire to understand. A thorough professionalism and an attention to detail, especially to shades of meaning and to fleeting impressions, is essential. Someone – we wish we could remember who – wrote: *'la vérité est dans les nuances'* (truth is in the nuances). How very true. There is no room here for cosmetics. It is not much use maintaining eye contact if this is perceived by the other person to reveal a glazed look and an invitation to collusion. The doctor has a need to feel effective, as much as the patient has a desire to be reassured. This may lead to short-term solutions and to superficial insights, a sort of psychological treading water. Collusion and care can thus become mutually exclusive. The role of rapport with homeless people has been illustrated by Shanks (1981). He interviewed a group of his patients obtaining socio-demographic information, this was repeated 6 months later. The discrepancy in the data was less than 1%. A colleague interviewed a different group, introducing himself as a hospital doctor doing research. His data showed over a third of data items were discrepant.

Clearly the responsibility for building up this trust is heavily weighted towards the doctor. He has more to do, more adjusting of attitudes to perform than the patient, who is a supplicant with problems that are both complex and obscure. To understand these the doctor has not merely to be on top of his *métier*, but he has to evaluate the situation that faces him and gauge the appropriateness of his response to it. It is our belief that people who are deprived or oppressed are generally very observant and astute as to the personality of the people they deal with. An eminent chest physician who has been interested in some aspects of the care of the homeless recently mentioned to us that when he was interviewing homeless patients, he felt that he was himself being interviewed! It has to be added that this evaluation is all the more potent because it is invariably wordless. How is the doctor to survive this appraisal and how is he to establish his credentials as someone who can be entrusted with the confidence of those who may be fragile, frightened or simply weighed down with guilt and shame?

The traditional received formula in such instances is to offer 'reassurance' and 'support' as though these are commodities in the keeping of the doctor, there to be dispensed as and when necessary pro re nata. This can become something of a culture, where the whole concept of what might happen after the consultation, and how far, and in what spheres, the doctor might influence the future course of the patient's life is very remote from what the doctor would see as his remit. Yet this attitude can have the most serious repercussions on the course of individual treatment, and even on the health of the general public. Two examples come readily to mind: the discharge into 'the community' of mentally ill homeless patients, and the notorious failure of effectively treating tuberculosis among the homeless (Ramsden et al., 1988), in whom it is prevalent. One can only point out the dangers, which are now clearly recognized in the USA, of the development of multi-drug resistant tuberculosis due to multiple failed treatments to appreciate that a major public health problem may well face us here as well. One must accept that this is an illustration of the inadequacies of our health services to understand the problems of this population or to respond to their needs.

One can think of the consultation as an 'enabling process' as opposed to a politically correct concept of giving the patient a voice to state his rights. The lack of distinction between these two seemingly similar ideas is at the root of what we consider to be the ineffectiveness of so many projects, voluntary or government funded, to come up with a convincing model of care in the community for the mentally ill. The sole purpose of the consultation could be said to lay a sound basis for the continuity of care, and hence for appropriate care to be followed through as far as it can be, so that one can be satisfied that it can be pursued no further by identifying the nature or causes of those limitations, be they social, economic or political factors, the doctor's resources, or the patient's personality. Little good is done to the cause of the homeless by well meaning but simplistic ideas about housing and integration. More attention needs to be devoted to understanding and addressing the individual needs of the vulnerable.

Clearly the structure of some services, in particular psychiatric, lend themselves poorly to be seen as a haven of care. A hospital setting and an appointment system for outpatients is so inappropriate as to verge on the grotesque. Their hierarchical structure and the constant change of personnel militate against the sort of continuity that is needed to build bridges and to lay foundations for a meaningful relationship between psychiatrist (and even more so, the nurse or the social worker) and those in their care. At Great Chapel Street Medical Centre (El-Kabir, 1982), funding had to be sought from a charity to fund the work of the psychiatrist along the lines we indicate. It has proved possible to establish continuity of care with many psychiatrically ill homeless people who had left previous psychiatric care, particularly those with schizophrenia (Joseph *et al.*, 1990).

The various types of provision of health services

The diversity of age, groupings and life-style suggests that no single approach to the health needs of the homeless is likely to be universally appropriate or successful. Historically general practice surgeries and clinics held in hostels provided medical care for the homeless. More recently a number of other approaches have been developed such as specialized general practice surgeries specifically designed to meet the needs of the homeless. A number of themes run through successful projects, and each approach has disadvantages as well as advantages. A variety of outreach services have developed, some with doctors going to sites where the homeless congregate, and others where social care and housing workers encourage sick individuals on the streets to attend local clinics. What has generally not been developed on a large scale is a planned and integrated arrangement of health care for all homeless people with effective links to social care and various forms of housing. Excellent care can be offered to large numbers of homeless people by general practice surgeries. They can be accessible and may become the point of access to a large number of services. Some general practitioners have been said to discriminate against the homeless, particularly by denying them registration, although in the authors' experience this is not common. Despite accessibility many homeless will not use these services for the reasons that have been alluded to above. There are also a few homeless people whose behaviour is so disruptive that they are difficult to cope with in a usual clinic setting. In order to widen availability of health care to those who would not otherwise utilize it, some general practitioners have for many years held clinics in day centres and hostels for the homeless. This works best when there is liaison between the centre staff and the medical services, and where the support of trustworthy staff can encourage the use of the services by reluctant people. We have found that patients will often develop a considerable degree of trust in the individual clinics, although they would still be cautious of seeing other doctors, particularly in a hospital setting. Some claim that such services increase the marginalization of the homeless by restricting their access to 'mainstream' services, although those who argue this rarely attempt to address the problems described above. Specialist clinics have evolved to care for the homeless and can function as a point of re-entry to services and society as a whole. Some have proved remarkably successful in gaining the trust of both patients and homeless networks, and have been able to orientate their services and style to their needs. For example, Great Chapel Street Medical Centre in Soho, London has open access to all services, including psychiatry as well as offering nurse, chiropody, dental and social work care. The centres can also gain expertise in the best use of social workers, housing and other resources, which may be needed to ensure effective care. They are probably most effective where there are particularly large populations of homeless people, including those sleeping rough. These conditions are most likely to be found in large inner cities. Outreach services can meet a further group of homeless people who rarely use day centres, hostels or other services. One study from a mobile clinic that visited various sites in London found that a third claimed to rarely use other services (Ramsden et al., 1989). Once trust had been established, people started to use the services, and a third of those visited started to use a nearby clinic for the homeless staffed by the same doctors within a month of the first consultation at the mobile surgery. Outreach services are most effective when the trust and rapport can be developed as a result of their operation effectively encourages patients to use services, as there are obvious limitations to the scope of medical care provided on the streets.

Homeless people often consult with a daunting combination of physical and psychiatric disorders, and on a number of occasions we have found that treatment is particularly difficult whilst the patient remains on the streets. Examples include leg ulcers, pulmonary tuberculosis, psychosis and severe 'flu'-like illnesses. Such patients are frequently reluctant to be admitted to hospitals, and in some cases, the hospitals themselves are reluctant to admit patients when 'social problems' form such a large component of the illness. In 1984 we started a sick bay, Wytham Hall, to admit such patients. Since then around 1400 patients have been cared for. It allows the treatment of complex problems, and many patients react to the relaxed and protected atmosphere by beginning to discuss their lives and consider changing the direction of their lives. All are offered housing on discharge, of a sort which is most likely to support the individual, and 2 years after discharge, about 40% remain in stable accommodation. The cure rate for tuberculosis has risen from about 25–30% without a sick bay to between 60–70%. In many ways the sick bay represents a synthesis of personal care, along with integrated social, housing and medical resources in a way that is often hard to achieve. Homeless people often use hospitals for their health care. Casualty departments particularly are used for primary care, and inpatient beds to care for those with a variety of conditions, particularly psychiatric, ortho-paedic and medical. There is often considerable frustration on both sides. Hospital doctors may feel they admit because they have no alternative and cannot make any real difference to the person's overall life. Discharge is difficult and all too often to inappropriate accommo-dation, and with poor or non-existant social follow-up. In many cases patients discharge themselves before treatment is completed. Home-less people frequently find the authoritarian atmosphere and loss of liberty distressing and even intolerable. A number of hospitals have started to develop links with primary care centres for the homeless and housing departments to overcome some of these problems and it is likely that close liaison between primary and secondary care can do much to improve the quality of care for homeless people.

Failure of projects

Whilst the above describes many initiatives and areas to develop, a relatively large number of projects over the past 20 years have ceased to exist or failed to develop beyond a quite limited scope. A number of themes underlie the success or otherwise of projects. Failure may result from a lack of clarity about the aims of the project or non-viable goals. These projects have suffered through poor groundwork to establish what resources were needed and have led to the service not being used by the homeless. Staff may have unrealistic expectations of what can be achieved, and rapidly lose heart. Some start or become isolated from others working in primary care and again become disillusioned. Successful projects usually start from a position of clear need, and may attract able staff who can carry the project through difficult times. Adaptation and change are also a feature, along with a willingness to shed rigid preconceptions about work patterns and job descriptions. In recent years new government money has become available for a variety of health initiatives for the homeless, but sadly it seems that the lessons of previous difficulties have yet to be learnt (or remembered) in a number of cases.

The need for integration

The starting point for the care of a homeless person begins with the first consultation. The scope of the consultation has been described during which areas of potential change in the person's life-style may be identified. People have problems with housing or may be unable to utilize available resources. They may need a supportive relationship to help negotiate difficult life situations. This at a stroke implies that social support, appropriate housing and psychological help should be available along with any continuing medical care. Addressing these broad and varied, but nonetheless urgent problems, is perhaps one of the weakest areas of our health system, particularly in inner cities where the single homeless are likely to be. Liaison between social service departments, general practitioners, hospitals, housing along with the voluntary sector is at best patchy. Resources are stretched and time limited. Carers are alas too often imprisoned in their roles and routines so that creative initiatives involving effective co-operation with other workers or agencies become difficult to initiate. One of the present ideals of community care is joint planning and the close liaison between health commissioning agencies and social services. It is too early to tell where this will lead, but already in some areas of London professional jealousies are resulting in limited co-operation with inevitable results. Resources are not the only issue, and imaginative schemes that break the cycle of ill health and homelessness are likely to turn out to be highly cost efficient. As an example, an average of £20 000 per patient (at 1993 prices) had been spent on unsuccessful hospital care for patients with tuberculosis subsequently admitted to our sick bay. Clearly the scope for economy as well as the good care of individuals with tuberculosis is consider-able if the cure rate can be doubled, as indeed we find could be the case at our sick bay.

At this point, perhaps we should describe our own vision of effective and integrated care. Hopefully it is not too naive. Each geographical urban area should make an assessment of the numbers of homeless, their accommodation, meeting points and the existing provision of care (which is often more extensive than is realized). Areas with high numbers of homeless, particularly street dwellers, may need a clinic focusing on the care of the homeless. This clinic should perhaps take the lead in co-ordinating information, liaising with secondary care and accident and emergency departments. Areas where care is efficient may need the encouragement of local general practitioners to expand their availability or perhaps the introduction of new services. Links need to be developed between social service and housing departments and flexible, 'fast track' assessments made possible. The slowness and formality of some assessments effectively exclude many homeless from using them, although on paper the services are available. The voluntary sector has much to offer, including day centres, outreach work, drug and alcohol support along with housing and is likely to be provided in a way that the homeless find acceptable. Some sort of sick bay provision will be needed, as would detoxification facilities. Finally links with more permanent housing facilities, particularly supportive housing and community based psychiatric support should be developed, although our experience suggests that much remains to be learned before psychiatric teams could be considered effective. However, perhaps what is needed most, before such a system could be set up and operate effectively, is the development of a new culture of care among its providers.

References

Balint, M. (1964). *The Doctor, his Patient, and the Illness.* 2nd edit. London: Pitman Publishers Ltd.

Editorial. (1989). Homelessness. *Lancet,* **ii,** 778–9.

El-Kabir, D. J. (1982). Great Chapel Street medical centre. *British Medical Journal,* **284,** 480–1.

El-Kabir, D. J. (1993). Quelques observation sur les sans-abris. *Les Temps Modernes. Paris.* **567,** 47–51.

Fischer, P. J. & Breakey, W. R. (1986). Homelessness and mental health: an overview. *International Journal of Mental Health,* **14,** 6–41.

Geddes, J., Newton, R., Young, G., Bailey, S., Freeman, C. & Priest, R. (1994). Comparison of prevalence of schizophrenia among hostels for homeless people in 1966 and 1992. *British Medical Journal,* **308,** 816–19.

Hewetson, J. (1975). Homeless people as an at-risk group. *Proceedings of the Royal Society of Medicine*, **68**, 9–13.

Joseph, P., Bridgewater, J., Ramsden, S. & El-Kabir, D. J. (1990). A psychiatric clinic for the single homeless in a primary care setting in inner London. *Psychiatric Bulletin*, **14**, 270–1.

Lodge Patch, I. C. (1971). Homeless men in London: demographic findings in a common lodging house sample. *British Journal of Psychiatry*, **118**, 313–17.

Marshall, E. J. & Reed, A. (1992). Psychiatric morbidity in homeless women. *British Journal of Psychiatry*, **160**, 761–8.

McAdam, J., Brickner, P. W., Glicksman, R., Edwards, D., Fallon, B. & Yanowitch, P. (1985). Tuberculosis in the SRO/homeless population. In P. W. Brickner, L. K. Scharer, B. Conanan, A. Elzy & M. Savarese (eds.), *Health Care of Homeless People*, pp. 155–79. New York: Springer Publishing Co.

Myerson, D. & Mayer, J. (1966). Origins, treatment and destiny of skid-row alcoholic men. *New England Journal of Medicine*, **275**, 419–25.

Patel, K. R. (1985). Pulmonary tuberculosis in residents of lodging houses, night shelters and common lodging houses in Glasgow: a 5-year prospective study. *British Journal of Diseases of the Chest*, **79**, 60–6.

Pendleton, D. A., Schofield, T. P. C. & Tate, P. H. L. (1982). *The Consultation: An approach to Learning and Teaching*. Oxford: Oxford University Press.

Powell, P. V. (1987). A 'house doctor' scheme for the primary health care for the single homeless in Edinburgh. *Journal of the Royal College of General Practitioners*, **37**, 444–7.

Ramsden, S. (1994). Epilepsy and Homelessness. MD thesis. University of London.

Ramsden, S., Baur, S. & El-Kabir, D. J. (1988). Tuberculosis among the central London single homeless. *Journal of the Royal College of Physicians*, **22**, 16–17.

Ramsden, S., Nyiri, P., Bridgewater, J. & El-Kabir, D. J. (1989). A mobile surgery for single homeless people in London. *British Medical Journal*, **289**, 372–4.

Reed, A., Ramsden, S., Marshall, J. *et al.* (1992). Psychiatric morbidity and substance abuse among residents of a cold weather shelter. *British Medical Journal*, **304**, 1028–9.

Scott, R., Gaskell, P. & Morrell, D. (1966). Patients who reside in common lodging houses. *British Medical Journal*, **2**, 1561–4.

Shanks, N. J. (1981). Consistency of data collected from inmates of a common lodging house. *Journal of Epidemiology and Community Health*, **35**, 133–5.

Shanks, N. J. (1988). Medical morbidity of the homeless. *Journal of Epidemiology and Community Health*, **42**, 183–6.

Tidmarsh, D. & Wood, S. (1972). Psychiatric aspects of destitution. In

J. K. Wing & A. M. Heuley (eds.), *Evaluating a Community Psychiatric Service. The Camberwell Register, 1964–1971*, pp. 328–40. Oxford: Oxford University Press.

Weller, M., Tobiansky, R., Hollander, D. & Ibrahimi, S. (1989). Psychosis and destitution at christmas. *Lancet*, **ii**, 1509–11.

Williams, S. & Allen, I. (1989). *Health Care for Single Homeless People*. Policy Studies Institute.

PART III

INTERNATIONAL PERSPECTIVE

12

European Perspectives

Introduction to European chapter

MAX MARSHALL

Reviews of homelessness and mental disorder in the UK inevitably draw comparisons with the situation in the USA (for example Scott, 1993). It is often assumed that the findings of any US study of homeless people (from the level of frostbite in New York to the rates of drug abuse in homeless women) are unquestionably generalizeable to UK populations. In fact close comparisons between the USA and UK are sometimes seriously misleading. In a Western democracy, the level of homelessness is essentially a product of social policy, and so too is the level of mental disorder amongst the homeless. In social policy terms, (for example, in the provision of subsidized housing, free health care, and state benefits) the UK now stands somewhere between American and European norms. Thus, the UK resembles the USA in that it has increasingly adopted a free market housing policy. On the other hand, the UK government remains committed (in public) to the European ethos of a national health service, and a reasonable level of state assistance to the unemployed and disabled.

Mental disorder in homeless women is a good example of an area where USA–UK comparisons may mislead, when differences in social policy are not taken into account. In the UK, local authorities are obliged to provide emergency accommodation to homeless families (usually a lone woman with children), and to rehouse such families as a priority. Whilst these families may face long periods in temporary accommodation (bedsits), they are eventually rehoused, and do not have to make use of emergency shelters or hostels. In the USA there is usually no obligation to rehouse homeless families. Hence it is commonplace to find women with children living in emergency accommodation. This difference in social policy has interesting epidemiological implications because homeless women

with children are much less likely to suffer from severe mental
disorder than single homeless women. Hence it is difficult to make
comparisons between US and UK studies of the rates of mental
disorder in homeless UK women as the studies draw on very different
populations.

The main reason for many specious USA–UK comparisons is
similarity of language rather than similarity of culture and social
policy. On these grounds a plausible case can be made that European
studies are of equal or greater relevance than USA studies. Yet UK
commentators have shown remarkably little interest in research
carried out by our European partners. This chapter attempts to
redress the balance by presenting the findings of relevant European
research that has remained largely uncited in English language
reviews. The amount of information presented is small in relation to
that which remains to be uncovered (for English readers). Nevertheless, the limited findings presented here demonstrate both the quality
of the research available, and the potential for furthering our
understanding of the causes of homelessness by cross-European
comparisons.

From Denmark, Brandt and Munk-Jørgensen, present a series of
studies of high epidemiological quality that have not previously been
discussed in the English language literature. From a UK point of view
the research has two interesting messages. First, even in societies with
highly developed welfare systems we see the problems of: homelessness amongst the young; accumulation of severely mentally ill in
lodging houses; and direct discharge of psychiatric patients from
hospitals to hostels. Secondly, unlike the UK, Denmark has not seen a
recent rise in the total numbers of homeless people, perhaps because
the state remains committed to providing low-cost accommodation to
those in need.

From Germany, Rössler and Salize again demonstrate that there is
a substantial body of relevant research that has not penetrated the
literature in English. As the authors point out, the interpretation of
the German findings is complicated by two special factors: the
problems of reunification, and the long-term effects of the Nazi policy
of exterminating people with severe mental disorders. Despite these
complicating factors, and the limitations of the available data, there is
evidence that Germany has seen an accumulation of people with
severe mental disorders in hostels for the homeless. It may be that

Germany is about to embark on a 'community care crisis' of the type so familiar in the USA and UK.

From the Republic of Ireland, Fernandez shows remarkable similarities with the situation in the UK. Both countries have seen a reduction in state provision of housing and both appear to have a growing homelessness problem. A unique aspect of the Irish situation however, is the rise in demand for housing caused by the country ceasing to be a net exporter of people.

In summary, a growing body of high quality research on homelessness and mental illness is beginning to emerge from other European countries. This research is particularly relevant for the UK because of its potential for showing how differences in social and community care policy affect the levels of homelessness amongst the mentally ill.

References

Scott, J. (1993). Homelessness and mental illness. *British Journal of Psychiatry*, **162**, 314–25.

Homelessness in Denmark

PREBEN BRANDT AND POVL MUNK-JØRGENSEN

Today we do not have poverty in Denmark, if poverty is defined as lack of money for food, clothing, or a place to live. But one of the consequences of poverty, homelessness, is well-known. It has been suggested that: 'a high standard of living in a community can produce its own problems as a by-product of the normal functions of the community' (Jonsson, 1967). Maybe that is why we find homelessness in Denmark although we are known to be a rich country with a good social welfare system.

But again it depends on definition. If homeless people are only those living in the streets, sleeping in parks, on pavements in the inner city, on railway stations, in basements, staircases, etc, few people are homeless in Denmark.

In Copenhagen[1], the capital of Denmark[2], about 100–500 persons sleep in such places every night, and only a few of them for longer periods.

Homeless people could also be defined as those who lack their own home, those living in institutions from where they can be discharged (i.e. psychiatric hospitals or prisons), or those living with friends for one or two nights, or living in lodging houses. On an estimate, 10–15 000 persons are homeless in Denmark. Of these 5–6000 homeless people are living in Copenhagen. Therefore, between 0.3% and 0.4% of the 3 500 000 adult inhabitants in Denmark are homeless.

It seems that the number of homeless has been stable in the last 20–30 years, however, in the same period the demographic changes in the group of homeless have been obvious. In Denmark it is still possible to meet the middle-aged or old alcoholic male, a character who 20 years ago made up 80–90% of the group of homeless, but today he is only one out of five. Instead the group has become younger. Even very young people are seen. There are both men and women, and in Copenhagen as well as in other capitals or large cities, you can meet the well-known group of 'bag-ladies'. Some are mentally ill, and among them are also young schizophrenics discharged from the mental hospitals. Alcohol and/or drug addicts are in the group, many are 'narco-prostitutes'.

Institutions for the homeless

According to the social security legislation, each county in Denmark is under an obligation to establish institutions for people 'who are homeless or not able to adjust to the ordinary way of living in the community'. These lodging houses are of a very different kind; some are best named as shelters, others are more like asylums (so called 'forsorgshjem') and finally, some function as boarding-homes.

In the shelters all homeless persons over 18 years can be offered a bed for a night or more. They do not meet any demands other than a very small payment for a stay. The staff is usually small and not trained in mental illness.

---

[1] Population in Copenhagen County: 603 883 inhabitants; in the municipality of Copenhagen: 466 129 inhabitants; in total 1 070 012 inhabitants.
[2] Denmark has a total population of 5.1 million.

Table 12.1. *Contribution of very young/older homeless men compared to contribution of very young/older homeless women*

Age (years)	Men (%)	Women (%)
24 and under	6	22
25 and over	94	78
	100	100

Source: Amstrådsforeningeni Danmark (1990).

In the other types of institutions, efforts are made to help the homeless back to 'a normal life'. In these institutions the homeless are in some way selected before they are let in. In some institutions they do not want drug addicts and in others they try to avoid severely mentally ill persons.

In Denmark there are 2300 lodging house beds, half of them in Copenhagen. Most of the institutions are run by religious organizations, but financed by the government.

Characterization of the homeless and the homeless mentally ill

In 1989 a 'one-day survey' was carried out on the initiative of the County Council Association among 2213 homeless people housed in lodging houses (Amstrådsforeningen i Danmark, 1990). The survey showed that the largest group of homeless (1100 persons) was 35–54 years old, and that the group of persons aged 18–34 years was sharply increased from 375 persons in 1976 to 800 in 1989. In the same period the group of persons aged 54 and over was halved.

The increase in number of homeless women was even more remarkable than the increase in the group of young homeless. The percentage of women in the lodging houses rose from 6% in 1976 to 20% in 1989. There seems to be a connection between the increasing number of young lodging house users and the growing number of homeless women. The homeless women were younger than the men (see Table 12.1). It was also in this group of young homeless that a growing number of persons with major mental disorders was found.

Previously in Danish literature about homelessness most of the homeless were described as having some kind of mental problems. In the investigation mentioned above the most common diagnoses were personality disorder, dementia and alcoholism. Only 2–3% had more severe functional mental illness.

A current report from a mainly rural county found that only a few percent of the users of the lodging houses have severe mental illness (Riis, 1987). But from another county (mainly rural, but including the third biggest town in Denmark) it was reported that 9% of the persons using the institutions for homeless were diagnosed as schizophrenics (Fyns Amt, 1991). From Copenhagen figures show that 14% of the users of the municipal lodging houses were diagnosed as schizophrenics (Brandt, 1987). A survey of 'the new group of homeless' i.e. the 18–35 year old users of lodging houses, carried out in Copenhagen in 1989, gave the result that 20% were diagnosed as having schizophrenia and 20% were diagnosed as having other kinds of schizophreniformic psychosis. (Brandt, 1992).

In Denmark we have unique possibilities of determining the number of mentally ill persons in the lodging houses, as all admissions to psychiatric hospitals and wards are registered in the psychiatric central register (Munk-Jørgensen et al., 1993). The present authors used these possibilities in a study of two Danish counties, namely Aarhus County, which covers a provincial area with about 600 000 inhabitants, of which about 260 000 people live in the town of Aarhus, and the county of North Jutland, which is a mainly rural county with about 490 000 inhabitants, of which about 160 000 people live in the town of Aalborg. Furthermore, the municipality of Copenhagen with about 470 000 inhabitants was included in the study (Munk-Jørgensen et al., 1992).

During 1 month in 1990 person identifiable information about all clients in contact with lodging houses in the two counties mentioned above and the municipality of Copenhagen were registered, in total 1008 persons. The information was linked with that in the Danish psychiatric central register, and it was found that 55% had formerly been admitted to a psychiatric hospital or ward. By way of comparison it may be mentioned that approximately 4% of the total Danish population has been admitted to a psychiatric hospital or ward (the figures are not sex and age standardized). No differences were seen between the clients living in Copenhagen and those attending the lodging houses in the two counties. Of the homeless formerly admitted to a psychiatric hospital, 12.6% were diagnosed as psychotics at their latest admission prior to the registration, 6% were diagnosed as having schizophrenia. By way of comparison, only 0.3–0.4% of the Danish population were admitted due to schizophrenia (the figures are not age and sex standardized). The remaining clients, from 12.6–55%, were mainly diagnosed as suffering from alcoholism, drug/substance abuse, neuroses and psychopathia. The study also showed that 23% of the homeless formerly admitted (12.5% of all the homeless) were discharged directly from the psychiatric hospital and wards to the shelters. If the observation period was extended to 1 month, it was found that 28.6% of the homeless formerly admitted (15.5% of all the homeless) were discharged directly from the psychiatric hospitals. It is, of course, impossible to presume that the homeless persons are actually mentally ill because they previously have been admitted to a psychiatric hospital, but a substantial number seem to be according to Brandt's (1992) investigations. Schizophrenia and organic psychoses are persistent conditions.

If the remarkably high and increasing incidence of psychotic patients in lodging houses is related to the high incidence of mentally ill in prisons (P. Kramp, personal communication), and the almost doubled standard mortality rate amongst newly diagnosed schizophrenics during the last 15 years (Munk-Jørgensen & Mortensen, 1992), mostly due to suicides (Mortensen & Juel, 1993), then it can be concluded that the organization of psychiatry in Denmark has most probably caused an adverse development for the mentally ill, although other factors might have added to this.

The young homeless

The group of young homeless living in the lodging houses in Copenhagen is the one most comprehensively described (Brandt, 1992). A total of 960 persons aged between 18–35 years (0.6% of all inhabitants in Copenhagen in the same age group) who, over a year, used a lodging house were investigated. Of these, 171 (18%) were women and 789 (82%) men. More than one third 358 (37%) were 26 years old or younger.

The average number of days the group spent in lodging houses was

110 days during 1 year, usually split up in to several periods. It was estimated that more than half of these young homeless persons were chronically homeless. If they were not in a lodging house they were living in the streets, in prison, in hospitals or they slept with friends. Only 16% received a social pension.

A representative sample of 129 persons were randomly selected from different lodging houses. They were all interviewed by the same psychiatrist to identify the kind of mental illness and abuse and to disclose their life-style and the events causing their homelessness.

Of those interviewed 17% were diagnosed as schizophrenics, and in all 43% got a diagnosis of psychosis, while 36% were diagnosed as having a personality disorder. Furthermore, 73% of those interviewed had a diagnosis of substance abuse; 19% were addicted to alcohol, 29% regularly used heroin intravenously, and 25% were addicted to alcohol and to different kinds of drugs. A little more than half of the persons who were diagnosed as schizophrenics were addicts as well, and nearly all of those with the diagnosis of personality disorder were addicts.

Four out of five with the diagnosis of schizophrenia had been hospitalized in a psychiatric hospital or ward, most of them several times. Besides, nearly all the young homeless had tried some kind of treatment and several of them had tried different kinds of treatment, but without positive results. In only 4% of the cases obvious reasons for the onset of homelessness, i.e. a single social event which led to loss of home, were found if the homeless persons' life-events just before onset of homelessness was studied retrospectively. As for the rest, it was reported that they had had severe psycho-social problems from early childhood and even sometimes before birth, for example in connection with alcohol-addicted parents.

It can be concluded that homelessness in youth is not a simple social problem, but is due to a lack of socialization, which gives these persons problems living in a complicated community and using its demand-making institutions.

Psychiatry in the streets

Copenhagen is one of the smaller capitals of the Western industrialized countries. Proportionally, we do not have a large number of people living in the streets. However, the problems of this group are very similar to what is reported from bigger cities (Isaac & Armat, 1990), and there will always be about 20–30 persons with severe mental illness living under very bad conditions, i.e. with dirty clothes, eating old food from their bags or from litter bins, sitting on the pavement in all kinds of weather.

In Denmark a debate about these mentally ill homeless people's right to live as they want has only just been opened. What we discussed is on the one hand the civil rights of the single homeless mentally ill and on the other hand the community's responsibility for ensuring everybody has any necessary treatment and a satisfactory social standard of living.

Since the beginning of 1992, a programme appealing to the homeless and homeless-threatened who are severely mentally ill and who reject treatment has been established in Copenhagen (P. Brandt, unpublished data). In the first year the programme was in contact with 37 persons and of these 19 had clearly got a better way of living, due to the programme.

It is obvious that what these people need is neither simple sheltering nor ordinary psychiatric treatment. It is also clear that the homeless psychotics who live in the streets will not go anywhere to ask for help and they will even usually start by refusing to accept any help offered.

Therefore, the programme is based on field-work in the streets and includes a wide spectrum of ways to act, including use of the mental civil law.

Research in mental illness among homeless

Comparison of reports from both Danish and foreign surveys about homelessness have problems due to a lack of consistency. The problems arise especially with the definition of homelessness and the identification of mentally ill persons among the homeless. Most Danish researchers define homeless people as people living in lodging houses, but even this causes problems due to the very different kinds of lodging houses present in Denmark. Also, identification of the mentally ill differs from one survey to another as the homeless are interviewed by different kinds of specialized persons, or identified from registers of formerly hospitalized psychiatric inpatients.

In spite of all the problems that complicate the research, it is evident that mental illness is common among homeless people and it seems to be an increasing problem that young chronic patients, especially those with a dual diagnosis, are left behind as homeless. As such they are not treated or are only getting a minimum or even interrupted treatment as revolving door patients. Furthermore, for some groups, e.g. homeless families and homeless women with children there has not been any research at all in Denmark.

References

Amtsrådsforeningen i Danmark (The Association of County Councils in Denmark) (1990). *Amterne og videreudviklingen af § 105-institutionerne. (The counties and the development of the Section 105-institutions).* København: Amstrådsforeningen i Danmark.

Brandt, P. (1987). Hjemløshed og psykisk lidelse. (Homelessness and mental illness) *Nordisk Psykiatrisk Tidsskrzift*, **41**, 295–301. (English abstract).

Brandt, P. (1992). Yngre Hjemløse i København. (Young homeless in Copenhagen. Doctoral degree thesis. Kovenhavn University. København: Fadl's forlag. (English abstract).

Fyns Amt (Fyns County) (1991). *Psykiatrien, Kommunerne og § 105-institutionerne.* (The Psychiatry, the Municipalities and the Section 105-institutions). København: Fyns Amt, Social- og sundhedsforvaltningen.

Isaac, R. J. & Armat, V. C. (1990). *Madness in the Streets.* New York: The Free Press.

Jonsson, G. (1967). Delinquent boys, their parents and grandparents. *Acta Psychiatrica Scandinavica*, **43** (supplement 195).

Mortensen, P. B. & Juel, K. (1993). Mortality and causes of death in first admitted schizophrenic patients. *British Journal of Psychiatry*, **163**, 183–9.

Munk-Jørgensen, P., Flensted-Nielsen, J., Brandt, P. et al. (1992). Hjemløse psykisk syge, en registerundersøgelse af klienter på herberg og forsorgshjem. (Psychiatric patients with no fixed abode. Registration of clients in hostels and care homes) *Ugeskrift for Læger*, **154**, 1271–5. (English abstract).

Munk-Jørgensen, P., Kastrup, M. & Mortensen, P. B. (1993). The Danish psychiatric register as a tool in epidemiology. *Acta Psychiatrica Scandinavica*, **Supplement 370**, 27–32.

Munk-Jørgensen, P. & Mortensen, P. B. (1992). Incidence and other aspects of the epidemiology of schizophrenia in Denmark 1971–1987. *British Journal of Psychiatry*, **161**, 489–95.

Riis, A. (1987). Forsorgshjem og distriktspsykiatri. En undersøgelse af klientprofilen på forsorgshjemmene i Vejle amt. (Welfare homes and district psychiatry. An investigation of the client profile in the welfare homes in the County of Vejle). *Ugeskrift for Læger*, **149**, 3216–20. (English abstract).

Endnote

The authors wish to point out that since the submission of this chapter, there has been a considerable body of further research on homelessness and related topics published in Denmark.

Continental European experience: Germany

WULF RÖSSLER AND HANS JOACHIM SALIZE

Introduction

In Germany, psychiatrists have historically taken an interest in the origins of homelessness. Early in this century they tended to ascribe psychopathological reasons for homelessness. In fact, two of the most famous German psychiatrists of this time, Wilmanns (1906) who developed the concept of 'Wandertrieb' (migration instinct) and Schneider (1934) who came out with his theory of psychopathic personality, were of this opinion. Unfortunately their work was used to legitimize the murder of thousands of homeless people during the Nazi regime. It was with this that the Nazis transformed the German mental health movement, which had it's heyday between the two wars (Haselbeck, 1985) into a massacre of the mentally disabled. However, theories of endogenous ætiologies of homelessness managed to survive the war (Ritzel, 1974; Garcia, 1986). An increased rate of pathological change in the brains of deceased homeless persons led Veith & Schwindt (1976) to hypothesize that homelessness was a symptom of psycho-organic syndromes. This concept was discussed very controversially (Locher, 1990). The Bodelschwingh institution in Bielefeld-Bethel, a well established centre for helping the homeless in Germany, conducted a large interdisciplinary study on ætiology and phenomenology of homelessness in 1977. Although the scientific design of this study had promised a profound empirical contribution to the debate on endogenous versus social factors in homelessness, there was unfortunately neither interdisciplinary synopsis nor interpretation of the results beyond the level of epidemiological statements. Sociological and medical findings were published separately (e.g. Goschler, 1983; Sperling, 1985), partly differing in description and interpretation (Locher, 1990).

Nevertheless at the present time the phenomenon of homelessness in the Federal Republic of Germany is mainly considered to be the result of an interaction between poverty, unemployment and social disintegration. Consequently, the old label 'Nichtseßhafte' (vagrants) is gradually being replaced by the label 'alleinstehende Wohnsitzlose' (single homeless). According to this concept uprooting, homelessness and vagrancy occur increasingly in times of economic crises, triggered by growing unemployment, a deficient housing market and an insufficient welfare system (Deutscher Verein für öffentliche und private Fürsorge, 1990). Thus, mental disorders are currently seen as one factor in a number of interacting variables resulting in homelessness.

One of the main reasons for the sporadic revivals of the discussion as to whether homelessness is caused by social or psychopathological reasons is the lack of valid empirical data on the relationship between homelessness, social distress and mental disorder. Unlike the UK or the USA, where research on homelessness and mental health is better established, the issue is still not adequately perceived in Germany. But the problem has grown in the last few years. As a result of the German reunification there are great difficulties in reforming the antiquated mental health care system of the former German Democratic Republic. In the so called 'new' federal states (of the former German Democratic Republic) large, insufficiently staffed and equipped psychiatric hospitals are still treating most of the chronically mentally ill. After being discharged, they do not find outpatient and rehabilitative services of Western standard (Rössler & Salize, 1994). If the communities fail to establish sufficient accommodation for these patients, they are at a significant risk of being dismissed into homelessness. Also the immigrants from Eastern Europe (whose number is steadily rising) run a heightened risk of social disintegration and mental strain with the worsening of the economic situation and the lack of cheap flats in Germany.

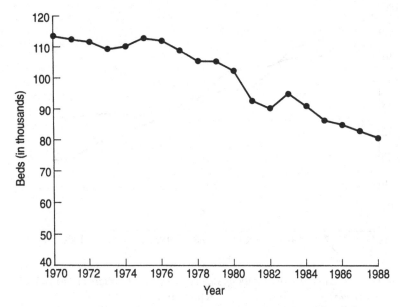

Figure 12.1. Reduction of psychiatric beds in the Federal Republic of Germany.

Historical development

The widespread neglect of the problem of mentally ill homeless in Germany in the post-war era was a symptom of the overall neglect of mental health care during this period. The reform of Germany's psychiatric care system started as late as the 1970s. One reason for this delay is the macabre consequence of the Nazi regime, where between 90 000 and 120 000 mentally ill people were murdered (Finzen, 1983). Therefore the large psychiatric hospitals in Germany did not suffer from overcrowding to the extent that psychiatric hospitals in other countries did. With a ratio of 1.6 psychiatric beds per 1000 population during the early 1970s the need for deinstitutionalization was not as urgent. Nevertheless there was a reduction of beds in mental health hospitals in Germany of approximately 30% within the last two decades (see Figure 12.1).

While in countries like the USA many chronically mentally ill were dismissed more or less directly into homelessness (Dennis *et al.*, 1991), there was enough accommodation for former long-term patients in Germany during the first period of deinstitutionalization. Frequently

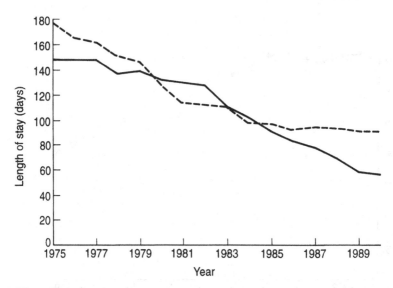

Figure 12.2. Decrease of mean length of stay in psychiatric hospitals in two federal states of Germany. – – –, Hessen; ———, Rheinland.

former tuberculosis clinics in the Black Forest, vacant due to medicine's successful conquest of this disease, were used for this purpose. These 'new' facilities received the status of homes for mentally ill, though they still resembled the traditional large psychiatric hospitals with their size and their location far away from the communities. Since these institutions could not be considered community based, this step of psychiatric reform was more like a transinstitutionalization than a deinstitutionalization (Kunze, 1977). Consequently, there were hardly any homeless mentally ill who were seen in public.

With the next reform steps the establishment of outpatient and rehabilitative services was intensified. Inevitably the remaining inpatient facilities had to face growing restrictions in funding. Between 1975 and 1989 the mean length of stay in psychiatric hospitals strongly decreased, in some federal states of Germany by as much as two thirds (Rössler & Salize, 1993; see Figure 12.2). Today the mean length of stay is approximately 70 days in Germany (Deutscher Bundestag, 1992).

Because of the dramatically growing inpatient admission rates due to the decreasing mean lengths of stay, the psychiatric hospitals were forced to cut social care offers for the chronically mentally ill. The hospitals' asylum function disappeared. One indication of this is the growing number of chronically mentally ill patients referred from inpatient treatment to social psychiatric mental health centres. In some areas this rate now amounts to 15–20% of all social psychiatric mental health centres' patients (Rössler *et al.*, 1993). Already at earlier stages of the reform in Germany there had been warnings that deinstitutionalization might become detrimental especially for the chronically ill (Kunze, 1977).

In the community, mentally ill patients are more exposed to economic and social stressors than they are behind the protective walls of the asylum, at least in this case. If the economic situation of a country gets worse, the mentally ill are among the first to suffer. The recent German reunification proved this to be true. In the former German Democratic Republic, many chronically mentally ill had opportunities to work in state owned enterprises, known as 'Volkseigene Betriebe (VEB)'. Because of the special conditions of Eastern Germany's economy VEBs could afford to employ a large number of mentally ill. When these companies were no longer competitive by the standards of the Western economy, the mentally ill lost their jobs. Unfortunately, there are no sheltered workshops or other rehabilitative services to which they can go. At the same time the mentally ill have difficulty finding housing accommodation since rent in Eastern Germany is rising at an explosive rate.

Current situation

The problem of the mentally ill homeless in Germany can no longer be concealed. It is acute. However, it is impossible to know the total number of homeless in Germany. Assessments have to rely on data from services for the homeless that record contacts. But only a few services participate. Moreover, there are homeless people who avoid any contact with care services. Estimations of the size of this group range from 'very little' to one third of all homeless.

Available data indicate a significant increase in the total number of homeless during the last few years. At the beginning of the 1970s, some 26 000 homeless persons were registered by the German Bundesarbeitsgemeinschaft für Nichtseßhaftenhilfe (Commission for Care for the Homeless). In 1978 the number increased to 32 000

Table 12.2. Studies on mental disorders among the homeless in Germany

Authors	Time	Population	Psychiatric morbidity	Alcoholism	Former psychiatric hospitalization (%)
Kluge (1972)	1968–1971	n = 1788 home and shelter users	1.3% psychosis	16.7%	5.2
Stadt Stuttgart (1976)			24%	40% alcoholism 44% at risk	
MAGS (1982)	1978/79	Services for homeless, Baden Württemberg	18%	46%	
Sperling (1985)	1976/77	Services for homeless, Bielefeld	1.8% schizophrenia 4.6% depression 15.6% attempted suicide	56% alcoholism 23.9% alcohol abuse	3.6
Stößel & Locher (1991)	February 1985	Home and shelter users, n 342, Kästorf	2.9% psychosis	34.7% alcoholism 32.2% at risk	
Kujat (1991)	Unknown	Shelter and homes, 224 beds, Hannover		70%	Many
Rieger & Wessel (1992)	1987	1800 outpatient contacts		30%	
John (quoted from Rieger & Wessel, 1992)	1988	In- and outpatient services for homeless, Bielefeld		60%	8
Hövelmann (quoted from Rieger & Wessel, 1992)	January 1990	400 places, homes and shelter, Bielefeld		67% (5–10% multi-morbidity)	
Eikelmann et al. (1992)	Nov–Dec. 1990	n = 52 shelter, Münster	9.6% schizophrenia 3.8% neurosis/ personality disorder	63.5%	36.5
Trabert (1995)	One and a half months in 1989	n = 40 males, specialized medical outpatient service for homeless, Mainz	5% psychiatric disorder 5% attempted suicide	17.5% alcoholism 25% alcohol abuse 5% drug addiction	

(MAGS, 1982). These figures, however, cannot be considered as complete, since they are based on voluntary reports from care services. In 1989, Iben estimated that 100 000 persons in Germany were without a home (0.17% of the total population of West Germany, which was not yet reunited with the Eastern part at that time) and another 200 000 persons were in provisional accommodation. Lately the federal state of Baden-Württemberg projected 16 600–17 400 homeless (LWV, 1993), which amounts to 0.17–0.18% of the total population of that part of Germany, as well. We can assume this figure to be a valid estimate for the 'old' federal states. Projections for the 'new' federal states are not possible at this time.

The institutionalized reform of German mental health care did not focus on the needs of homeless people. The large community support programmes that carried out an evaluation of mental health care did not take them into account (Rössler *et al.*, 1987; BMJFFG, 1988).

Reliable empirical data not being available, the number of mentally ill among the German homeless people cannot be ascertained. Researchers have only recently conducted a few isolated studies on mental disorders among the homeless. These studies in most cases are limited to recording morbidity rates and account for regional conditions. Table 12.2 summarizes the results of some of these studies.

All German studies suffer from the same problems that other international studies on this issue do. Results can therefore hardly be generalized or compared with those of other studies.

In spite of some studies claiming representativeness (Veith & Schwindt, 1976; Sperling, 1985) all of them fail to meet this methodological standard. All study populations are highly selective, as they include only those homeless who frequent one or two of all types of services (mainly shelters and homes) offered for them.

Almost all studies are cross-sectional. Apart from the general limitations of cross-sectional studies, in this case seasonal variations of service utilization also cannot be controlled.

In many studies researchers complain that the homeless tend to be unco-operative. Generally homeless people are difficult people to work with. Being afraid of adverse consequences, the homeless tend to refuse inquiries or dissimulate problems much more than other patient groups (especially concerning items such as previ-

ous convictions, psychiatric treatments, venereal diseases, con-
sumption of alcohol etc).

Assessment methods are disparate. Although standardized diag-
nostical interviews have become generally accepted during the
last few years (Susser *et al.*, 1989), psychiatric assessment is
frequently still conducted by insufficiently trained interviewers.
Psychiatric morbidity rates in many studies rely only on observations or impressions of service staff members (MAGS, 1982). In
Sperling's (1985) study psychiatric examinations were done by
specialists in internal medicine.

Co- and multi-morbidity has not been sufficiently assessed. Even
data on co-morbidity of mental disorders and alcoholism are
often lacking, as Table 12.2 shows. Methodologically however, it
is even more difficult to assess and interpret coincidences of
physical and mental disorder in an adequate manner. The above
mentioned debate on endogenous versus social ætiologies of
homelessness is continuously stimulated by badly supported or
too extensively interpreted findings in this field.

All studies are below the standards required to use multi-factorial
analysis methods. Many possible influencing factors are often
merely described and not recorded in a standardized manner. It
is therefore not possible to analyze them using multi-variate
models.

The care system for homeless in Germany

The provision of care for the homeless in Germany is regulated by the
federal social welfare law (Par.72 BSHG). The following services are
provided:

1. *Social welfare offices.* The local social welfare agencies responsible
   check the legal claim for public assistance of homeless people and
   deliver income support.
2. *Advisory services for homeless.* These services counsel, distribute
   clothing and refer to special services if the homeless are in need of
   specialized help. In some federal states of Germany, homeless
   people can apply for income support at these services, which pay it
   directly. Some advisory services offer medical or legal advice for a
   few hours every week.

3. *Shelters.* Shelters provide overnight accommodation. This help is short-term. Shelters only allow homeless to stay nights and their stay is limited to a few days. Usually shelters offer no specialized help or advice.
4. *Residential homes.* These facilities provide long-term accommodation. Residents care for themselves. Institutional care is not offered except during office hours by social workers.
5. *Rehabilitative homes.* These facilities are usually run by social workers and allow homeless people to take temporary residence. The main purpose is the rehabilitation of homeless people, but persons with their own income can live there as well, without having to give up their entire wages.
6. *Drop-in centres.* Drop-in centres provide meals and a heated day-room. Some also have showers and washing machines. Frequently legal and medical advice is offered.
7. *Hotels and boarding-houses.* Due to the intensified general housing shortage new institutions have been established all over Germany that offer simple accommodation for the homeless. These houses are private and profit-oriented.

This overview shows that mental health care is provided only in a few institutions – and even then only as a part of general medical advice. In many cases the most care that can be delivered is a referral to a specialized service. Besides these quantitative deficits there also exists a qualitative limitation that is a result of the structure of the German welfare and health care systems. Both of these systems are strictly separated from each other, and are in themselves dispersed into a wide range of different small institutions and services. Therefore, the provision of mental health care within the overall service for the homeless is not only financially, but also structurally limited. However, medical care in Germany is not restricted to members of health insurance companies (as it still is in the USA), but is practically free of charge for everybody. If a non-insured patient is in need of medical help, all treatment is paid by social welfare. Using medical care services, however, requires initiative of one's own and the knowledge that one is in need of help. Unfortunately homeless people are often lacking both habits.

Conclusions

The problem of mentally ill homeless people in Germany is, above all, a problem of care. The need for mental health care among the homeless cannot be quantified due to a lack of information. Nevertheless what we do know suggests that this need is considerable. General services for homeless people carry the main load of mental health care of their clientele. However, they are not adequately equipped or staffed for this purpose. They are not able to deliver any form of care beyond a subsistence level. So these institutions are in most cases underqualified when they have to deal with people suffering from mental disorders. The most urgent problem is the alcohol problem. However, the idea that present services for the homeless in Germany can substitute for specialized care in the field of alcoholism amounts only to wishful thinking (Rieger & Wessel, 1992).

Professionals are conscious of this problem, because they experience it daily (Kujat, 1991). However, most new concepts or plans for the further development of care for the homeless do not take into account the mental health of this group (LWV, 1993). If reform plans refer to this problem, the only recommendation is to improve outpatient care of the homeless in order to ease the burden of inpatient services for those with alcohol problems (Deutscher Verein für öffentliche und private Fürsorge, 1990).

This is not sufficient. Plans that do not consider mental health needs will not be effective in helping care for the growing number of homeless people. Data available indicate even now that there is a substantial need for mental health care for these people.

Exactly what services the mentally ill homeless need and how they can be combined with the existing mental health care system and the care system for the homeless cannot yet be determined with our present knowledge. Further investigations are needed. The results of international study on this issue will not fill the gap. The historical development already described in this chapter suggests that the mentally ill homeless in Germany might differ from those in countries such as the USA or UK. We can hypothesize that the rate of persons directly dismissed from inpatient treatment to homelessness in Germany is smaller. However, there might be a relatively large group of persons with mental disorders that reject treatment and avoid utilizing the welfare and health care agencies.

References

BMJFFG (Bundesminister für Jugend, Familie, Frauen und Gesundheit) (State Department of Youth, Family, Women and Health) (1988). *Empfehlungen der Expertenkommission der Bundesregierung zur Reform der Versorgung im psychiatrischen und psychotherapeutisch-psychosomatischen Bereich auf der Grundlage des Modellprogramms Psychiatrie. (Suggestions made by the Federal Government's Commission of Experts on Reform in the Psychiatric and Psychotherapeutic-psychosomatic Fields as Based on the Model Programme of Psychiatry)*. Bonn: BMJFFG.

Dennis, D. L., Buckner, J. C., Lipton, F. R. & Levine, I. S. (1991). A decade of research and services for homeless mentally ill persons: where do we stand? *American Psychologist*, **46**, 1129–38.

Deutscher Bundestag (1992). *Antwort der Bundesregierung auf die Große Anfrage der SPD zur Situation der psychisch Kranken in der Bundesrepublik Deutschland. (The Federal Government's Response to the Question Posed by the Social Democratic Party (SDP) Regarding the Situation of the Mentally Ill in the German Federal Republic)*. Bonn: Drucksache 12/4016.

Deutscher Verein für öffentliche und private Fürsorge (1990). *Hilfe für alleinstehende Wohnungslose (Nichtseßhafte). (Aid for the Homeless)*. Frankfurt/Main: Eigenverlag des Deutschen Vereins für öffentliche und private Fürsorge.

Eikelmann, B., Inhester, M. L. & Reker, T. (1992). Psychische Störungen bei nichtseßhaften Männern. Defizite in der psychiatrischen Versorgung. (Mental disorders in homeless men. Inadequacy in Psychiatric Care). *Sozialpsychiatrische Informationen*, **2**, 29–32.

Finzen, A. (1983). *Auf dem Dienstweg. Die Verstrickung einer Anstalt in die Tötung psychisch Kranker. (In the Line of Duty. The Involvement of an Asylum in the Killing of the Mentally Ill)*. Rehburg-Loccum: Psychiatrie-Verlag.

Garcia, C. (1986). Karl Wilmanns und die Landstreicher. (Karl Wilmanns and the vagrants). *Nervenarzt*, **57**, 227–32.

Goschler, W. (1983). Die alleinstehenden Wohnungslosen. (Homeless people). *Gefährdetenhilfe*, **25**, 7–14.

Haselbeck, H. (1985). Zur Sozialgeschichte der offenen Irrenfürsorge – Vom Stadtasyl zum Sozalpsychiatrischen Dienst. (On the social history of mental health care – the change from urban asylums to social-psychiatric services). *Psychiatrische Praxis*, **12**, 171–9.

Iben, G. (1989). Armut der Obdachlosen und Nichtseßhaften. (Poverty and the homeless). *Blätter der Wohlfahrtspflege*, **11/12**, 316–20.

Kluge, M. (1972). Nichtseßhaftigkeit aus der Sicht einer Arbeiterkolonie. (Homelessness from the viewpoint of a worker's commune). *Gefährdetenhilde*, **14**, 5–8.

Kujat, H. (1991). Der "immer wiederkehrende Patient" – aus der Sicht einer Einrichtung der Nichtseßhaftenhilfe. (A service for aiding the homeless and its view on the "perpetual patient"). *Sozialpsychiatrische Informationen*, **2**, 35–7.

Kunze, H. (1977). Psychiatrie-Reform zu Lasten der chronisch psychisch Kranken? Entwicklungstendenzen der stationären Versorgung chronisch psychisch Kranker in England, den USA und der Bundesrepublik Deutschland. (Psychiatric reform at the cost of the chronically mentally ill? Tendencies on the Development of hospital care of the chronically mentally ill in England, USA and the Federal Republic of Germany). *Nervenarzt*, **48**, 83–8.

LWV (Landeswohlfahrtsverband Württemberg-Hohenzollern und Landeswohlfahrtsverband Baden) (1993). *Fortschreibung der Kommunalen Konzeption zur Hilfe für alleinstehende Wohnungslose (Nichtseßhafte) in Baden-Würtemberg. (More on the Community Concept of Aid for the Homeless in Baden-Würtemberg, Germany)*. Stuttgart, Karlsruhe: LWV Württemberg-Hohenzollern/Baden.

Locher, G. (1990). *Gesundheits-/Krankheitsstatus und arbeitsbedingte Erkrankungen von alleinstehenden Wohnungslosen. (The Health Situation and the Work-related Illnesses of Homeless Persons)*. Bielefeld: Verlag Soziale Hilfe.

MAGS (Ministerium für Arbeit, Gesundheit und Sozialordnung Baden-Württemberg) (State Department for Health and Social Affairs, Baden-Württemberg) (1982). *Hilfen für Gefährdete und Nichtseßhafte in Baden-Württemberg. (Services for the Homeless and Those Threatened with Homelessness in Baden-Württemberg)*. Stuttgart: MAGS.

Rieger, J. & Wessel, T. (1992). Ambulante und stationäre Nichtseßhaftenhilfe: Endstation Armut – wohnungs- und arbeitslose Abhängigkeitskranke ohne Chance? (Outpatient and hospital aid for the homeless: destination poverty. Homeless and unemployed mentally ill persons suffering from an addiction – have they got a chance?) In G. Wienberg (ed.), *Die vergessene Mehrheit*, pp. 159–67. Bonn: Psychiatrie Verlag.

Ritzel, G. (1974). Entwicklung und gegenwärtiger Stand der psychiatrischen Nichtseßhaftenforschung. (The development and present state of psychiatric research on the homeless). *Psychiat. clin.*, **7**, 26–49.

Rössler, W., Häfner, H., Martini, H., an der Heiden, W., Jung, E. & Löffler, W. (1987). *Landesprogramm zur Weiterentwicklung der außerstationären psychiatrischen Versorgung Baden-Württemberg – Analysen, Konzepte, Erfahrungen. (Programme for the further Development of Community Mental Health Care in Baden-Württemberg –Analyses, Concepts, Experiences)*. Weinheim: Deutscher Studienverlag.

Rössler, W., Fätkenheuer, B. & Löffler, W. (1993). *Soziale Rehabilitation Schizophrener – Modell Sozialpsychiatrischer Dienst. (Social Rehabilitation of Schizophrenics – A Model for Socio-psychiatric Services)*. Stuttgart: Enke Verlag.

Rössler, W. & Salize, H. J. (1993). *Planungsmaterialien für die psychiatriche*

Versorgung. (*Data and Guidelines for Planning Mental Health Care*). Weinheim: Deutscher Studien Verlag.

Rössler, W. & Salize, H. J. (1994). Longitudinal statistics of mental health care in Germany. *Social Psychiatry and Psychiatric Epidemiology*, **29**, 112–18.

Schneider, K. (1934). *Die psychopathischen Persönlichkeiten.* (*Psychopathic Personalities*). Leipzig: Thieme Verlag.

Sperling, M. (1985). Medizinische Untersuchungen an 109 Nichtseßhaften Männern. (*Medical Examinations of 109 Homeless Men*). Medizinische Fakultät der Westfälischen Wilhelms-Universität: Inaugural-Dissertation. (Medical thesis for Wilhelms University in Westfalia).

Stadt Stuttgart (1976). *Hilfe für Gefährdete und Nichtseßhafte in Stuttgart.* (*Aid for the Homeless and Those Threatened with Homelessness in Stuttgart*) Stuttgart: Stadt Stuttgart.

Stößel, U. & Locher, G. (1991). Gesundheit und Krankheit bei alleinstehenden wohnungslosen Männern: Eine Sekundäranalyse von Daten einer diakonischen Einrichtung in der Bundesrepublik Deutschland. (Health and illness among homeless men: a secondary analysis of data gathered by a diakonic organization in the Federal Republic of Germany). *Soziale Präventivmedizin*, **36**, 327–32.

Susser, E., Struening, E. L. & Conover, S. (1989). Psychiatric problems in homeless men. Lifetime psychosis, substance use, and current distress in new arrivals at New York City Shelters. *Archives of General Psychiatry*, **46**, 845–50.

Trabert, G. (1995). Soziales Umfeld beeinflußt Gesundheitszustand. *Deutsches Ärzteblatt*, **92**, A.748–A.51.

Wilmanns, K. (1906). *Zur Psychopathologie des Landstreichers.* (*Psychopathology of Vagrants*). Leipzig: J. A. Barth-Verlag.

Veith, G. & Schwindt, W. (1976). *Von den Krankheiten der Nichtseßhaften.* (*On the Illness of the Homeless*). Bielefeld-Bethel: Beiträge aus der Arbeit der von Bodelschwinghschen Anstalten in Bielefeld-Bethel. Heft 16. (Number 16).

Homelessness: an Irish perspective

JOSEPH FERNANDEZ

This chapter on homelessness in Ireland is based largely on the study of and the work carried out among the homeless in Dublin. Although not typical of homelessness in Ireland, these studies and reports suggest some common themes applicable to issues related to homelessness across various centres. This chapter does not look at the rural homeless in Ireland.

Domestic perspectives

Identifying the homeless

Following the implementation of the Housing Act (Department for the Environment, 1988), an assessment of housing need was conducted by the Department of the Environment in 1989, wherein 987 homeless people were enumerated around the country. Disquiet among voluntary agencies about this serious undercounting prompted a refinement in methodology during subsequent assessments. Thus, 2751 individuals were found to be homeless nationwide in 1991; an increase of almost 180% on the previous figure (National Campaign for the Homeless, 1992) and 2667 individuals nationwide in 1993 (Department for the Environment, 1993).

The Republic of Ireland is populaced by approximately 3.5 million individuals (Central Statistics Office, 1993) and of these 5000 are believed to be homeless of whom 750 are young people (National Campaign for the Homeless, 1992). However, this finding excludes: (a) approximately 7400 travellers who move between halting sites countrywide (Barry & Daly, 1986) and technically have no fixed abode; (b) over 28 600 approved applicants on our housing lists (Department for the Environment, 1993) with approximately 32 000 child dependants; (c) over 4500 long-stay psychiatric inpatients (Health Research Board, 1993) who meet the criteria for homelessness specified in the Housing Act (Department for the Environment, 1988); and (d) a further unquantifiable number of 'hidden' homeless, e.g. single adults working as live-in domestics.

The present group of homeless includes: adult males and females at a ratio of approximately 4:1, an increasing number of children at a ratio of almost 1:1, and occasionally entire families.

Factors contributing to homelessness in the Republic of Ireland

Social factors

Notwithstanding strategies to down-size public perceptions of the problem (Gallagher, 1994) the average number of unemployed on the Live Register in 1993 was around 294 000 individuals (Central Statistics Office, 1994) or over 18% of the workforce, the second highest unemployment rate in the European Community (Statistical Office of the European Communities, 1994). Many are long-term unemployed and this 'subversive level of unemployment' (Connell, 1993, p. 2) is believed to lead to poverty and, in some cases, to homelessness.

Emigration

Emigration has for long served as a safety valve for Ireland's unemployment problem. However, given recent economic trends the world over, the number of people emigrating from the Republic (expressed as the net migration rate) has changed dramatically from minus 46 000 individuals in the year ending mid-April 1989 (National Economic and Social Council, 1991) to plus 2000 individuals in the year ending mid-April 1992 (Dáil Éireann, 1993) leading in the latter instance to an inward movement of migrants and/or returning emigrants. This has led to a growing demand for accommodation.

Lack of accommodation

The availability of low-cost rented accommodation is now being reduced by conversion and refurbishment into high-cost units (Kasinitz, 1984). People displaced from their low-cost accommodation are forced to consider other residential options. The latter include emergency accommodation in hostels and night shelters, sharing with friends and relatives, or 'squats' or 'sleeping rough'. Some homeless mentally ill are known to show either self-injurious or property-destructive behaviour to gain admission to hospital or to prison.

Closure of Casual Wards

The closure of 'Casual Wards' in rural areas has also added to the current homeless problems. County Homes were the progeny of Workhouses established countrywide, around the mid-1800s. In the course of their development, an area was set aside in County Homes, which came to be known as the casual or night-lodgers ward (Doherty, 1982). As late as 1949, County Homes were used as repositories for the chronically sick, the aged, mental defectives, the

blind, deaf mutes, casuals, unmarried mothers and children (Inter-
Departmental Committee, 1949). By the late 1960s, provisions were
made to unscramble the needs of many of the disadvantaged groups
in County Homes. In 1968, recommendations called for the redesig-
nation of County Homes as Geriatric Hospitals and casuals were
excluded from concern. The latter were seen to constitute a 'social
problem ... not an appropriate problem for consideration in connection with the care of the aged' (Department of Health, 1968, p. 32).

Conditions for the homeless did not improve following the reorganization of the national health-care system in the 1970s. The McKinsey Report (McKinsey & Co, 1974), which contributed to this
reorganization made no mention of the homeless and responsibility
for this 'social problem' was allocated to neither the Special Hospital
Care Programme nor the Community Care Programme within the
new area Health Boards.

Disinvestment in public housing

Progressive disinvestment in Local Authority housing is another
factor that has compounded the current problem of homelessness.
Thus, 7002 public housing units were completed nationwide in 1984
compared to 1482 units in 1992 (Department for the Environment,
1991, 1993). The government's decision to raise the level of housing
starts to 3500 a year nationwide – beginning in 1993 – does not reflect
the need of the Eastern Planning Region (including Dublin and its
dormitory surrounds), which contains 38% of the national population (Central Statistics Office, 1993).

Poverty, morbidity and the 'underclass'

The inter-relationship between long-term unemployment, poverty
and physical and psychological morbidity has been documented
(Nolan, 1990; Whelan et al., 1991) and the evidence augurs poorly for
marginalized individuals. Murray (1984) has promulgated the view
that long-term unemployment and poverty impact on the creation –
in deprived inner city areas – of an 'underclass' characterized by
widespread drug abuse, casual violence, petty crime, illegitimacy,
child neglect, work avoidance, welfare dependence, apparent con-
tempt for conventional values and homelessness.

Murray's observations (1984, 1989) were confined to developments in the USA and in the UK. However, related concerns are reflected in a study conducted by McKeown (1991) in the north inner city of Dublin, wherein it was noted that: (a) the admission rate of children into care was four times higher than the national average, (b) the admission rate to public psychiatric hospitals was three times the national average, (c) the attendance rate for the treatment of drug abuse was three times the national average per head of population and (d) the crime rate was four times the Dublin Metropolitan Area average and eight times the national average.

Homeless children

The Committee on Reformatory and Industrial Schools (1970) recommended that monolithic institutions then catering for children who were being reared 'in care' be replaced by smaller home-style units, with the result that 1500 institutional places were lost by 1983. Individuals above the age of 16 years were discouraged from leaving care facilities under the provisions of the antiquated Children Act of 1908. Notwithstanding this, the visibility of homeless children started increasing, notably in cities around Ireland, and by 1983 it was felt that a young homeless class was emerging (National Youth Policy Committee, 1984). The Children Act of 1908 has been replaced by the Child Care Act (1991) in which the legal definition of a child has been raised to 18 years and legal responsibility for the accommodation needs of homeless children is placed on area Health Boards. It is too early to evaluate the impact of this legislation on youth homelessness but the increasing use of 'bed and breakfast' accommodation is not felt to represent a legitimate response to the needs of this group.

Surveys conducted around the country in 1987 revealed the presence of 712 homeless children nationwide below the age of 18 years (Streetwise National Coalition, 1988). Media concern about the lack of detention facilities for juvenile offenders – many of them homeless – is matched by related concern about the lack of adolescent psychiatric residential facilities for the same population (Streetwise National Coalition, 1991). However, very little is known about the prevalence of psychiatric morbidity among homeless children in the Republic of Ireland.

Homeless females

Females are believed to be victims of their unequal position in society and homeless females epitomize this discrepant situation (Kennedy, 1985). Older homeless females are known to live in direct access hostels while younger females either stay with friends or remain in unstable and unsuitable relationships (Austerberry & Watson, 1983) until a major domestic crisis and/or repeated physical violence force them to seek help (Bell, 1989).

Homeless women are known to experience high rates of psychiatric morbidity (Marshall & Reed 1992; Scott 1991; also see Chapter 5). In recent years the admission rate of homeless females to urban psychiatric hospitals has increased; against a background of disproportionate under-provision for this group in direct access hostels, refuges and night shelters (Kelleher et al., 1992). It is felt that the number of homeless females identified in psychiatric hospitals in any given year is an underestimate. Homelessness in females tends to be 'hidden', as many of them are inclined to stay with friends and relatives and to use their latter address as one of convenience.

Homeless families

Very little is known about the extent or severity of psychological distress among homeless families in the Republic of Ireland.

The prison service

There is a consensus that more mental illness is arriving in the prison system (Royal College of Psychiatrists, 1993). The practice of diverting mentally ill homeless petty offenders from custody to treatment, though widely used elsewhere (Joseph & Potter, 1990; Cooke, 1991), has yet to be accorded formal acceptance in the Republic of Ireland.

Deinstitutionalization in urban settings

Strategies aimed at rehabilitation and the discharge of patients to community living were in vogue long before the formal recommendations of successive Commissions of Inquiry on Mental Handicap and Mental Illness (Department of Health, 1965, 1966). However, the climate in which *The Psychiatric Services – Planning for the Future* (Department of Health, 1984) came to be conceptualized and accompanying shifts of responsibility to facilitate resource management provided the impetus for 'resettlement' and the present dismantling of antiquated institutions. Unlike the Italian experience (Endean, 1993) it is not possible to establish a clear relationship between the discharge of patients from psychiatric hospitals and the incidence of homelessness, except in Dublin (Leahy & Magee, 1976). However, from the late 1980s onwards, the waters get muddied (Fernandez, 1983).

Thus far, policies aimed at dismantling institutions have ensured that positive bias is exercised in making available such sheltered or supervised accommodation as exists to the 'new deserving poor', namely those old, long-stay patients who are deemed capable of being relocated outside of hospital. Given this, it is felt that many long-term homeless mentally ill are forced to resort to emergency social accommodation for their permanent abode. For the latter, remaining homeless is a decision mediated not by 'personal choices' but by a lack of statutory responses to their need. Deinstitutionalization and the concomitant reduction in bed numbers had led – as elsewhere – to policies and practices that emphasize preclusive admissions and accelerated discharges. In consequence, the younger homeless mentally ill of today have long histories of brief intermittent patient-hood rather than of prolonged institutional residence.

An answer to Leff's (1993) query about where today's homeless come from could perhaps be found among the foregoing interlocking structural conditions, which are believed to exacerbate individual vulnerabilities. Regrettably, some politicians view homelessness as a psychiatric problem rather than a consequence of policies that marginalize people and exclude the poor from housing. Psychiatric services cannot be unconditionally expected to cater for the casualties of other interlocking systems (Fernandez, 1994). Given this, the issue of homelessness needs to be locked firmly into the political arena and psychiatric aspects of this problem should ideally be tackled together with the general problem (Birley, 1990). Though government must provide the right framework to facilitate social change, the role of the churches in Ireland cannot be ignored (Editorial, 1989). Church leaders have recently begun to question the perceptions of the government and the laity on social justice (e.g. Connell, 1993), while reassessing their own role in building family and community values. Demands from church leaders for the government 'to do something' about almost everything does not, in the Republic of Ireland, betray their 'inability to do much about anything' (Editorial, 1989, p. 2), but will necessitate a focused and concerted lead from the centre.

A survey in Ireland

A prospective survey was conducted from 1 January through to 31 December 1978 in St. Brendan's Hospital, Dublin. A total of 425 psychiatric admissions (313 male and 112 female) were referred for review but 169 admissions (106 male and 63 female) were excluded, as they did not meet specified criteria, or had left hospital before they could be assessed (Fernandez, 1984, 1985). A total of 256 admissions (207 male and 49 female) were included in the survey. Relevant findings have been summarized in Table 12.3, wherein the characteristics of this group, including gender-specific differences are evident.

Outcome of the Irish initiative

On 1 April 1979, the Programme for the Homeless was initiated, to run in tandem with the concurrently established Assessment Service and Geriatric Service in St. Brendan's Hospital. Operationally is was anticipated that:

1. Homeless patients who needed help in an emergency would be screened by the Assessment Service.
2. Homeless females who needed hospitalization, would be treated in the admission wards of the hospital's three catchment area teams on a rotational basis.
3. Homeless males over the age of 65 years would be referred to the Geriatric Service.

4. Homeless males who met the criteria for 'homelessness' would be referred to the Programme.
5. If admission was considered necessary, this would be to the programme's Admission Unit.
6. Patients discharged from the Admission Unit would, in the first instance, be returned to their customary residence in the city's direct access hostels.
7. Such patients would be offered the option of attending the programme's Day Centre in the grounds of the hospital. The latter facility would also be available to those for whom day care was felt to be more appropriate than hospitalization.

Unless stated otherwise, all hospital based facilities described hereafter and the outcomes specified, refer only to homeless males.

Characteristic problems noted when dealing with homeless persons include the following:

1. Some patients use aliases when entering hospital, leading to multiple hospital charts under different names; difficulty in obtaining medical records from other hospitals and follow-up problems thereafter.
2. Given the solitary nature of our patients' life-styles and their lack of social networks, it is often impossible to obtain any collateral history. Hence, one has to rely solely on any given patient's version of events, without an opportunity for further validation.
3. Many patients are anxious to leave hospital before their treatment is satisfactorily concluded; for fear of losing temporary rented accommodation they may have, or because of equally significant concerns about an interruption in their welfare entitlements following hospital entry. For these patients, leaving hospital – sometimes against medical advice – is often seen by them as a necessary strategy for survival in the community.

The admission unit: outcome

Figure 12.3 summarizes the impact the hospital based components have had on the annual admission rates of homeless males from 1979/80 onwards, relative to those over the 4 years prior to the introduction of the Programme and supporting services.

Table 12.4 summarizes other relevant data relating to:

Table 12.3. *Prospective survey of homeless patients (1978)*

Main findings	Males (%)	Females (%)
1. Age on entry[a]		
(a) 18–30 years	20.9	28.6
(b) 31–50 years	62.6	53.6
(c) 51–65 years	16.5	17.8
2. Median age on entry (in years)[a]	40.5	37.0
3. Marital status[a]		
(a) Single: unmarried	73.9	64.3
(b) Single: separated/divorced	3.5	21.5
(c) Single: widower/widow	2.6	7.1
(d) Married	19.1	7.1
(e) No data available	0.9	Nil
4. Having no dependants[a]	89.6	64.3
5. Having relatives but no contact with them[a]	80.0	89.3
6. Occupation[a]		
(a) Unskilled manual/factory workers	60.0	50.0
(b) Semi-skilled workers	21.8	10.7
(c) Skilled workers	13.0	7.1
(d) Retired from work with a pension/disability benefit	3.4	Nil
(e) Housewives	—	17.9
(f) No stated occupation (M) or in an unregistered profession (F)	0.9	14.3
(g) No data available	0.9	Nil
7. Currently unemployed[a]	91.3	71.4
8. Length of unemployment prior to hospitalization[a]		
Range in months	0.5–375	1.5–101[b]
Median in months	24.5	40.5[b]
9. Having a current medical card[a]	17.4	39.3
10. History of multiple admissions to psychiatric hospitals in the past[a]	70.4	85.7
11. Entered hospital voluntarily[c]	90.0	77.5
12. Compulsorily hospitalized[c]	10.0	22.5
13. Stated reason for admission[c]		
(a) Psychiatric problems	45.0	30.6
(b) Psychiatric ± medical ± social problems	48.8	59.2
(c) Medical ± social problems	6.2	10.2
14. Primary problem/condition that needed attention[c]		
(a) Alcohol dependence	46.0	4.1
(b) Schizophrenic/affective and other psychoses	33.3	34.7
(c) Mainly social problems	7.2	10.2
(d) Alcohol + drug dependence	4.3	Nil
(e) Depressive disorder	2.9	14.3
(f) Dementia	1.9	Nil
(g) Epilepsy	1.9	Nil
(h) Mainly medical problems	1.5	Nil
(i) Personality disorder (in those not belonging to any of the above subgroups)	1.0	36.7

Table 12.3. (*cont.*)

Main findings	Males (%)	Females (%)
15. Welfare benefits[a]		
(a) On welfare benefits	55.6	39.3
(b) Not on any benefits	17.4	10.7
(c) No information forthcoming or no data available	27.0	50.0
16. Length of hospitalization[c]		
(a) Range of days	0.5–293	0.5–345
(b) Median in days	9.1	10.5
17. Mode of discharge[c]		
(a) Discharged by staff	81.0	61.2
(b) Absconded from hospital or self-discharged	12.6	22.5
(c) Still in hospital during survey	3.0	8.2
(d) No data available	3.4	6.1
(e) Died during survey	Nil	2.0
18. Number of admissions during 1978[a]		
(a) Range of admissions	1–7	1–5
(b) Median number of admissions	4	3
(c) Percentage of patients having only one admission during 1978	60.9	60.7

[a] $n=115$ male and 28 female patients.
[b] These figures refer to only 14 females. The remaining 14 patients in this group were excluded (a) by virtue of their being 'housewives' or 'ex-housewives' who were not in employment since their marriage, separation or widowhood, or (b) because some patients could not recall when they last worked, or (c) because some were in an unregistered profession.
[c] $n=207$ male and 49 female admissions.

1. The range of annual admissions per patient.
2. The median number of admissions per patient. This shows a significant drop from the base-line of four admissions annually, prior to the inception of the Programme (see Table 12.3, no 18b), but appears to be reverting towards base rate over the latter years.
3. The number of patients who had only one admission annually dropped from an average of 70% during the first 7 years of the Programme to 59.06% during the latter 7 years.
4. On average, the Programme had approximately 42 'new contact' referrals annually who had to be hospitalized. If one excludes those patients who entered the Programme in 1979/80 when all entrants would have represented new contacts, the number of new contacts dropped from an average of 50 new contacts annually

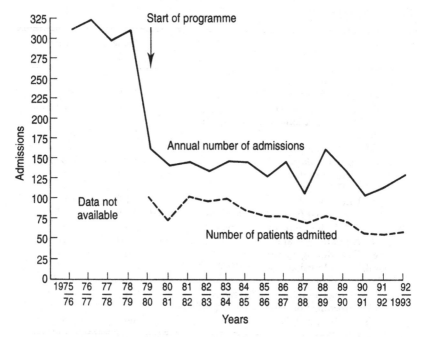

Figure 12.3. Annual admission rate (homeless men).

over the first 6 years thereafter to around 25 new contacts annually over the last 6 years.

When translated into service related issues, the foregoing figures suggest that the annual number of admissions per patient is increasing, while the number of new contacts is decreasing. The latter finding is not surprising given the fact that (a) some new contacts were deflected from hospitalization through our Day Care facility and (b) the criteria for inclusion in the Programme had to be raised from the year 1989/90 onwards, to include a stay of 3 months in direct access hostels in the city, so as to prevent an off-loading (of overnight or short-stay) hostel occupants on to our Programme.

The day centre: operational aspects

Patients discharged from our Admission Unit are encouraged to attend at our Day Centre in the hospital grounds, which has full

Table 12.4. *Programme for the homeless (admission unit): Audit of admissions (1979/80 to 1992/93)*

	Years													
	79/80	80/81	81/82	82/83	83/84	84/85	85/86	86/87	87/88	88/89	89/90	90/91	91/92	92/93
Range of admissions	1-8	1-8	1-6	1-6	1-5	1-7	1-6	1-9	1-5	1-8	1-7	1-7	1-6	1-9
Median re: admissions	1	1	1	1	1	2	2	2	2	3	1	1	3	3
Percentage of patients with one admission annually	67.96	60.53	79.81	76.77	70.87	67.03	67.07	58.02	67.6	57.83	58.21	57.38	60.34	54.09
New contacts	103	+42	+78	+46	+60	+39	+34	+38	+29	+30	+33	+19	+22	+16

Table 12.5. *Programme for the homeless: Outcome data (1/4/79 to 31/3/93)*

	Number of patients
(A) Patients serviced	
Through Admission Unit and Day Centre	589 (1937 admissions)
Through Day Centre with no admission	+51
Total	640
(B) Known deaths	53 (8.28%)
(C) Re-united with family and/or returned to former domicile	20
(Ireland × 8; England & Wales × 9; Italy × 1; South Africa × 1; India × 1).	
(D) Replaced/retained in institutional settings	46
(E) Placed in community based supervised settings	46
(F) Placed in the community (+ Day Centre support)	54
Dublin Corporation flats	24
Other city flats/bedsitters	28
Supervised lodgings	2
(G) Screening for tuberculosis	
Tuberculosis discovered in	15 (2.34%)

nursing cover from 8.00 a.m. to 8.30 p.m. each day. Facilities and services available in the Day Centre include the following: meals, medication, contact with medical staff, follow-up of other outstanding matters e.g. medical tests, appointments in other city hospitals and contact with welfare agencies, a 'Follow-up Service' in the community to track infrequent attenders, a 'Money-Management Service' for those who are unable to handle their finances, along with emergency dockets for accommodation in city hostels, facilities for bathing and 'launderette' facilities.

The day centre: outcome

It was originally intended to cater for 36 attenders at our Day Centre. However, unanticipated uptake has ensured that the average number of day attenders ranges from 70 upwards and, in more recent months, this number has risen further. The high and regular attendance rate endorses the need to ensure that homeless mentally ill who are being maintained in the community are routinely provided with access to comprehensive day care facilities; a recurring theme, made evident by examination of different aspects of the needs of our population.

Outcome data

Table 12.5 summarizes outcome data relating to all individuals who passed through the two hospital based components of our Programme. Attention is drawn to the high mortality rate of our patients, i.e. 8.28%, and this refers only to 'known deaths'. Thus, few of the homeless patients in our Programme are felt likely to achieve sufficient seniority to avail themselves of psychiatric services for the elderly.

Data presented at (D), (E) and (F) in Table 12.5 represent a snapshot of placements at the time these were made. The extreme mobility of our population, even among those retained in institutional settings, does not guarantee their current presence in the stated locations. However, all attempts have been made to ensure that patients were not counted-in more than once in the groups reported.

Incidence of tuberculosis

Results of the National Tuberculosis Survey in the Republic of Ireland indicate that the incidence rate of tuberculosis in the 26 Counties at 21.37 new cases per 100 000 population is the highest in Western Europe and is twice that of Great Britain and Northern Ireland (Stinson *et al.*, 1988; Fogarty, 1991). Data presented at (G) in Table 12.5 indicate that tuberculosis was detected in 2.34% of our homeless population. When patients are known to be infected and infective, provisions exist to ensure their removal, but none to guarantee that they remain in specialist hospitals for treatment of their condition, until they are free from infectivity. This poses a particular problem in the management of subgroups of the homeless mentally ill, notably those with a history of alcohol and drug dependence.

High prevalence rates for tuberculosis have also been reported in the USA among homeless populations; notably among homeless urban alcoholics. A linear relationship is believed to exist between the prevalence of tuberculosis and the length of homelessness, with substance abusers including alcoholics, emerging as the most vulnerable (Brickner *et al.*, 1984).

Community based components

Apart from the two hospital based components, i.e. the Admission Unit and the Day Centre, our Programme now has three community components which include (a) a High-Support hostel with 24 hour nursing cover for ten residents and eight day attenders, (b) a Rehabilitation Programme that caters for 22 residents and 10 day attenders and (c) a supervised group home for five residents.

Outcome data relating to our patients over the last 14 years (see Table 12.5 (D)) indicate that 7.19% of programme participants had to be retained in institutional settings because of their presumed 'inability to survive' outside of hospital or because of 'dangerousness'. If this decision was appropriate in only 10% of these cases, the recommended guidelines for 'new long-stay' beds (Department of Health, 1984), would be seriously breached in urban catchment areas where the prevalence of homelessness is high.

Day care and accommodation needs

The unexpectedly high attendance rate at our Day Centre has been mentioned earlier. Likewise, the closure of our hospital's inpatient unit for those suffering from alcohol addiction, without the parallel provision of detoxification services for homeless alcoholics, has led to a situation wherein outpatient detoxification often has to be conducted in the Day Centre for ex-patients who reside in direct access hostels.

Other difficulties in our Programme relate to the range, the availability and the quality of accommodation deemed necessary to cater for existing demands. Night shelters and direct access hostels offer a necessary, though temporary, solution to the problems of individuals who insist on asserting their autonomy in a palpably destructive fashion. Voluntary organizations that provide and staff the majority of hostel and shelter beds in the country would be among the first to acknowledge that such hostels are part of the problem of homelessness and not one of its solutions, since their availability is felt to deter statutory services from providing appropriate residential alternatives in the community (Fernandez, 1993).

Nor, for that matter, does a solution to the problem lie in the provision of unsupervised accommodation, helpful though this option may be for a minuscule number capable of independent living. For the majority, it is felt that graded, supervised, sheltered community settings are necessary, with access to day facilities and a range of properly funded and co-ordinated ancillary services (Talbot & Lamb, 1984).

Under the provisions of the Health Act of 1953, area Health Boards are required to provide institutional assistance, i.e. access to both hospital and to community based alternatives, to persons who are unable to provide shelter and assistance for themselves. The Housing Act (Department for the Environment, 1988) gives Local Authorities the enabling power – but does not oblige them to provide emergency and long-term accommodation for homeless persons, as defined by the Act. This confusion about responsibility for the shelter needs of the homeless mentally ill needs to be resolved. Likewise, statutory services would do well to examine the limits of their respective responsibilities and harmonize attempts at service delivery – lest Community Care 'deserve the odium now attached to the worst practices of former times' (Wing, 1990, p. 822).

'Planning for the future'

Planning for the Future (Department of Health, 1984), which addresses the present and anticipated needs of the mentally ill in the Republic of Ireland, devoted a mere 26 lines in its 138 pages to the needs of the homeless. The conceptionalization offered fuels the unsubstantiated belief that the local universe of the homeless is populaced mainly by 'vagrant alcoholics' (Department of Health, 1984, p. 111) when there was compelling local evidence (O'Hare, 1978, 1983) to suggest that in this group, diagnoses of schizophrenia (33.8%) and other psychoses (15.6%) outweighed that of alcoholism and alcoholic psychosis (32.3%). The only recommendations made were that 'Health Boards should co-operate with voluntary organizations in providing special services for homeless alcoholics' (Department of Health, 1984, p. 119), and that 'some homeless people will need to avail [themselves] of the alcoholism service and day facilities provided by the psychiatric service' (Department of Health, 1984, p. 111).

Changes in legislation catering for the mentally ill and derivative recommendations are long overdue. Unless there has been a radical reappraisal of the needs of the homeless mentally ill over the last

decade, it is improbable that initial misperceptions will serendipitous-
ly translate into adequate provision.

Conclusion

When Community Care was being proselytized, a theme repeatedly
emphasized was the provision of community based alternatives to
institutional care (Department of Health, 1966, 1984). An equally
important theme, namely the provision of adequate funding to
support proposed developments, was less forcefully presented. The
former theme has now evolved into a major symphonic work
(Murphy, 1991) while the latter is barely audible.

Recent evidence suggests that the percentage of the public health
services budget allocated to psychiatric care in the Republic of
Ireland has fallen from 13.5% in 1971 to 10.1% in 1992 and is
estimated to have dropped further to 9.8% in 1993 (Institute of
Public Administration, 1993). Psychiatrists and their colleagues who
work in the public sector derive comfort from neither the statistical
validation of known misery, nor the curiously confusing commenta-
ries on the funding of services (Editorial, 1990; Walsh, 1994). Public
psychiatric patients have for long been placed on the lowest rung of
the ladder of health-need, and the homeless mentally ill who form a
subset of this group are inevitably left holding the ladder, while their
domiciled and politically more valuable peers are facilitated to
ascend.

References

Austerberry, H. & Watson, S. (1983). *Women on the Margins*. London:
    City University Housing Group.
Barry, J. & Daly, L. (1986). *The Travellers' Health Status Study*. Dublin:
    The Health Research Board.
Bell, J. (1989). *Women and Children First*. Dublin: National Campaign for
    the Homeless.
Birley, J. (1990). Blame homelessness, not the hospitals. *The Guardian*, 14
    March, p. 21.
Brickner, P. W., Filardo, T. Iseman, M., Green, R., Conanan, B. &
    Elvy, A. (1984). Medical aspects of homelessness. In *The Homeless
    Mentally Ill*, H. R. Lamb (ed.), pp. 243–55. Washington, DC:
    American Psychiatric Association.

Central Statistics Office (1993). *Census 91*, vol. 1. Dublin: Stationery Office.

Central Statistics Office (1994). *Economic Series, Monthly, February.* Dublin: Stationery Office.

Child Care Act (1991). *An Act to Provide for the Care and Protection of Children and for Related matters.* Dublin: Stationery Office.

Committee on Reformatory and Industrial Schools (1970). *Report on the Reformatory and Industrial Schools System.* Dublin: Stationery Office.

Connell, D. (1993). *Address of His Grace, Archbishop Desmond Connell DD, on the Occasion of the Public Launch of Crosscare, September.* Dublin: Catholic Social Service Conference.

Cooke, D. J. (1991). Treatment as an alternative to prosecution: offenders diverted from treatment. *British Journal of Psychiatry*, **158**, 785–91.

Dáil Éireann (1993). Dáil Éireann, Debates, 4 May, vol. 430, p. 45.

Department for the Environment (1988). *Housing Act.* Dublin: Stationery Office.

Department for the Environment (1991). *A Plan for Social Housing.* Dublin: Stationery Office.

Department for the Environment (1993). *Housing Statistics Bulletin. September Quarter.* Dublin: Stationery Office.

Department of Health (1965). *Commission of Inquiry on Mental Handicap. A Report.* Dublin: Stationery Office.

Department of Health (1966). *Commission of Inquiry on Mental Illness. A Report.* Dublin: Stationery Office.

Department of Health (1968). *The Care of the Aged.* Dublin: Stationery Office.

Department of Health (1984). *The Psychiatric Services – Planning for the Future. A Report.* Dublin: Stationery Office.

Doherty, V. (1982). *Closing down the County Homes.* Dublin: Simon Community.

Editorial (1989). The British underclass. *The Sunday Times.* News Focus: Opinion, 26 November, p. B2.

Editorial (1990). Capital funding for psychiatry. *Irish Journal of Psychiatry*, **11**, 2.

Endean, C. (1993). Italy retreats from community care for the mentally ill. *British Medical Journal*, **306**, 605.

Fernandez, J. (1983). Who cares for the NFA's? *Proceedings of the Conference on Homelessness, September 1983.* Dublin: Simon Community.

Fernandez, J. (1984). In Dublin's fair city: the mentally ill of no fixed abode. *Bulletin of the Royal College of Psychiatrists*, **8**, 187–90.

Fernandez, J. (1985). On planning a service for the homeless mentally ill in Dublin. *International Journal of Family Psychiatry*, **6**, 149–63.

Fernandez, J. (1993). Tide of suffering on indifferent streets. *The Sunday Times* (Irish edit.), Platform: Opinion, 19 September, sect. 4, p. 5.

Fernandez, J. (1994). Psychiatric services for the homeless mentally ill. *Health Services News*, **6**, 14.

Fogarty, J. (1991). Chemoprophylaxis for tuberculosis: a review. *Irish Doctor*, **4**, 931–4.

Gallagher, J. (1994). Unemployment: The crisis, the clichés, the 'cures'. *The Irish Times*, 15 January, p. 6.

Health Research Board (1993). *The Irish Psychiatric Hospitals and Units Census 1991*. Dublin: The Health Research Board.

Inter-Departmental Committee (1949). *Report on County Homes*. Dublin: Stationery Office.

Institute of Public Administration (1993). *Health Expenditure in Ireland*. Health Fact Sheet 7/93. Dublin: Institute of Public Administration.

Joseph, P. L. & Potter, M. (1990). Mentally disordered offenders – diversion from custody. *Health Trends*, **2**, 51–3.

Kasinitz, P. (1984). Gentrification and homelessness: the single room occupancy and inner city revival. *Urban and Social Change Review*, **17**, 9–14.

Kelleher, C., Kelleher, P. & McCarthy, P. (1992). *Focus on Hostels: Patterns of Hostel Use in Dublin*. Dublin: Focus Point.

Kennedy, S. (1985). *But Where Can I Go? Homeless Women in Dublin*. Dublin: Arlen House.

Leahy, A. & Magee, D. (1976). *A Medical Service for Single Homeless People in the City of Dublin*. Dublin: Trust.

Leff, J. (1993). All the homeless people – where do they all come from? *British Medical Journal*, **306**, 669–70.

McKeown, K. (1991). *The North Inner City of Dublin: An Overview*. Dublin: Daughters of Charity.

McKinsey & Co. (1974). *Restructuring the Department of Health and Public Service: The Separation of Policy and Execution*. Dublin: Stationery Office.

Marshall, J. E. & Reed, J. L. (1992). Psychiatric morbidity in homeless women. *British Journal of Psychiatry*, **160**, 761–8.

Murphy, E. (1991). Community mental health services: a vision for the future. *British Medical Journal*, **302**, 1064–5.

Murray, C. (1984). *Losing Ground: American Social Policy 1950–1980*. New York: Basic Books Inc.

Murray, C. (1989). Underclass. *The Sunday Times*, Magazine Section, 26 November, pp. 26–46.

National Economic and Social Council (1991). *The Economic and Social Implications of Emigration*. Dublin: National Economic and Social Council.

National Youth Policy Committee (1984). *Final Report*. Dublin: Stationery Office.

National Campaign for the Homeless (1992). *Promises, Promises. An Assessment of the Effectiveness of the Housing Act 1988 in Housing Homeless People in Ireland*. Dublin: National Campaign for the Homeless.

Nolan, B. (1990). *Public Provision, Insurance and Health Service Utilization in Ireland*. Dublin: The Economic and Social Research Institute.

O'Hare, A. (1978). *Mental Illness and the Homeless.* Dublin: Simon Community.

O'Hare, A. (1983). Provision of care for the mentally ill homeless in Ireland. *Irish Journal of Psychiatry,* **4,** 12–23.

Royal College of Psychiatrists (1993). *Report on the Position of Psychiatry in the Republic of Ireland, 1992.* CR 23. London: Royal College of Psychiatrists.

Scott, J. (1991). Resettlement units or asylum? *Abstracts of Proceedings of Meetings of the Royal College of Psychiatrists. Psychiatric Bulletin,* **Supplement 4,** 61.

Statistical Office of the European Communities (1994). Unemployment in the European Union. In *Unemployment, Monthly, March.* Luxembourg: Eurostat.

Stinson, J., Kelly, P., Howell, F. & Clancy, L. (1988). National tuberculosis survey (1986). *Irish Medical Journal,* **81,** 7–10.

Streetwise National Coalition (1988). *A National Survey of Young People Out of Home in Ireland.* Dublin: Streetwise National Coalition.

Streetwise National Coalition (1991). *At What Cost? A Research Study on Residential Care for Children and Adolescents in Ireland.* Dublin: Focus Point.

Talbot, J. A. & Lamb, H. R. (1984). Summary and recommendations. In H. R. Lamb (ed.), *The Homeless Mentally Ill,* pp. 1–10. Washington, DC: American Psychiatric Association.

Walsh, D. (1994). Letters to the Editor. *Irish Medical Times,* 11 February, p. 4.

Whelan, C. T., Hannan, D. F. & Creighton, S. (1991). *Unemployment, Poverty and Psychological Distress.* Dublin: The Economic and Social Research Institute.

Wing, J. K. (1990). The functions of asylum. *British Journal of Psychiatry,* **157,** 822–7.

13

Lessons from America: semantics and services for mentally ill homeless individuals

Leona L. Bachrach

It has been noted that, in the practice of medicine, words have a profound effect on the conceptualization of patients' needs, the planning of services and the evaluation of programmes and systems of care (Robb-Smith, 1978). The field of psychiatry is no exception. In fact, the words used to formulate mental health policy and promote service planning in the USA often have imprecise referents and frequently reflect a vagueness of concept that may be harmful to the care of patients (Hardin, 1957; Campbell, 1981; Bachrach, 1985, 1988b,c, 1994b; Talbott, 1985; Fink, 1988). This has, at times, caused serious problems for the most severely mentally ill individuals; and it extends to those within this population who, in addition to suffering from major mental illnesses, are also homeless.

Following Hardin's (1957) advice that 'language should periodically be put on trial', this chapter discusses some semantic issues that affect our concepts of treatment for, and our delivery of services to, these vulnerable individuals. Primary attention is given to those problems that interfere with our efforts to delimit the mentally ill homeless population and to provide services that respond to its unique requirements. Although the major focus here is on service development within the USA, many of the derivative lessons are applicable to other countries where, with the implementation of deinstitutionalization policy, mentally ill homeless people are becoming increasingly visible (Schmidt, 1992).

The meaning of homelessness

The word 'homeless' is often used as if there is agreement about its meaning, when, in fact, it refers to a variety of events (Bachrach,

1992; US General Accounting Office, 1992; and see Chapter 3). Morrison (1989) has documented some of the confusion surrounding this word by applying various definitions found in the research literature to a population of psychiatric patients living in short-stay residences in San Francisco. His finding that homelessness rates ranged from 22% to 57% of the total study population depending on the specific definition employed led him to conclude that 'homelessness is by no means a unitary concept; definition is key'.

Indeed, confusion over the meaning of homelessness is sufficiently widespread in English-speaking countries that some advocacy groups in Great Britain have introduced the concept of 'houselessness' in contradistinction to 'homelessness' (Bailey, 1977). While 'houselessness' may be understood to imply a simple lack of physical residence such as one might incur if his or her home is destroyed by fire or a natural catastrophe, 'homelessness' is reserved for conditions of more generalized deprivation. The implication here is that a simple lack of shelter is, by itself, not sufficient to render an individual homeless: that a degree of social isolation or disaffiliation is equally essential to the definition.

The absence of physical residence thus represents but one part of a two-part equation that underlies the concept of homelessness; the absence of resources and community ties – of sufficient social margin to reverse this physical condition – is the other. In fact, Liebow (1993) has reported that some homeless persons prefer to consider themselves 'familyless' rather than 'homeless', thus stressing the disaffiliation portion of the equation over the absence of housing.

Although the vast literature on homelessness in the USA acknowledges in a general sense that both parts of the equation are essential to the definition of homelessness (Bachrach, 1992), research and other working definitions found within that literature are somewhat less fastidious. There is a distinct gap between the theoretical and the practical; and, generally speaking, working definitions are based primarily on place of residence. More subtle variables that might reflect some degree of social isolation are largely ignored, even though this is a variable that is acknowledged to affect the service needs of mentally ill individuals greatly (Susser *et al.*, 1990). In a practical sense, then, disaffiliation is treated as a minor, if not extraneous, term in the equation.

This uni-dimensional focus on whether an individual is domiciled or undomiciled is, however, but one of several difficulties that we encounter in attempting to define homelessness; the need to establish temporal parameters is also frequently overlooked. Thus, although it would seem obvious that we must ask how long the disaffiliation and absence of housing must endure for a person to be declared homeless, most working definitions are cross-sectional: they ask whether an individual is undomiciled at the moment that he or she is being screened for inclusion in research or is being considered for placement in a particular programme.

That such inattention to the durational aspects of homelessness may provide a biased view of the population is reflected in the results of research conducted in Tucson, Arizona. A study of individuals using psychiatric emergency services in that city demonstrated that the number of homeless people in a research population can be increased by 50% when a slight longitudinal refinement is introduced into the definition of homelessness (Santiago *et al.*, 1988). Thus, 22% of people using psychiatric emergency services could be classified as homeless if asked where they were living at the time of admission, but 33% could be so classified if asked whether they had lived on the streets, in a shelter, or in an automobile at some time during the preceeding 3 months. Although the investigators in that study called for standardization in defining homeless people, little progress has been made in this regard to date.

To add to this confusion, having a home does not constitute a variable with binary values: housed or not housed. Rossi *et al.* (1987) have, for example, distinguished people who are 'literally' homeless from those who are precariously housed and thus at immediate risk for becoming homeless. Roth & Bean (1986) have also developed a three-part typology of homelessness based on service use patterns within shelters for homeless people.

It is little wonder that service planners and providers often find themselves at cross purposes when they speak about the 'homeless population'! In the USA many conferences have been held, and numerous grants have been conferred, toward the end of improving the life circumstances of homeless individuals, with little if any concern expressed over the subtle differences that characterize the persons so designated. Furthermore, even though 'homeless' is an adjective with a variety of referents, policymakers do not appear at all constrained from planning services for 'homeless people' as if they are all alike.

Such practical indifference to the diversity of homeless individuals stands in direct contrast to a basic principle of programme planning in mental health: that services must be specifically fashioned for carefully designated and circumscribed target populations (Bachrach & Lamb, 1989).

Mental illness and homelessness

These problems that attend our imprecision in defining homelessness are compounded when we attempt to plan services for the mentally ill portion of the homeless population; for defining mental illness, particularly chronic or long-term mental illness, contributes its own set of special issues. Under the best of circumstances, there is a distinct absence of consensus regarding who is chronically mentally ill (Bachrach, 1988b); under conditions of homelessness this problem is vastly exaggerated (Snow *et al.*, 1988; Barrow *et al.*, 1989). As Snow *et al.* (1986) have noted, certain behaviours and characteristics prevalent among homeless people, such as inappropriate affect and appearance, depressed mood, agitation and unresponsiveness, may in fact be 'adaptive responses to the arduous nature of life on the streets or patterned manifestations of a subculture or way of life different from the larger normative order'. Moreover, as Baxter & Hopper (1982) have asserted, it can be extremely difficult to establish the presence of psychopathology in individuals who are suffering extreme physical deprivation: with 'several nights of sleep, an adequate diet, and warm social contact, some of their symptoms might subside'.

Establishing valid criteria for identifying mentally ill homeless persons is thus an extremely complex endeavour. However, what is even more damaging to conceptual clarity in this instance is a frank reluctance on the part of many service planners and caregivers to give credence to the existence of mental illness as a major variable affecting the lives of some homeless people (Snow *et al.*, 1986; Culhane, 1991; Mossman & Perlin, 1992; Liebow, 1993). There is a widely held perception that poverty is the defining characteristic of homelessness, and that its ramifications are so powerful that it somehow neutralizes the consequences of mental illness (Snow *et al.*, 1986; Adelson, 1991; Enda, 1993). There is also a closely related notion that separating those homeless individuals who are mentally ill from those who are not is an invidious process that is tantamount to 'blaming the victim' (Alters, 1986).

Two American psychiatrists, Cohen & Thompson (1992), have

written a Commentary for the *American Journal of Psychiatry*, in which they passionately argue that the dichotomy between the general homeless and mentally ill homeless populations is 'illusory'. Although I identify with many of the issues of conscience and social responsibility raised by these authors, common sense, and certainly my own observations of homeless people in different parts of the world both inside and outside the USA, persuade me that there are dangers inherent in this kind of inclusiveness. Thus, although on a personal level I care deeply about homeless people of all descriptions and do not wish to minimize the needs of any of them, I feel compelled to separate my professional and personal concerns in order to be responsive to the special needs of those who are mentally ill. Even though these individuals certainly share some characteristics with other homeless people, they possess unique service requirements that tend to get overshadowed if they are not separated out as a special population. I believe, moreover, that we do all homeless people, whether mentally ill or not, a great injustice when we lump them together and fail to respond to their categorical needs.

This point has been made most persuasively in the popular literature by Baum & Burnes (1993a,b) and in the professional literature by Lamb (1992), authors who, in my judgement, present unimpeachable evidence for the need to differentiate the two populations. However, lest readers of this chapter feel that I am excessively pedantic in calling for such a conceptual separation, I would note that there are distinct practical advantages to separating the two populations that deserve consideration, a point well-illustrated in the matter of residential service planning.

The goal of stable housing

There is now a substantial literature that emphasizes the notion that the best cure for homelessness among mentally ill people lies in providing them with housing, particularly stable housing (Kanter, 1989; Bachrach, 1992; Dugger, 1992). Proponents of this view basically argue that, once mentally ill individuals have been provided with permanent residence, their problems will ease, and their life situations will improve materially.

Now, I appreciate the fact that such a prescription may be appropriate for those members of the *general* homeless population who have suffered temporary crises or economic set-backs and who experience a minimum of attendant disaffiliation (although it is probably more appropriate for some parts of this population than it is for others). However, when the goal of stable housing is extended to *mentally ill* homeless people, it becomes simplistic and, for at least some portion of the population, potentially dangerous.

The simple and sad fact is that, even after mentally ill individuals have been provided with housing, they will still be mentally ill. They require more than a mere residential assignment to overcome their disabilities and to cope with their problems in living; they also need an array of other services ranging from psychiatric and medical care, counselling and rehabilitative interventions to case management, social support, recreational opportunities and financial planning (Wolch *et al.*, 1988; Lamb, 1990; Stokes, 1993). Very often, other basic subsistence requirements, such as access to clothing and food, must also be arranged for these persons (Belkin, 1992). Although non-mentally ill homeless people may at times require similar services, the specific programme content and measures for engaging the two populations must be quite different (Susser *et al.*, 1990).

It is for this reason that Lamb & Lamb (1990) have written about the importance of 'coming face to face with the clinical reality' of mentally ill homeless people and about what we must do to provide these individuals with 'support, protection, treatment, and rehabilitation'. In this catalogue of needs, housing emerges as one of many service requirements that mentally ill homeless individuals have, one that must always be integrated with and balanced against their other service needs.

However, service integration of such complexity requires patience and imagination, qualities that are sometimes difficult to realize in goal-oriented societies like that of the USA where pragmatic, 'quick-fix' solutions are often the order of the day (Freedman, 1967). American mental health service planners are frequently disposed to reduce complex events to single variables; and historically, housing has been an area singled out for this purpose. Our early efforts at deinstitutionalization had a distinctly residential focus: far more attention was devoted to where a mentally ill persons would live – either inside or outside a psychiatric hospital – than to what specific clinical and supportive services he or she would be offered (Bachrach, 1994a).

We are once more in the position of understating the critical importance of interventions other than housing as we develop services for mentally ill homeless persons, a problem that is fuelled by our failure to separate these individuals conceptually from those homeless persons who are not mentally ill. Our current emphasis on providing *stable* housing exacerbates the problem, for the very fact of mental illness may interfere with some homeless people's ability to handle the kind of permanence that is implied in the concept of stability.

Geographic mobility

There is now evidence that some severely mentally ill homeless people are highly mobile: they simply move about a great deal (Lamb, 1982; Appleby & Desai, 1987; Bachrach, 1987, 1992; Mercier *et al.*, 1992; Dixon *et al.*, 1993; Wolch, *et al.*, 1993). Although some professional writers appear reluctant to acknowledge the full extent of mobility within this population (Bachrach, 1987), a number of popular journalists have reported on the prevalence of this circumstance and captured its significance (Bachrach, 1990).

In fact, three broad varieties of mobility are found among mentally ill homeless persons. First, there is substantial movement into and out of the homeless population, so that some individuals may be regarded as 'permanently' homeless and others as 'episodically' homeless (Arce *et al.*, 1983).

Secondly, there is considerable diurnal and seasonal movement of the population within circumscribed geographical areas. Although some mentally ill homeless people live more or less continuously in one place, many others branch out within the community as services become available to them or as their specific needs for food, shelter and health care shift.

Thirdly, many mentally ill homeless people exhibit patterns of gross mobility over wide geographical areas and move, with greater or lesser regularity, from one city or region to another (Bachrach, 1987, 1988a).

The antecedents of mobility among these individuals are complex; inadequately investigated, they are certainly appropriate areas for intensive study. It appears, however, that some portion of the restlessness that characterizes mentally ill homeless persons relates to sociologically entrenched patterns of coping (Stokols & Shumaker, 1982). Some individuals in the population, for example, recall childhoods in which the standard familial response to crisis was to move to a new location (Harris & Bachrach, 1990). For others in the population the experience of residential mobility during childhood is positively correlated with adult homelessness (Susser *et al.*, 1987).

It is likely, however, that sociological factors commonly interact with complex clinical factors to exacerbate restlessness and promote residential instability among at least some mentally ill homeless persons. Corin (1990) has provided a thoughtful description of the need that some mentally ill individuals have to relate to others 'without having to be personally committed in personal interactions'. They often desire to be close to other people even as they wish to maintain a distance from them. Residential instability may be one means of responding to such a need.

Lamb's (1982) description of patients he has called 'new drifters' underscores this point. These individuals typically wander from community to community in search of a 'geographic solution to their problems; hoping to leave their problems behind, they find that they have simply brought their difficulties to a new location ... [Some] drift in the community from one living situation to another, and some, though they remain in one place, can best be described as drifting through life'. Lamb has explained the movement of these individuals as resulting both from a 'desire to outrun their problems, their symptoms, and their failures', and from great difficulty in achieving closeness and intimacy.

Indeed, we know that there are some mentally ill homeless people who remain highly mobile even while they are undergoing treatment and beginning to get involved with the system of care (Harris & Bachrach, 1990). An in-depth study of 25 homeless mentally ill women in the District of Columbia has shown that, after assignment to a special case management programme, 19 were still in treatment after 2 years, even though they had changed residences frequently – an average of 5.5 moves per woman over the study period. The median tenure for their residential stays was only 3.8 months, with a range of 0.7 to 8.0 months per stay. And although many of the moves were local – perhaps a shift to another room in the same house or to another residential facility in the same system of care – the goal of stable housing was not being realized, even though permanent housing placements were certainly available to these women (Harris & Bachrach, 1990).

We must thus question the wisdom and validity of using residential stability as an indicator of programme outcome for mentally ill homeless people. Planning for this population must be seen as a more complicated endeavour, a fact that is easily minimized when we fail to differentiate the general homeless and the mentally ill homeless populations. Unlike many non-mentally ill homeless persons who may potentially use stable housing as a stepping stone to societal integration, a sizeable number of mentally ill homeless people appear to experience a need not to 'stay put' even under the most benign clinical conditions, at least at the beginning of treatment (Harris & Bachrach, 1990).

It is essential that we learn more about both the sociology and the clinical antecedents of restlessness among mentally ill homeless people if we are to serve them in a meaningful and appropriate manner. Until we understand this phenomenon more completely – until we are able to explain more fully why this apparent restlessness occurs – we are well-advised to view residential placements in a broader context and de-emphasize the primacy of stable housing as a programme goal.

There is precedent in American mental health planning for blurring the boundaries of service populations. Dinitz & Beran wrote in 1971 that American community mental health had moved 'well beyond traditional mental health's focus on psychopathology' and become a 'boundaryless and boundary-busting system' with 'a boundaryless goal: the improvement of the quality of life of the whole man, and every man, in his total environment'. Unfortunately, despite its genuine intent to serve the mental health needs of all people in an egalitarian manner, this conceptual blending led to the design of community mental health services in which those people who are generally most in need – those who are the most defenceless – were often shoved aside in the planning process and left to fend for themselves (Hansell, 1978; Bachrach & Lamb, 1989; Bachrach, 1994a). We have not yet completely solved this problem, and we run the risk of compounding it in our service planning for mentally ill homeless persons today.

Discussion and concluding comments

Although this chapter has focused largely on residential planning to illustrate the importance of viewing the general homeless and mentally ill homeless populations as separate entities, other domains may be used towards the same end. For example, treatment planning, counselling programmes, vocational skills training and job placements must all be approached differently for these two populations. It thus appears that, in the last analysis, it helps neither the general homeless nor the mentally ill homeless population to consider their differences to be 'illusory'.

There is, in fact, an element of tragedy in the history of policy development for mentally ill homeless people in the USA. Some individuals in official positions have at last begun to recognize the dangers inherent in grouping the general homeless and mentally ill homeless populations together. However, the process has been long and arduous, one in which both moral ground and many opportunities for financial support have been lost (Bragg, 1994). Thus, after many years of federal inattention to the problems of homelessness in the USA, President Clinton has finally announced a demonstration initiative to provide categorical funding and resources for mentally ill homeless people living in the District of Columbia. Because funding streams will be separated, they will no longer need to compete with non-mentally ill homeless people for resources (DeParle, 1993). The problem is, however, that there is far too little money attached to this initiative to make a difference at this time, a situation that has prompted Secretary of Housing and Urban Development Cisneros to assert that the number of dollars spent is 'less important' than the philosophy that is being put forth (DeParle, 1993).

What lessons, then, may we derive from the observations presented here? It would seem that the first and most basic lesson lies in the area of semantics. Not only must we begin to define the general homeless and mentally ill homeless populations with greater precision; we must also focus on separating them conceptually as we promulgate policy and plan services.

A second lesson is that our research and other working definitions of mentally ill homeless people must be derived from the conceptual frameworks that we profess. It is not enough to give lip service to the notion that these individuals are disaffiliated; unless we incorporate the idea of social isolation into our working definitions of this population they will continue to be regarded as having a single major problem: the lack of housing. Had we heeded this lesson in the past, we might have paid more attention to the fact that engaging in social network development and repair (Harris & Bergman, 1985) is at least as important a variable in serving mentally ill homeless people as is the provision of housing. We might also have been similarly disposed to regard stable housing as at best a distant, not an immediate, programme goal for many members of this population.

Finally, we must acknowledge the fact that 'boundary-busting', however appealing it may be to social activists and idealistic programme planners, carries certain risks for target populations. When we fail to define the boundaries of these populations with care, we are apt to level our service offerings and minimize the needs of those individuals who are the most difficult to serve. Our decades-old experience with deinstitutionalization and our more recent efforts in programme planning for mentally ill homeless persons should by now have alerted us to the fact that one-size-fits-all approaches do not work to the advantage of mentally ill individuals, and we must strive to become more precise in developing programme goals for all in this population, including those who are homeless.

References

Adelson, J. (1991). The ideology of homelessness. *Commentary*, **91**, 32–6.
Alters, D. (1986). Roots of homelessness debated at conference. *Boston Globe*, 28 March, p. 16.
Appleby, L. & Desai, P. N. (1987). Residential instability: a perspective on system imbalance. *American Journal of Orthopsychiatry*, **57**, 515–24.
Arce, A. A., Tadlock, M., Vergare, M. H. & Shapiro, S. H. (1983). A psychiatric profile of street people admitted to an emergency shelter. *Hospital and Community Psychiatry*, **34**, 812–17.
Bachrach, L. L. (1985). *Slogans and Euphemisms: The Functions of Semantics in Mental Health and Mental Retardation Care*. Austin, TX: Hogg Foundation for Mental Health.
Bachrach, L. L. (1987). Geographic mobility and the homeless mentally ill. *Hospital and Community Psychiatry*, **38**, 27–8.
Bachrach, L. L. (1988a). Transient patients in a western state hospital. *Hospital and Community Psychiatry*, **39**, 123–4.
Bachrach, L. L. (1988b). Defining chronic mental illness: a concept paper. *Hospital and Community Psychiatry*, **39**, 383–8.
Bachrach, L. L. (1988c). Community mental health centers and other semantic concerns. *Hospital and Community Psychiatry*, **39**, 605–6.
Bachrach, L. L. (1990). The media and homeless mentally ill persons. *Hospital and Community Psychiatry*, **41**, 963–4.
Bachrach, L. L. (1992). What we know about homelessness among mentally ill persons: an analytical review and commentary. In H. R. Lamb, L. L. Bachrach, & F. I. Kass (eds.), *Treating the Homeless*

Mentally Ill., pp. 13–40. Washington, DC: American Psychiatric Association.

Bachrach, L. L. (1994a). Residential planning: concepts and themes. *Hospital and Community Psychiatry*, **45**, 202–3.

Bachrach, L. L. (1994b). The semantics of mental health service delivery. Paper presented at the Annual Meeting of the Ontario Psychiatric Association, Toronto, 28 January.

Bachrach, L. L. & Lamb, H. R. (1989). What have we learned from deinstitutionalization? *Psychiatric Annals*, **19**, 12–21.

Bailey, R. (1977). *The Homeless and Empty Houses*. London: Penguin Books.

Barrow, S. M., Hellman, F., Lovell, A. M., Plapinger, J. D. & Struening, E. L. (1989). *Effectiveness of Programs for the Mentally Ill Homeless*. New York: New York State Psychiatric Institute.

Baum, A. & Burnes, D. W. (1993a). *A Nation in Denial: The Truth About Homelessness*. Boulder, CO: Westview Press.

Baum, A. & Burnes, D. W. (1993b). Facing the facts about homelessness. *Public Welfare*, **51**, 20–27, 46, 48.

Baxter, E. & Hopper, K. (1982). The new mendicancy: homeless in new York City. *American Journal of Orthopsychiatry*, **52**, 393–408.

Belkin, L. (1992). Treating the sick can mean clothing them too. *New York Times*, 24 November, pp. B1, B2.

Bragg, R. (1994). Homeless seeing less apathy, more anger. *New York Times*, 25 February, pp. A1, B2.

Campbell, R. L. (1981). The language of psychiatry. *Hospital and Community Psychiatry*, **32**, 849–52.

Cohen, C. I. & Thompson, K. S. (1992). Homeless mentally ill or mentally ill homeless? *American Journal of Psychiatry*, **149**, 816–23.

Corin, E. E. (1990). Facts and meaning in psychiatry: an anthropological approach to the lifeworld of schizophrenics. *Culture, Medicine and Psychiatry*, **14**, 153–88.

Culhane, D. P. (1991). Images of the homeless. *Hospital and Community Psychiatry*, **42**, 200. (Letter).

DeParle, J. (1993). U.S. offers "model" plan for Capital homeless. *New York Times*, 21 September, p. A15.

Dinitz, S. & Beran, N. (1971). Community mental health as a boundaryless and boundary-busting system. *Journal of Health and Social Behavior*, **12**, 99–108.

Dixon, L., Friedman, N. & Lehman, A. (1993). Housing patterns of homeless mentally ill persons receiving assertive treatment services. *Hospital and Community Psychiatry*, **44**, 286–8.

Dugger, C. (1992). Memo to Democrats: housing won't solve homelessness. *New York Times*, 12 July, p. E9.

Enda, J. (1993). Studies: poverty at root of homelessness. *Philadelphia Inquirer*, 16 November, p. A2.

Fink, P. (1988). The power of semantics. *Psychiatric News*, 2 September, pp. 3, 7.

Freedman, A. M. (1967). Historical and political roots of the Community Mental Health Centers Act. *American Journal of Orthopsychiatry*, **37**, 487–94.

Hansell, N. (1978). Services for schizophrenics: a lifelong approach to treatment. *Hospital and Community Psychiatry*, **29**, 105–9.

Hardin, G. (1957). The threat of clarity. *American Journal of Psychiatry*, **114**, 392–6.

Harris, M. & Bachrach, L. L. (1990). Perspectives on homeless mentally ill women. *Hospital and Community Psychiatry*, **41**, 253–4.

Harris, M. & Bergman, H. C. (1985). Networking with young adult chronic patients. *Psychosocial Rehabilitation Journal*, **8**, 28–35.

Kanter, A. S. (1989). Homeless but not helpless: legal issues in the care of homeless people with mental illness. *Journal of Social Issues*, **45**, 91–104.

Lamb, H. R. (1982). Young adult chronic patients: the new drifters. *Hospital and Community Psychiatry*, **33**, 465–8.

Lamb, H. R. (1990). Will we save the homeless mentally ill? *American Journal of Psychiatry*, **147**, 649–51.

Lamb, H. R. (1992). Perspectives on effective advocacy for homeless mentally ill persons. *Hospital and Community Psychiatry*, **43**, 1209–12.

Lamb, H. R. & Lamb, D. M. (1990). Factors contributing to homelessness among the chronically and severely mentally ill. *Hospital and Community Psychiatry*, **41**, 301–5.

Liebow, E. (1993). *Tell Them Who I Am: The Lives of Homeless Women*. New York: The Free Press.

Mercier, C., Fournier, L. & Peladeau, N. (1992). Program evaluation of services for the homeless: challenges and strategies. *Evaluation and Program Planning*, **15**, 417–26.

Morrison, J. (1989). Correlations between definitions of the homeless mentally ill population. *Hospital and Community Psychiatry*, **40**, 952–4.

Mossman, D. & Perlin, M. L. (1992). Psychiatry and the homeless mentally ill: a reply to Dr. Lamb. *American Journal of Psychiatry*, **149**, 951–7.

Robb-Smith, A. H. T. (1978). International nomenclature of diseases. *Australian and New Zealand Journal of Medicine*, **8**, 445–7.

Rossi, P. H., Wright, J. D., Fisher, G. A. & Willis, G. (1987). The urban homeless: estimating composition and size. *Science*, **235**, 1336–41.

Roth, D. & Bean, J. (1986). New perspectives on homelessness: findings from a statewide epidemiological study. *Hospital and Community Psychiatry*, **37**, 712–19.

Santiago, J. M., Bachrach, L. L., Berren, M. R. & Hannah, M. T. (1988). Defining the homeless mentally ill: a methodological note. *Hospital and Community Psychiatry*, **39**, 1100–102.

Schmidt, W. E. (1992). Across Europe, faces of homeless become more visible and vexing. *New York Times*, 5 January, pp. 1, 8.

Snow, D. A., Baker, S. G. & Anderson, L. (1988). On the

precariousness of measuring insanity in insane contexts. *Social Problems*, **35**, 192–6.

Snow, D. A., Baker, S. G., Anderson, L. & Martin, M. (1986). The myth of pervasive mental illness among the homeless. *Social Problems*, **33**, 407–23.

Stokes, S. L. (1993). Telling the Truth about Homelessness. *Washington Post*, 1 February, p. A17. (Letter).

Stokols, D. & Shumaker, S. A. (1982). The psychological context of residential mobility and well-being. *Journal of Social Issues*, **38**, 149–71.

Susser, E., Goldfinger, S. M. & White, A. (1990). Some clinical approaches to the homeless mentally ill. *Community Mental Health Journal*, **26**, 463–80.

Susser, E., Struening, E. L. & Conover, S. (1987). Childhood experiences of homeless men. *American Journal of Psychiatry*, **144**, 1599–601.

Talbott, J. A. (1985). Some assorted nits and picks. *Psychiatric News*, 1 March, pp. 2, 13.

US General Accounting Office (1992). *Homelessness: HUD's Interpretation of Homeless Excludes Previously Served Groups*. GAO Report RCED-92-226. Washington, DC: Government Printing Office.

Wolch, J. R., Dear, M. & Akita, A. (1988). Explaining homelessness. *Journal of the American Planning Association*, **54**, 443–53.

Wolch, J. R., Rahimian, A. & Koegel, P. (1993). Daily and periodic mobility patterns of the urban homeless. *Professional Geographer*, **45**, 159–69.

14

Homelessness and mental health: lessons from Australia

HELEN HERRMAN AND CECILY NEIL

Introduction

The extent of serious mental illness among single homeless people, broadly defined, is similar in Australia to that found elsewhere in the Western world (Scott, 1993). During the 1980s in Australia the problems of ill and disaffiliated people became increasingly apparent to service agencies. The problems have been less visible than in other parts of the world, hidden to a large degree in special accommodation houses, cheap boarding houses and shelters or crisis accommodation centres (Doutney *et al.*, 1985; Herrman *et al.*, 1989; Teesson & Buhrich, 1990, 1993; Virgona *et al.*, 1993). Even so, national reports estimate that thousands of Australians, and in particular many thousands of young people, live without adequate shelter (HREOC, 1989; Neil *et al.*, 1992).

A relatively high proportion of homeless people have a mental illness, but many do not. The problem of homelessness, for those with or without severe mental illness, is influenced by the social and housing issues that affect all marginalized people. At the same time it is important to recognize among the homeless those who would benefit from psychiatric treatment, and the barriers to care that exist (Bachrach, 1987). Furthermore, homelessness among mentally ill people may be seen in part as a reflection on inadequacies in the delivery of health, welfare and housing services to those with severe mental disorder, many of whom develop multiple disabilities and handicaps, and to their families and other caregivers.

Homelessness was defined recently in an Australian government report as: 'that state in which people have no access to safe and secure shelter of a standard that does not damage their health, threaten their personal safety, or contribute to their marginalisation by the absence either of cooking facilities or facilities that permit adequate personal hygiene'. This definition gives weight to the absence of the most basic features of a 'home', and encompasses those living on the street, in squats, in refuges and shelters. It also encompasses those moving about between relatives and friends, since 'such accommodation is necessarily temporary, usually insecure and fails to offer ... protection and support' (HREOC, 1989, p. 7). Those living in rooming houses and intermittently in small inner city hotels may be considered homeless if such places fail to offer any sense of 'permanency' or protection from others. Local authors (Chamberlain & MacKenzie, 1992) have differentiated absolute homelessness, in which people are without a proper roof over their heads, and several degrees of relative homelessness. The first relative degree of homelessness is that experienced by people moving between various forms of temporary or medium-term shelter such as refuges, hostels, or the homes of friends. The second degree is that experienced by people living permanently in single rooms in situations in which their personal safety is threatened, or in which lack of infrastructure may increase their marginalization. The third degree of homelessness is that experienced by people who are housed, but inadequately housed in terms of commonly accepted norms in Australia.

In the face of current trends in the labour and housing markets in Australia, the housing situation confronting vulnerable people is likely to deteriorate in the foreseeable future. If this occurs, people with longstanding mental illness are in danger not only of becoming homeless, but of being displaced into absolute or first degree relative homelessness. Melbourne and Sydney are the two largest Australian cities and each has a population of over three million people. Survey findings (Doutney *et al.*, 1985; Herrman *et al.*, 1989; Teeson & Buhrich, 1990, 1993; Virgona *et al.*, 1993) suggest that individuals who are marginally accommodated have severe mental disorders in proportions similar to those among homeless people more narrowly defined, both locally and abroad. In other words, the group of people who are marginally accommodated in Melbourne and Sydney is likely to include many people, both with and without mental illness, who would be shelterless in some of the cities in the USA. Relevant to this are differences in the Australian social conditions and policies that affect the supply of cheap housing and access of chronically mentally ill persons to shelter (Herrman, 1992). The inner-city areas in Australia still have an adequate supply of cheap housing. In addition, disabled people receive a pension or benefits sufficient to allow rental of a room or flat for a single person, unless, for instance, the person has a substance abuse problem and spends money on alcohol or drugs. However, economic conditions in Australia are changing and creating a 'new poor' at risk of homelessness. Areas with cheap accommodation are being eroded by the development of housing for the affluent, and government policies are restricting the eligibility for and levels of benefits. The demand for public housing is increasing at a faster rate than supply. There is a real danger that each group in the homeless population may be pushed another rung down the accommodation ladder, and more of the most vulnerable people will be left without shelter.

Resultant problems are likely to be exacerbated by the fact that a reduced provision of institutional care in Australia since the 1960s has not been complemented by adequate provision of appropriate housing and community care for those people with mental illness who have difficulty coping with everyday life. During the 1980s, the federal government launched a number of policies designed to assist people with disabilities to stay in the community. However, services of this nature tend to facilitate care in the home, not care in the community (Rosenman, 1992, p. 44).

> [A]ny movement away from institutional care to community care of this nature, to be effective, is dependent on there being an adequate supply of appropriate and affordable accommodation within the community for those who require some assistance to live independently. If this is not available, community care offers little to the person who is inadequately housed, and in need of assistance to live independently – although the person unable to access affordable and appropriate accommodation may well be the one most in need of assistance.
>
> (Neil et al., 1992, p. 198)

Some specialized accommodation options exist for those living outside institutions who are neither living with family nor friends, nor capable of fully independent living. Such special-purpose accommodation is in short supply, however, and often inappropriate to the needs or realistic preferences of those without housing. The situation is exemplified by the struggle to find appropriate accommodation for a person being discharged from a psychiatric hospital. At the same time, some state governments are moving increasingly towards user-pay principles, leading in the current economic climate to the suggestion that 'it is the articulate, those with higher incomes and those with less demanding behaviour who have the best chance of accessing government programs, whilst others of equal need are forced into substandard private provision' (Victorian Council of Social Service and the Office of the Public Advocate, 1992, p. 13).

Local economic conditions and social welfare policies may be seen in this way to create a changeable 'threshold' for true or absolute homelessness among isolated people with severe mental illness. This view is supported by recent work in the USA challenging the impression that homeless mentally ill people are shelterless by choice. Two prospective follow-up studies reported good clinical and social outcomes for individuals provided with accommodation and on-site mental health care and day care (Lipton *et al.*, 1988; Caton, 1990); and assertive case management helped women who wished to move around to remain in contact with services and be adequately housed (Harris & Bachrach, 1990). The majority of 208 long-stay patients discharged from mental hospitals in Sydney and elsewhere in New South Wales to supported community accommodation between 1984 and 1987 were functioning well and had remained in the accommo- dation over some years (Andrews *et al.*, 1990).

In this chapter we will consider factors that may change this threshold, as well as those that may affect the entry to and exit from a broadly defined homeless state. Social and housing policies, and the ways in which services for people with severe mental illness are organized, are all likely to be relevant. Individuals are differently affected according to many aspects of their own background, personality and situation. The needs of people soon after the onset of an illness and with a close and perhaps affluent family for support, are different from those of a destitute person alone after several years of episodically worsening disorder. The management and prevention strategies possible will depend on the attitude and behaviour of those working in and planning the services, the resources provided and the social policy climate.

Contributions of mental illness to the origins and maintenance of homelessness

Homeless people commonly experience a number of social, health and criminal problems. Homelessness for any individual may be

determined by a combination of broad social trends, family circumstances and individual attributes (Susser *et al.*, 1988). Post-war
changes in homeless populations are commonly associated with
broad social changes. These include changes in the population
structure, a growing scarcity of housing, increased levels of unemployment and changes in welfare and psychiatric services. The
process of 'deinstitutionalization' of the mentally ill has affected each
generation differently over the past 30 years. In Australia, as in other
countries, this process has been implemented overall without adequate treatment or support or residential alternatives, and appears to
have interacted with the political economy to contribute to homelessness among the mentally ill. Policies have taken little account
furthermore, of the needs of families, and of the factors that may
enhance the ability and willingness of families to provide care. The
breakdown of family links tends to increase the chances of homelessness for an individual with severe mental illness.

While wider factors may be involved, attention to risk factors at the
individual level may reverse, or prevent, a drift towards homelessness.
Homeless mentally ill people frequently have a history of childhood
family separation or institutional care (Susser & Struening, 1987),
and are often socially isolated (Thornicroft & Breakey, 1991). A
Melbourne survey of homeless and disaffiliated people found high
rates of overlap in individual respondents between substance dependence and the mood and psychotic disorders (Herrman *et al.*, 1989).
Similar rates of dual diagnosis were found in other recent surveys
using standardized diagnostic instruments (Koegel *et al.*, 1988).
Co-morbidity of mental disorders and of mental and physical
disorders may well be an important factor in the genesis of homelessness, as may cognitive impairment. Over 40% of a cohort of homeless
men resident in a large shelter in Sydney showed at least mild
cognitive impairment and more than one in four showed severe
impairment (Teesson & Buhrich, 1993).

In the relationship between risk factors and homelessness, the
direction of causality may be unclear. For instance, drug abuse, social
isolation and mental disorder are all plausible consequences as well as
causes of homelessness. In addition, it is usually difficult to date the
onset of homelessness for any individual (Susser *et al.*, 1988). In the
Melbourne study, *life charts* were constructed from the information
obtained at interview, which was often rich although retrospective,
and from state records of service use. For many respondents evidence
of severe mental disorder preceded sustained periods of homelessness

or marginal accommodation, even when residence in these settings was episodic. Only a small number of respondents appeared to have become mentally ill after becoming homeless (Herrman *et al.*, 1992). The findings support suggestions that the occurrence of one or more severe mental disorders is a risk factor for homelessness and disaffiliation (Lamb & Lamb, 1990). Homelessness may follow an accumulation of problems, including mental illness, that severely limit function and choice.

Findings from the Melbourne survey were indicative in a number of other respects. Almost half the respondents received diagnoses of current mental disorders and over 70% received diagnoses of life-time disorders. Women formed a small minority, and the rates of disorder were at least as high as those for men, consistent with information available from Sydney (Virgona *et al.*, 1993) and the USA (Bachrach & Nadelson, 1988). The prevalence of life-time and current disorders in all categories was as high in young as in older men. These findings also accord with widely reported observations that while the number and proportion of mentally ill people among the homeless have increased significantly over the last 20 years, the proportion of young chronically ill has apparently increased as the proportion of older substance abusers has decreased (Bachrach, 1984; Koegel *et al.*, 1988; Scott, 1993). There has been a marked shift in age distribution towards the young among single homeless people overall (Susser *et al.*, 1988). The relatively high prevalence of disorder in the younger men in Melbourne may be related to selective factors in the survey, to a cohort effect, or to recovery or death of older men with a history of mental disorder (Herrman *et al.*, 1990). Important questions remain, however, about the effects of changing systems of mental health care, and of welfare and housing policies, on the course and outcome of the various disorders, and on the likelihood of individuals living impoverished and isolated lives. We do not know how many of the people, including the young adults and women, represented by those interviewed will still be living in these settings in 20 years time, and how this could be influenced by the provision of various kinds of services.

Provision and use of mental health services

In Australia, the problems of the care of those with severe mental illness and the direction of changes in service provision are similar to those found elsewhere in the Western world. A National Mental Health Policy and Plan were released in 1992 (Singh, 1992; Whiteford *et al.*, 1993). They emphasize a balance of community and hospital care, with enough flexibility and continuity of care to provide treatment and support suitable for each individual. The difficulties lie in adjusting services to the needs of the different areas, and in the provision of an adequate supply and range of accommodation and family support in the community. State governments fund psychiatric services, increasingly in the 'mainstream' of general health care, and the Commonwealth government subsidizes consultation fees for private practitioners. A problem for the state psychiatric services, and hence by and large for the services for those with severe mental illness, is the difficulty in recruiting and retaining psychiatrists in the face of the opportunities for private practice (James, 1993).

Good management of severe mental illness is similar in principle whether or not the patients are homeless; and is likely to contribute to the prevention of homelessness. At the same time, service providers need to be aware of factors particular to the management of homeless people. The provision of a decent place to live is a primary need, complemented by access to appropriate levels of treatment and support. While mentally ill homeless people exhibit high mobility (Bachrach, 1987), the Melbourne study defined a substantial core of relatively stable people (Herrman *et al.*, 1989), as have studies in the UK (Marshall & Gath, 1992). Both of these features are relevant to service provision. Providers may assume that standard care has little to offer the drifting person for whom homelessness represents some form of actively sought anonymity. This assumption is likely to overlook the lack of choice that many people have in this situation (Burns, 1989; and see above); and to underestimate the influence of the style and organization of service provision on the accessibility of mental health care to homeless people.

Studies of service use by single homeless people in the USA have been concerned mainly with *specialist mental health services*. Between 20% and 40% of the persons surveyed in these studies have had a past history of psychiatric hospitalization (compared with 40% of respondents in Melbourne) and another 15% had contact with outpatient psychiatric services only. The higher rates of hospitalization have applied in those studies that consider admissions for drug or alcohol abuse. Very few of the people with a history of hospital stay have had recent contact with outpatient or community mental health services (Gelberg *et al.*, 1988).

Homeless people presenting to an emergency service may be substantially less likely than domiciled people with similar morbidity to be admitted (Burns, 1989). These observations require replication in Australia and elsewhere. From the opposite perspective, state funded psychiatric hospital services tend to have a high proportion of homeless people among those admitted for acute treatment. In 1991 an Australian researcher interviewed 269 patients newly admitted to the psychiatric wards at the Royal Brisbane Hospital, which has a catchment area covering half of the inner city's suburbs. The study found that 27% (50 men and 22 women) had either used a shelter for the homeless, had no fixed address, or had had one or more changes of address in the 3 months previous to their admission. Of the total, 14% (or almost one in five men and almost one in ten women) had been shelter users or literally homeless (Quinn, 1993).

It is clear that changes in any single service type or setting, or provision of health services alone, are unlikely to alleviate the problems of homeless people with mental illness. One logical response has been the establishment of specialized service programmes with potential to 'engage the disengaged' and provide a range of basic and specialized services (Levine, 1984; Gelberg *et al.*, 1988) including assertive outreach mental health services. The latter have been successful in engaging numbers of people in care and in maintaining adequate levels of housing (see Chapter 11). Outreach services have developed in areas of Sydney, Melbourne and other cities (Teesson & Hambridge, 1992; N. Buhrich, M. Teesson & L. Jayes, unpublished results). In different parts of Melbourne, such services have been established as specialized mental health treatment teams for homeless people, and as part of assertive community services for those with severe mental illness. Assessment is now in progress of how effectively these different approaches serve the varying needs of the local populations.

The use of *primary care services* by homeless mentally ill people has received less attention in the USA where the contribution of this service sector is relatively small, but more attention in the UK (Powell, 1988; Reuler, 1989; and see Chapter 11). In Australia a survey of Sydney boarding house occupants suggested that the primary care physician was, by a long way, the main carer for many isolated mentally ill people (Harris *et al.*, 1987). The respondents in the Melbourne survey of homeless people reported high rates of current contact with primary and mental health services. We do not know the quality and frequency of these contacts, but do know that relatively few people were taking prescription medication (Herrman et al., 1992).

These observations suggest a different and perhaps complementary response to the provision of services to homeless mentally ill people. Many of the homeless people surveyed do make contact with health services. Despite relatively stable location for a sizable group, many people with severe disorders do not maintain that contact. The important question then becomes what factors make these contacts helpful and lasting; both for the stably located groups and for the probably more difficult to engage transient and shelterless people. It is likely that doctors and other professionals in primary health care could have a greater role in management of homeless (and other) people with severe mental illness than they generally have at the moment in Melbourne and other places. In particular, these practitioners could become a focus for other services, or perhaps more realistically link with outreach services, to provide access to a range of preventive, crisis and support services in a variety of hospital and community settings. Incentives for primary care practitioners to participate in this work may be combined with more focused training in community mental health care at undergraduate and postgraduate levels, and with service changes. Access to psychiatric treatment in local hospital and community settings, and an adequate range and supply of supported accommodations are the minimum requirements.

However, a number of factors limit access to these service components, including restrictions in the hours of operation, location and flexibility of the mental health services. Support workers in generic services lack training in understanding people with mental illness, and often have little back-up in crisis situations from the specialist services, especially after hours. This reflects the 'poorly developed intersectoral links between mental health and general health, social and disability services present[ing] a range of barriers to continuity of care... Social justice reforms with social and income support, and labour market programs which address the needs of people with disability have only recently recognised the specific needs of people with psychiatric disability' (National Health Strategy, 1993; pp. 9–10). Information systems are not sufficiently developed to facilitate the continuity and integration of service delivery (National Health Strategy, 1993, pp. 10).

The fragmentation of services particularly affects people with dual disabilities. There is a critical lack of service and care for people with co-existing serious mental illness and problematic drug or alcohol use. Of particular importance are the apparently conflicting views of the problem among service providers in different health and welfare sectors and the impact of administrative divisions, which increase the difficulties of people with these dual problems. The social policy of 'harm minimization' may, if developed within the mental health domain provide a crucial first step in addressing critical needs for services (McDermott & Pyett, 1994). There is also a need for culturally-sensitive facilities that cater for the language and cultural differences of people from non-English speaking backgrounds (Morrissey *et al.*, 1991; Minas *et al.*, 1993; Jablensky, 1994), and Aborigines and Torres Strait Islanders (McKendrick *et al.*, 1992).

In addition, there are a number of features of some mental health services in Australia that specifically affect adolescents, which may have profound implications for the ability of young people with psychiatric disabilities to avoid or escape from homelessness. These include the fact that adolescent psychiatric units often have long waiting periods, traditionally require the family to be involved, and mostly require young people to have secure accommodation before treatment is offered. Many adolescent services do not assist young people over the age of 16, while adult services tend to be inappropriate for this age group, and state adolescent psychiatric units are often unable to provide a service for young people with aggressive behaviour (Hearn, 1993). Young people with severe mental disorders surveyed in supported housing in Melbourne were mostly out of contact with any mental health services (Reilly *et al.*, 1994). The Homeless Agencies Resource Project is the collaborative response of the youth housing services and adolescent psychiatry services of north-east Melbourne, taking adolescent psychiatry services information and expertise to youth housing services (Pawsey & Fuller, 1993).

Impact of housing provision and service links on ability of people with psychiatric illness to avoid or escape homelessness

These problems have, at best, led to a tendency for people with longstanding or episodic mental illness to be lost to the system. At worst, the fragmentation of services has enabled people, especially those with dual disabilities, to be excluded from services, each service seeing the provision of assistance as the responsibility of the other. Lack of continuity of care or, indeed, at times, any care, is likely to increase the number of people with mental illness who become homeless or are at risk of homelessness.

The problems of service provision discussed above not only affect the drift into homelessness, they also make it very difficult for someone with mental illness who has become homeless to escape. There is an acute shortage of exit points for homeless people in general in Australia (Fopp, 1992). The problems are compounded for people with mental illness by the fact that government and community groups have never fully resolved the question of who has the ultimate responsibility for the accommodation of people with special needs (Neil *et al.*, 1993). Most services for homeless people are currently managed by community groups. There has, however, been little negotiation between the community-managed housing sector and the government concerning the extent to which the former is now expected to undertake the provision of accommodation to those who, in the past, may well have been institutionalized, especially where the behaviour of the latter is disruptive or threatening (Neil *et al.*, 1993). To the extent that the community-managed housing sector has assumed responsibility for accommodating and supporting 'difficult' tenants, this has tended to be by default, rather than the outcome of negotiation, agreement, careful targeting and planning.

Perhaps as a result, no housing sector has been appropriately resourced to undertake this function. In addition, the social and community service sector's growth has been such that adequate training and career paths for staff have not been provided (Nyland, 1992, pp. 144–5). Very few accommodation services have the resources to provide appropriate care and support for people with psychiatric illnesses if their illness is not controlled, and cannot be expected to broaden their role unless additional resources are provided (Chesterman, 1988, p. 81).

When people with mental illness *are* accepted by such services, the absence of back-up psychiatric services in a crisis can create a risk for either the client or other residents. Disruptive behaviour may, at best, be unsettling for other residents (Rymill, 1992, pp. 27–8 and 34–5). In extreme situations this can lead to people being barred from accommodation and other services. This means that those with possibly the greatest support needs may be left to absolute homelessness. There is anecdotal evidence that groups responsible for community-managed medium-term supported accommodation for young people exclude those with psychiatric disabilities because they believe that their workers lack the skills to handle situations that might arise. This same lack of experience makes services unlikely to be able to differentiate between those people who may display disruptive behaviour and those who may not, and may therefore tend towards making a blanket exclusion.

People with psychiatric disabilities may only obtain access to particular forms of accommodation, generally those without security of tenure that are least likely to provide an environment that can facilitate a person's exit from homelessness, and therefore his or her ability to cope with mental illness. While 'drifting' appears to be associated with some illnesses, it may well be that a partial explanation of this behaviour is the services providers' selection process, especially where shared medium-term accommodation is involved, and other tenants have a say in the selection process.

Even where access to accommodation is obtained, people with mental illness do not always receive the support they need to live independently. Co-ordination between agencies offering generic support and those offering specialist psychiatric support is often poor. As noted by Neil *et al.* (1992, pp. 35–6), a number of service providers are reluctant to acknowledge the probable extent of mental illness in the homeless population. There is an understandable sensitivity to blaming the victim, and thereby stigmatizing an already disenfranchised population (Bassuk *et al.*, 1984). However, this outlook, coupled with lack of training, has at times prevented housing workers in the social and community services sector from acknowledging the need of some of their clients for specialist services. At the same time, partly because of the lack of clearly negotiated responsibilities of community-managed housing groups in the overall provision of social services, specialist services frequently ignore community-managed housing groups and generalist support workers who may have contact with their clients, other than to criticize their perceived reluctance to provide accommodation for people with psychiatric or drug-related disabilities.

The problems of co-ordination are exaggerated by the fact that community-managed housing organizations may have to find their way through a maze of possible services to help some of their clients access the type of assistance they need. Further, the growth of the community management of services has led to a degree of conflict between specialist, professionally-oriented, community-based government agencies and community-managed organizations that supply generic support. The former are concerned that professional sensitivities are being ignored, and the latter fear that clinical care will dominate the life of their clients.

There is now a greater recognition of the need for a holistic approach on the part of specialist government agencies, as well as on the part of community-managed housing groups, and therefore of the need for more intersectoral linkages. However, there is still a general lack of intersectoral co-ordination, and, indeed, of mutual respect, common language and level of understanding between generic service providers and providers of specialist services (Sawyer *et al.*, 1992).

Prospects for the future

Changing policies associated with the provision of psychiatric services

The National Mental Health Policy statement in 1992 (see pp. 250) proposed a number of major changes including the development of an integrated network of specialist psychiatric services and their delivery within the mainstream system of health care. The policy marks the health sector's movement away from providing 'whole of life' services. A community-oriented approach is advocated, involving the establishment of a new relationship between mental health services and the wider housing sector, an increase in the range and amount of supported accommodation, and decentralization of the 'mainstreamed' mental health services, so that the removal of people from community, family and cultural networks is minimized.

If successfully implemented, the agreed national policy promises to resolve many of the problems of mental health service provision. These changes could have a profound effect on reducing the vulnerability of people with mental illness to homelessness. The mainstreaming of health services in particular could have a number of significant advantages for people with mental health problems. It could help overcome the past marginalization and stigma of people with mental illnesses, and, as well, to break down the perception that people with severe mental illness are the sole responsibility of the mental health services. Improved community awareness and access to community health services could lead to the tendency to seek help earlier, and thus to better outcome for some people. The impediments to continuity of care are likely to be reduced, and its acceptability to clients increased. The tendency may be lessened for people with psychiatric disabilities to be concentrated in particular residential locations near the former centralized services. There is likely to be increased support for carers, self-help groups and consumer advocacy, and access to more support for non-mental health workers.

The restructuring of services that is taking place, however, is by no means complete. Further, there are dangers that in the process of implementing these policies, a number of unintended consequences may emerge that are detrimental for people with mental illness and at risk of homelessness. A reduction could occur in access to general health services, including drug and alcohol services. In a number of areas mainstream services themselves are inadequate. In addition, the behaviour patterns of some vulnerable people may contribute to them failing to receive the type of attention they need from busy and unprepared mainstream services. Equally, homeless people may not see the mainstream services available as appropriate to their needs. There is also a danger of an unintended reduction in the relative funding of services required by certain people with mental illness in an economic climate that stresses cost-effectiveness.

While the community-based provision of government services can tend to reinforce existing inequalities unless carefully planned and resourced (Ife, 1993), the community-managed provision of services also has its risks. First, it can enable a government to absolve itself from the responsibility of ensuring social equity. Secondly, the mistaken belief that community-based provision of services through the non-government sector offers a low-cost option for the provision of services can result in inadequate funding, which, in turn, can make it impossible for such services to succeed. Thirdly, while it has a number of major advantages, the transfer of responsibility for the general support services to community-managed organizations can present a number of barriers to realizing social equity and accountability. These services may be funded on the basis of principles that are neither well-targeted nor equitable, size may make some smaller agencies economically inefficient, even in situations where economic inefficiency cannot be justified in terms of the agencies' social goals (see Neil *et al.*, 1993), and poor management standards with respect to both administration and service delivery have been observed in some community-managed groups. There are also dangers when structural changes occur at a time of economic recession. The tensions likely between professional groups and community groups in the process of increasing the community-based provision of services tend to be exacerbated. The same tensions are likely to hinder informal co-ordination between government departments.

These are all areas where vigilance is required to ensure that, as intended, people with psychiatric disabilities at risk of homelessness benefit rather than lose from the service restructuring currently taking place.

Other changes required in the provision of supported accommodation options to build on service provision changes

Before significant improvement can be made in helping those who become homeless exit from that state, negotiation is required between the community-managed housing groups and the government about the provision of supported housing. Once the extent to which the community sector is to assume this role has been resolved, the sector needs adequate resources, including money, training and sufficient autonomy, to be able to do the job properly (Neil *et al.*, 1993). An important issue that must be resolved is the extent to which generic service providers are to be given access to clinical information. Then it is urgent to address the issue of training of generic support workers for homeless people. It is important for support workers to be able to recognize those clients in need of specialist services, and to be familiar with the range of specialist services to which they can help clients gain access.

There is a need for conscious effort to improve the level of understanding between providers of generic support to homeless people and providers of specialist services. Some consideration, for example, might be given to secondment of health workers to youth support services, or to an extension of the idea of the guidance of youth workers by clinicians in rural areas.

There is also a need to rethink rules and policies on access to accommodation, especially with respect to issues such as drug use on the part of those with mental illness. Further rethinking may be required regarding both the appropriate responses to tenants' failure to meet such obligations as rent payment, and the types of accommodation that should be provided. In particular, there is a need for:

- An increase in the number of single bedroom units in medium-term supported accommodation projects so other tenants already under stress do not have to accept responsibility in crisis situations for someone whose behaviour is disruptive or threatening.
- More projects that provide accommodation specifically for people with challenging behaviour, and have limited expectations of the residents (McDonald, 1993).

Improved and simplified funding policies to allow more flexible arrangements, and the increased availability of multi-disciplinary outreach teams from the mental health services appear to be essential. To ensure that the mainstreaming of services does not lead to the reduced accessibility of these services for their clients, generic service providers need to advocate strongly for a growth in the number of outreach teams, and work closely with such teams where they are available. The wide availability of crisis services that can provide accommodation managers with support in emergencies is also essential.

Improved co-ordination between the different sectors responsible for housing and supporting people with psychiatric disabilities is important. Australian experience has highlighted the fact that policies with respect to community-managed social housing should never be developed without consideration of other social service provision policies. As Hamilton (1991, p. 14) points out, the sector 'needs to be an equal partner in integrated planning on [a] regional/demographic needs base'. Once appropriate policies have been evolved, diverse approaches to the provision of housing are required, matched to local needs.

Conclusion

Australia has a system of comprehensive health insurance and state funded mental health services, which are currently being integrated and linked into local systems of health and social services. Recognition of the plight of homeless mentally ill people has been part of the impetus for a national approach to reform of mental health services. However, economic recession and policies of economic rationalism make the necessary reforms difficult to implement and in themselves are likely to result in more mentally ill people becoming homeless and shelterless. The genuine attempts to respond to need and to emphasize preventive approaches continue. Areas of particular interest in this regard include the promotion and support of primary medical practitioners in the care of people with serious mental illness, and recognition of the needs of families and other caregivers.

Vital to service developments at this point are recognition of the role of community psychiatrists and other key clinicians and support workers in local service developments, and negotiation of the role and resourcing of the various housing support sectors. Service research and evaluation are required. Services need to be responsive to community needs, and at the same time public education is required about the scale of the problem, and about the service and policy changes that are likely to help. Professional advocacy, and support for self-help and family support groups, are important in the face of the continuing stigma of mental illness.

References

Andrews, G., Teesson, M., Stewart, G. & Hoult, J. (1990). Follow-up of community placement of the chronic mentally ill in New South Wales. *Hospital and Community Psychiatry*, **41**, 184–8.
Bachrach, L. L. (1984). The homeless mentally ill and mental health services: an analytic review of the literature. In H. R. Lamb (ed.), *The Homeless Mentally Ill*, pp. 11–53. Washington, DC: American Psychiatric Association.

Bachrach, L. L. (1987). Issues in identifying and treating the homeless mentally ill. In *Leona Bachrach Speaks: Selected Speeches and Lectures*, pp. 43–62. No. 35 in *New Directions for Mental Health Services*, series, ed. H. R. Lamb, San Francisco: Jossey-Bass.

Bachrach, L. L. & Nadelson, C. C. (1988). *Treating Chronically Mentally Ill Women*. Washington, DC: American Psychiatric Press.

Bassuk, E. L., Rubin, L. & Lauriat, A. (1984). Is homelessness a mental health problem?' *American Journal of Psychiatry*, 141, 1546–50.

Burns, T. P. (1989). Community care and rehabilitation. *Current Opinion in Psychiatry*, 2, 273–7.

Caton, C. (1990). Solutions to the homeless problems. In C. Caton (ed.), *Homeless in America*, pp 174–90. Oxford: Oxford University Press.

Chamberlain, C. & MacKenzie, D. (1992). Understanding contemporary homelessness: issues of definition and meaning. *Australian Journal of Social Issues*, 27, 274–97.

Chesterman, C. (1988). Homes away from homes: final report of the national review of the supported accommodation assistance program. Canberra: Australian Government Printing Service.

Doutney, C. P., Buhrich, N. Virgona, A., Cohen, A. & Daniels, P. (1985). The prevalence of schizophrenia in a refuge for homeless men. *Australian and New Zealand Journal of Psychiatry*, 19, 233–8.

Fopp, R. (1992). *Homelessness: Implications for State Housing Authorities*. Melbourne: Ministerial Advisory Committee on Homelessness and Housing.

Gelberg, L., Linn, L. S. & Leake, B. D. (1988). Mental health, alcohol and drug use, and criminal history among homeless adults. *American Journal of Psychiatry*, 145, 191–6.

Hamilton, C. (1991). The crisis of change. Paper presented at the ACOSS (Australian Council of Social Services) National Congress. Melbourne, October 1991.

Harris, M. & Bachrach, L. (1990). Perspectives on homeless mentally ill women. *Hospital and Community Psychiatry*, 41, 253–4.

Harris, R., Maley, M. & Szajnoha, A. (1987). Chronically Mentally Ill in Boarding Houses, A Discussion of Service Utilisation. Project report. University of New South Wales: Community Medicine Department.

Hearn, R. (1993). *Locked up Locked Out. The Denial and Criminalisation of Young People's Mental Health Crisis*. Melbourne: Victorian Community Managed Mental Health Services Inc. (VICSERV).

Herrman, H. (1992). A survey of homeless mentally ill people in Melbourne, Australia. *Hospital and Community Psychiatry*, 41, 1291–2.

Herrman, H., McGorry, P., Bennett, P. & Singh, B. (1990). Age and severe mental disorders in homeless and disaffiliated people in inner Melbourne. *The Medical Journal of Australia*, 153, 197–205.

Herrman, H., McGorry, P., Bennett, P. van Riel, R. & Singh, B. (1989). Prevalence of severe mental disorders in disaffiliated and homeless people in inner Melbourne. *American Journal of Psychiatry*, **146**, 1179–84.

Herrman, H., McGorry, P., Bennett, P., Varnavides, K. & Singh, B. (1992). Use of services by homeless and disaffiliated individuals with severe mental disorders. In B. Cooper & R. Eastwood (eds.), *Primary Health Care and Psychiatric Epidemiology*, pp. 143–59. London, New York: Tavistock/Routledge.

HREOC (Human Rights and Equal Opportunity Commission) (1989). *Our Homeless Children*. Canberra. The Burdekin Report. Canberra: Australian Government Publishing Service.

Ife, J. (1993). Community-based services: opportunity or con trick. In P. Saunders & S. Graham (eds.), *Beyond Economic Rationalism: Alternative Futures for Social Policy*. Proceedings of a joint conference with the Department of Social Work and Social Administration, University of Western Australia, 27 November 1992. Social Policy Research Centre Reports and Proceedings No 105.

Jablensky, A. (1994). Whither transcultural psychiatry? A comment on a project for a national strategy. *Australasian Psychiatry*, **2**, 59–61.

James, N. Mcl. (1993). On the perception of madness. *Australian and New Zealand Journal of Psychiatry*, **27**, 192–9.

Koegel, P., Burnam, A. & Farr, R. K. (1988). The prevalence of specific psychiatric disorders among homeless individuals in the inner city of Los Angeles. *Archives of General Psychiatry*, **45**, 1085–92.

Lamb, H. R. & Lamb, D. M. (1990). Factors contributing to homelessness among the chronically severely mentally ill. *Hospital and Community Psychiatry*, **41**, 301–5.

Levine, I. S. (1984). Service programs for the homeless mentally ill. In H. R. Lamb (ed.), *The Homeless Mentally Ill*, pp. 173–200. Washington, DC: American Psychiatric Association.

Lipton, F. R., Nutt, S. & Sabatini, A. (1988). Housing the homeless mentally ill: a longitudinal study of a treatment approach. *Hospital and Community Psychiatry*, **39**, 40–5.

Marshall, M. & Gath, D. (1992). What happens to homeless mentally ill people? Follow up of residents of Oxford hostels for the homeless. *British Medical Journal*, **304**, 79–80.

McDermott, F. & Pyett, P. (1994). Co-existent psychiatric illness and drug abuse: a community study. *Psychiatry, Psychology and Law*, **1**, 45–52.

McDonald, P. (1993). *Confronting the Chaos*. Melbourne: The Salvation Army Crossroads Housing and Support Network.

McKendrick, J. H., Cutter, T., McKenzie, A. & Chiu, E. (1992). The pattern of psychiatric morbidity in a Victorian urban Aboriginal general practice population. *Australian and New Zealand Journal of Psychiatry*, **26**, 40–7.

Minas, I. H., Silove, D. & Kunst, J. P. (1993). Mental Health for Multi-cultural Australia: A National Strategy. A Report by the

Victorian Transcultural Psychiatry Unit, St Vincent's Hospital, Melbourne.

Morrissey, M., Mitchell, C. & Rutherford, A. (1991). *The Family in the Settlement Process.* Canberra: Australian Government Publishing Service.

National Health Strategy (1993). *Help Where Help is Needed. Continuity of Care for People with Chronic Mental Illness.* National Health Strategy Issues Paper No 5. Canberra: National Health Strategy.

Neil, C. C. & Fopp, R. with McNamara, C. & Pelling, M. (1992). *Homelessness in Australia: Causes and Consequences.* Melbourne: CSIRO.

Neil, C. C., Pelling, M., Ashley, J. & McNamara, C. (1993). Community management of public housing stock in Australia. Paper presented at the ENHR Conference, Budapest, 7–10 September.

Nyland, J. (1992). The role of funding bodies in in-service training for the non-government sector. In P. Saunders & D. Encel (eds.), *Social Policy in Australia: Options for the 1990s,* vol. 3: *Contributed Papers.* Proceedings of the National Social Policy Conference, Sydney, 3–5 July 1991. Social Policy Research Centre Reports and Proceedings, No. 98. Kensington: University of New South Wales.

Pawsey, R. & Fuller, A. (1993). The homeless agencies resource project. *Youth Studies Australia,* **Autumn**, 45–7.

Powell, P. V. (1988). Qualitative assessment in the evaluation of the Edinburgh primary health care scheme for single hostel dwellers. *Community Medicine,* **10**, 185–96.

Quinn, J. (1993). Are the Homeless Mentally Ill Different From Other Mentally Ill People? Thesis, University of Queensland.

Reilly, J., Herrman, H., Clarke, D. M., Neil, C. C. & McNamara, C. L. (1994). Psychiatric disorders in and service use by young homeless people. *Medical Journal of Australia,* **161**, 429–32.

Reuler, J. B. (1989). Health care for the homeless in a national health program. *American Journal of Public Health,* **79**, 1033–5.

Rosenman, L. (1992). Community care: social or economic policy? In P. Saunders & D. Encel (eds.). *Social Policy in Australia: Options for the 1990s,* vol. 1: *Plenary Sessions.* Proceedings of the National Social Policy Conference, Sydney, 3–5 July 1991. Social Policy Research Centre Reports and Proceedings No. 96. Kensington: University of New South Wales.

Rymill, A. (1992). *Making the Links.* Adelaide: Department of Family and Community Services/South Australian Mental Health Service/Commonwealth Department of Health, Housing and Community Services.

Sawyer, M., Meldrum, D., Tonge, B. & Clark, J. (1992). *Mental Health and Young People.* Hobart: National Clearinghouse for Youth Studies.

Scott, J. (1993). Homeless and mental illness. *British Journal of Psychiatry,* **162**, 314–24.

Singh, B. (1992). Mainstreaming psychiatric services. *Medical Journal of Australia*, **156**, 373–4.
Susser, E. & Struening, E. L. (1987). Childhood experiences of homeless men. *American Journal of Psychiatry*, **144**, 1599–601.
Susser, E., Lovell, A. & Conover, S. (1988). Unravelling the causes of homelessness and of its associations with mental illness. In B. Cooper & T. Helgason (eds.), *Epidemiology and the Prevention of Mental Health Disorders*, pp. 228–39. London: Routledge.
Teesson, M. & Buhrich, N. (1990). Prevalence of schizophrenia in a refuge for homeless men: a five-year follow-up. *Psychiatric Bulletin*, **14**, 597–600.
Teesson, M. & Buhrich, N. (1993). Prevalence of cognitive impairment among homeless men in a shelter in Australia. *Hospital and Community Psychiatry*, **44**, 1187–9.
Teesson, M. & Hambridge, J. (1992). Mobile community treatment in inner city and surburban Sydney. *Psychiatric Quarterly*, **63**, 119–26.
Thornicroft, G. & Breakey, W. R. (1991). The COSTAR Programme. 1: Improving social networks of the long-term mentally ill. *British Journal of Psychiatry*, **159**, 245–9.
Virgona, A., Buhrich, N. & Teesson, M. (1993). Prevalence of schizophrenia among women in refuges for the homeless. *Australian and New Zealand Journal of Psychiatry*, **27**, 405–10.
Victorian Council of Social Service and the Office of the Public Advocate (1992). *Double Disadvantage. Housing for People with a Disability in Victoria*. Melbourne: Victorian Council of Social Service and the Office of the Public Advocate.
Whiteford, H., MacLeod, B. & Leitch, B. (1993). The national mental health policy: implications for public psychiatric services in Australia. *Australian and New Zealand Journal of Psychiatry*, **27**, 186–91.

PART IV

POLICY AND EVALUATION

15

Implications of social policy

David Kingdon

Whilst there may continue to be some disagreement about the precise nature and extent of mental illness amongst homeless people, commentators generally view social and health policy as playing the major part in its causation and consequently it has the potential to alleviate it. Bassuk *et al.* (1984) have said that explanations for the marked increase in the numbers of homeless people include unemployment and the economic recession, deinstitutionalization of mental patients, unavailability of low-cost housing, reduced disability benefits and cutbacks to social service agencies. Policy developments may be viewed therefore as directly responsible for the increased incidence of mental illness in homeless people. Alternatively, changes occurring in society, for example, the reduction in importance of the extended family and increase in divorce rates, may not have evoked the necessary policy response to minimize adverse effects.

Housing

People with mental illness will be particularly vulnerable to being made homeless. In a competitive market for homes, those with severe and enduring mental illness will be disadvantaged by their lack of employment, disabilities consequent on their illness and stigmatization. Securing accommodation may therefore be difficult and maintaining it equally problematic for much the same reasons. In turn, housing difficulties are life events and circumstances predisposing to relapse and persisting disability. Of particular consequence therefore, has been the availability of low-cost housing in the public or private rental sector. Both areas are known to have reduced over the past decade (recently reviewed comprehensively by Everton, 1993). This has occurred in part because of the encouragement of owner-occupation, now supported in the UK by both major political parties. The gentrification of urban areas and possibly rising house and rental prices in the late 1980s may have been other factors. So, whilst the number of homes has probably increased more rapidly overall than the population, social changes, particularly the trend towards smaller household sizes, has led to increases in the numbers presenting to local authorities as homeless.

Housing policy in most countries has amongst its key aims the minimization of homelessness. In the UK, the intention to provide for the vulnerable was embodied in the Housing Act 1967, the Housing and Homeless Person's Act 1976 and the Housing Act 1985. Part 3 of this latter Act states that a local authority has the duty to secure suitable accommodation if someone is homeless, or threatened with homelessness within 28 days; is in priority need; and is not intentionally homeless. Priority need includes single people who are vulnerable as a result of mental illness. The Housing Act 1988 increased the role of housing associations and a new Special Needs Management Allowance was introduced to enable them to produce a wider range of special needs housing including that for people with mental illness.

Employment and social security

Employment policy can have effects on the availability of work for people with mental illness and therefore their ability to maintain or obtain housing as well as less specific effects on their mental state. Policy on welfare benefits is also a relevant factor with effects on homelessness. The National Assistance Act 1948 in the UK set a framework that considered the needs of vulnerable groups such as those who were mentally ill. In 1989, hostel residents were transferred from receiving support payments for 'board and lodging' to a combination of housing benefit and income support. This brought homeless people into the same benefits framework as other people but has proved complicated, in some circumstances (Everton, 1993), to administer in practice. Similarly, the change in housing benefit rules in 1988, which affected its availability to those under the age of 25, has been cited as having diverse effects. Theoretically, this may have had a tendency to reduce homelessness in promoting more efficient use of limited housing stock and resources generally by discouraging young people from leaving the parental home until they are in a position to financially maintain themselves. Alternatively, the view expressed by homelessness agencies (Everton, 1993) is that homelessness is increasing because young people are continuing to leave home but the reduction in benefits and the level of unemployment has meant that they are unable to obtain accommodation. In the USA, changes in welfare arrangements whereby people with mental illness became eligible for Aid to the Disabled (now Supplemental Security Income) in 1963, are believed to have had an impact on the deinstitutionalization process (Talbott & Lamb, 1984). This was further accentuated in the USA with the introduction of Medicaid, which allowed a shift of half or more of costs to federal government when patients transferred from state mental hospitals to nursing homes. Similarly in the UK, most patients transferred from hospital to nursing and residential homes became the funding responsibility of the Department of Social Security from the early 1980s and this had a similar effect.

Difficulties met by homeless mentally ill people in obtaining benefits may result from the complexities of social welfare systems combined with the cognitive and social disabilities associated with mental illness. Paranoid symptomatology and the profound distrust of authority that many homeless people experience, further complicates an already problematic situation. Citizen's advice bureaux, welfare rights specialists and even computer packages can assist where available.

Emergency shelters

A response to homelessness over many decades has been the development of emergency shelters. In New York City, Bassuk & Lauriat (1986) reported there to have been 2 shelters before 1980 and 18 in 1986 and they asked the question: 'Are emergency shelters the solution?' Their answer was that: 'Emergency shelters are an essential short-term solution to the plight of the homeless. They save lives. The trouble is that many shelters do little more ... Shelters [are] becoming permanent institutions that have replaced the almshouses and mental institutions of past decades' (Bassuk & Lauriat, 1986, p. 134). Some shelters in the USA have developed 'wards' staffed by psychiatrically trained personnel; in the UK, the attachment of community psychiatric nurses to shelters is increasingly common. In New York City, the situation has apparently forced the reopening of a decommissioned hospital to provide care to homeless mentally ill people.

The Resettlement Units Executive Agency (RA), part of the Department of Social Security, is currently responsible for the direct management of 15 resettlement units throughout the UK providing 1136 bedspaces. These are direct access hostels managed by the RA under the Supplementary Benefits Act 1976. Their own surveys had demonstrated a high prevalence of health problems including mental disorder amongst people using the units. The RA, which used to run a total of 22 units some years ago, is actively disengaging from the business and expects to cease directly managing its hostels by 1996. Instead figures available for 1993 showed that it provided both capital and revenue funding for a further 1912 bedspaces in various parts of the country. These additional bedspaces, which are not directly managed by the RA, are increasing as the RA decreases the number of bedspaces that it does directly manage.

Legislation and the criminal justice system

Legislative and criminal justice system policies may also have a significant impact. New York's efforts to remove homeless mentally ill people from the streets involuntarily to give medical and psychiatric attention – Project HELP (New York City Homeless Emergency Liaison Project) – is one illustration of this (Mechanic & Rochefort, 1992) although it must be noted that only 2% of those assessed were detained. Most state commitment laws use the criterion for detention that the person assessed must be in danger of causing serious harm to him or herself or others. In New York, this was interpreted as being 'within the foreseeable future' rather than the standard test of 'imminent danger'. Legal challenges overturned this in a number of cases and other obstacles to the programme included the overcrowding of municipal units, long lengths of stay and attempts by the city to transfer large numbers of patients to state facilities at a time when they were dramatically reducing in number. Finally, community facilities were not available to provide back-up. Criteria under mental health legislation in the UK, except for Northern Ireland, is wider than in the USA as it allows for involuntary admission for reasons of health or safety or the protection of others. This has recently been reaffirmed in a Government circular and in the revision of the Code of Practice for the Mental Health Act (1983). However, in practice, there is little evidence that its use has been any more widespread amongst homeless people than in other countries with more restrictive legislation.

Policing policy might also make an impact on street homelessness but again there is no evidence of changes in policy, although local interpretation by individual forces may differ over time. Police involvement with mentally ill people is substantial but under-researched. In Los Angeles 20% of emergency calls to police are believed to be related in some way to psychiatric problems (Walker, 1991). The police force there developed a 'mental evaluation unit' that now receives 1000 referrals a month. In the UK, a National Schizophrenia Fellowship survey in 1990 reported the provision of care by police to be more highly rated by carers that they received responses from than that by doctors, psychiatrists, social workers or community nurses (National Schizophrenia Fellowship, 1990).

Many homeless mentally ill people spend time in police custody and prison. In the UK, a recent joint Department of Health and Home Office report (1992) *Review of Health and Social Services for Mentally Disordered Offenders and Others Requiring Similar Services*, made a number of recommendations highlighting the need for *local* assessment of the service needs of mentally disordered offenders to take account of the need for local and medium secure hospital provision at all levels and non-secure provision. This includes efficient development of court diversion schemes and transfer of mentally disordered offenders, where appropriate, to community support or hospitals and the general development of links between the criminal justice system and health and social services. Both appear to be occurring and in 1992/3 transfers to hospital increased substantially.

Primary health care

Most mental illness is managed by non-specialists in mental health. In the UK, this predominantly means by the primary health care team (PCHT: see also Chapter 11). Much inevitably depends on the attitude of PHCTs to how accessible they make their services and how effectively they provide services for homeless people generally, and those who are mentally ill in particular. However, some leverage can be applied through policy and management channels to improve services and, crucially, develop understanding by PHCTs of the difficulties faced by mentally ill people when they are about to, or have become, homeless. Access to specialist care for most people is by referral from the PHCT and this means that initial assessment, treatment and emergency care is given prior to contact being established with specialist services. The PHCT will usually have records and often acquaintance with the individual that can be a source of valuable information for specialists. Even more importantly, anxieties about the process of referral to mental health services can be alleviated and any complications or disruptions in this process can be resolved. The PHCT in effect acts as advocate and provides an introduction for the person to services that elicit apprehension in most people. For those who need it most, people with severe mental illness who are also homeless, this smoothing of the path into specialist care is usually not available. Many homeless people are not registered with a PHCT. Where they are, this is often only temporary, previous records are unavailable and time or circumstances frequently makes the development of a positive therapeutic relationship difficult. Contact with specialist services may therefore occur in difficult circumstances, through Accident and Emergency services or the criminal justice system.

In the UK, two pilot projects were established in 1986 in the City and east London and Camden and Islington areas to improve primary health care available to homeless people. Multi-disciplinary teams were set up, each with a salaried general practitioner (GP), who visited places where homeless people congregated, seeking where possible to secure admission of homeless people to GPs lists. Evaluation of the scheme in 1989 suggested some drawbacks to this separate approach to the homeless and modifications have been made to the scheme, which was expanded in 1991, to integrate it more with mainstream services.

Mental health services

The rising recognition of mental illness amongst homeless people has coincided with the decrease in hospital bed numbers. Numbers of residents in mental hospitals in the USA reached 559 000 when the population was 165 million (339/100 000) in 1955 and fell to 100 000 out of a population of 250 million (41/100 000) in 1987. In the UK, there were 143 000 mental hospital beds (320/100 000) dropping to 20 000 (43/100 000) mental hospital beds (45 000 hospital beds overall) in 1992. However, much of this drop is accounted for by trans-institutionalization; in the USA, there is estimated to be 1.5 million people in nursing homes and mental illness amongst nursing home residents has been demonstrated to be 30–75% (dependent on definition). Furthermore, 300 000–400 000 mentally ill people are housed in non-traditional institutions – halfway houses, board-and-care homes and other community residences. In the UK, rises from 179 500 to 289 900 in nursing and residential homes occurred between 1978–9 and 1990–91 and similar proportions have been estimated to have mental illness. The numbers in residential accommodation specifically for mentally ill people has risen from 5600 to 12 840 over the same period. A recent review (Mental Health Task Force, 1994) of 'bed spaces' in residential and hospital accommodation has found that the overall numbers have remained at approximately 80 000 throughout the 1980s but in about 1000 locations at the start, 2500 at the end, with a marked reduction in the proportion in mental hospitals. The proportion of those with mental illness amongst homeless people over 20 years has probably remained unchanged (Leff, 1993).

Despite public conviction that deinstitutionalization is responsible for the numbers of people with mental illness amongst the homeless population, the effects of these changes are certainly not clear cut. The first publicized closure of a mental hospital in the UK – Banstead, Surrey in 1986 – did give rise to concern with reports of patients scattered around the UK including moves to bed and breakfast lodgings in seaside towns without support being arranged from local services (Bassuk & Lauriat, 1986). But systematic follow-up studies of long-stay patients who have been discharged from hospital have generally shown that very few are added to the numbers of homeless people (Double & Wong, 1991; Leff, 1993). The reduction of beds could nevertheless reduce access to patients who have never become long-stay either because they are of a younger generation or because short-term hospital admission previously maintained them in hostels or their own homes. This has been described as a particular problem in inner cities. The evidence that numbers of resident inpatients who have stayed under 1 year in hospital, has remained constant at around

21 000 (in England) since 1986 tends to counter this argument. However, further investigation is to occur as part of the changes being made to London's health services.

So, much change has occurred in the settings where mental health services are provided but also the ways in which it is provided. There have been marked increases in the numbers of staff providing services – in England, numbers of community psychiatric nurses have risen to 3600 from 1083, and consultant psychiatrists to 1670 from 1174 over a similar period from the late 1970s to the early 1990s. But, as occurred in the USA, many of these community based staff have turned their attention away from the more severely mentally ill. Services also do not appear to have adequately followed up or been sufficiently flexible in the care package offered to patients so that severely mentally ill people have fallen through the safety net of care (Talbott & Lamb, 1984). The introduction of methods of case management and assertive outreach have begun to make an impact on this.

Fischer & Breakey (1986) have said that: 'In relation to the chronically mentally ill, prevention of homelessness seems to be the key. Mental health services need to be expanded and augmented to protect patients from falling through the cracks of the system' (Fischer & Breakey, 1986, p. 28). The degree of mental illness amongst homeless people could be viewed as one quality indicator for mental health services. General developments in the integrated provision of mental health services should make an impact on the numbers of people who are homeless and mentally ill – at least in theory. In the USA, the extension of coverage under the Health Care plans being developed by President Clinton for introduction between 1995 and the end of the century are relevant, although how relevant remains to be seen. In England, the development of the Mental Illness Key Area prioritized under the Government's health strategy, *The Health of the Nation: A Strategy for Health in England* (1992) is intended to bring about greater focus on the needs of severely mentally ill people and purchasing of services for them has been specifically highlighted in guidance to Health Authorities (DH/SSI, 1994). This has been reinforced by the establishment of a Mental Health Task Force with a remit to oversee the development of effective and comprehensive local mental health services to replace the mental hospitals as they close over the next decade. More specific but concise guidance detailing ways of assessing and meeting the needs of homeless people has been given by Access to Health (1992).

The development of services that are flexible and responsive is a challenge to all involved in their provision. Case management methods have been introduced in many services internationally with this intention. In England, the introduction of the 'Care Programme Approach' (Department of Health, 1990) for implementation nationally has been designed to reduce the potential for patients accepted by specialist mental health services losing contact with services inappropriately. Essentially it requires services to provide individuals with a 'keyworker' who co-ordinates assessment, management and review of the individual's needs. It promulgates multi-disciplinary working and the negotiation of care plans with users of services and their carers. It also specifically requires health authorities to ensure that appropriate community services, including housing, are available before a person is discharged from a psychiatric unit. The principles involved are generally accepted; implementation is gradually occurring as resistance to re-targeting of resources on those most at need is overcome and clarification of some initial misunderstandings of the circular's requirements occurs (North *et al.*, 1993).

Housing and other social policies are fundamental to the reduction of homelessness generally but Bachrach (1992, p. 460) has warned that: '... residential planning is sometimes raised to such primacy that the population's other requirements are virtually ignored...'. Co-ordination of the widely dispersed responsibility for people who are homeless and mentally ill is necessary although remarkably difficult. The variety and number of statutory and non-statutory agencies involved in any one geographical area can be quite overwhelming to those attempting to co-ordinate policy – and far more to those on the receiving end of it. Planning however, needs to be for the individual not for an undefined mass, and where they are not where we want them (Bachrach, 1992). In the USA, a Federal Interagency Council on Homelessness created an interdepartmental Task Force on Homelessness and Severe Mental Illness, which released a national strategy report in 1992 (Hospital & Community Psychiatry, News Section, 1992). This proposed action in promoting systems integration; expanding housing options and alternative services; improving outreach efforts and access to existing programmes; generating knowledge and disseminating information about the homeless mentally ill population (see Chapter 13).

In the UK, the Department of Health established an Inner London

Homeless Mentally Ill (HMI) initiative in 1990. This followed the recognition of significant levels of mental illness amongst homeless people and followed the success of an initial pilot project. Its aim was to provide specialist mental health services to people 'sleeping rough' with the intention of bringing them back, as far as possible, into contact with mainstream services. Five multi-disciplinary teams have been set-up and seven staffed hostels have been established accepting referrals from the teams. Accommodation for longer-term support is being established gradually. A 'Rough Sleepers Initiative (RSI)', commenced soon after the establishment of the HMI by the Department of the Environment, and provides accommodation for street homeless people generally. Furthermore, 900 additional hostel bed-spaces are being directly provided, with around 2900 places in more permanent accommodation, to which people in hostels can move, being developed by the Housing Corporation. The RSI is also funding voluntary bodies to provide outreach and resettlement work. Both initiatives are being evaluated and lessons learnt as they progress – initial results have demonstrated that the teams are making contact with the population targeted. They are engaging and maintaining contact with approximately three quarters of their clients.

Elsewhere in the UK, specialist mental health teams or posts have been established, often utilizing the Mental Illness Specific Grant (available since 1991) in, for example Newcastle, Birmingham, Cambridgeshire, Essex, Oxfordshire, East Sussex and Newham with some 1300 homeless people reported to have benefited. Varying patterns have evolved. In Nottingham, a team provides liaison between the non-statutory and statutory sectors with a range of Local Authority, Health Service and Voluntary Sector provision available, particularly for those with alcohol problems (Nottingham Hostels Liaison Group, 1991). Development of mutual understanding between statutory and non-statutory sectors has involved the former developing much more flexible ways of operating and the latter an understanding that identifying homeless people as mentally ill should not be viewed as a 'labelling issue' (Bachrach, 1992) but one that allows appropriate care to be offered.

Conclusions

When homeless people have been asked about their needs, food, shelter and general medical care usually come before mental health care, if the latter is included at all. Policies need to address these expressed needs. But there also needs to be provision of appropriate mental health care designed to prevent people from becoming homeless and mentally ill and to assist them in maintaining their independence once other basic needs are being met.

There is a longstanding tradition of local responsibility for care for the homeless. Such responsibility can lead to services that are tailored to local need because of more individualized assessment of needs. In most areas, the local mental health teams are in the best position to provide the range of services needed by the relatively small numbers of homeless people with mental health problems in consultation with them. Policies need to be focused on creating services that recognize their needs with staff that have the basic level of training needed to address them. This may involve management specification through purchasing contracts to ensure targeting of services. In a few inner city areas specialist workers or teams are needed to reach patients – assertively, not aggressively – and reintroduce them to mainstream services where possible. A few will need continuing support from the specialist teams or workers. Likewise specialist hostels are needed in some areas, direct access hostels are essential in the short-term but cannot be expected to provide longer term mental health care.

Interest in homelessness and mental illness by policymakers has dramatically increased in the past 5 years (Manderscheid & Rosenstein, 1992). Early signs are that this may be having an impact on numbers and availability of services. Evaluative studies are underway and will report in the near future.

Acknowledgements

Acknowledgements are due to colleagues from the various different government departments involved for their comments on early drafts of the above.

References

Access to Health (1992). *Purchasing and Poverty*. London: Access to Health.

Bachrach, L. (1992). What we know about homelessness among mentally ill persons: an analytical review and commentary. *Hospital and Community Psychiatry*, **43**, 453–64.

Barham, P. (1992). *Closing the Asylum*. Harmondsworth: Penguin.

Bassuk, E. L. & Lauriat, A. (1986). Are emergency shelters the solution? *International Journal of Mental Health*, **14**, 125–36.

Bassuk, E. L., Rubin, L. & Lauriat, A. (1984). Is homelessness a mental health problem? *American Journal of Psychiatry*, **141**, 1546–50.

Department of Health (1990). *Joint Health/Social Services Circular: Health and Social Services Development: 'Caring for People'. The Care Programme Approach for People with a Mental Illness Referred to the Special Psychiatric Service*. Heywood, Lancs.: Department of Health. (Joint circular: HC(90)23, LASSL(90)11).

Department of Health and Home Office (1992). *Review of Health and Social Services for Mentally Disordered Offenders and Others Requiring Similar Services. Final Summary Report*. London: HMSO. (Cm 2088).

DH/SSI (Department of Health/Social Services Inspectorate) (1994). *Health of the Nation. Key Area Handbook: Mental Illness*, 2nd edit. London: HMSO.

Double, D. B. & Wong, T. I. (1991). What has happened to patients from long stay psychiatric wards? *Psychiatric Bulletin*, **15**, 735–6.

Everton, J. (1993). Single homelessness and social policy. In K. Fisher & J. Collins (eds.), *Homelessness, Health Care and Welfare Provision*, London: Routledge.

Fischer, P. J. & Breakey, W. R. (1986). Homelessness and mental health: an overview. *International Journal of Mental Health*, **14**, 6–41.

Hospital and Community Psychiatry, News Section (1992). Federal task force develops national strategy to improve services to homeless mentally ill. *Hospital and Community Psychiatry*, **43**, 523–4.

Leff, J. (1993). All the homeless people – where do they all come from? *British Medical Journal*, **306**, 669–70.

Manderscheid, R. W. & Rosenstein, M. J. (1992). Homeless persons with mental illness and alcohol or other drug abuse: current research, policy, and prospects. *Current Opinion in Psychiatry*, **5**, 273–8.

Mechanic, D. & Rochefort, D. A. (1992). A policy for inclusion for the mentally ill. *Health Affairs*, **11**, 128–50.

Mental Health Task Force (1994). *Survey of English Mental Illness Hospitals*. London: NHSE (National Health Service Executive).

National Schizophrenia Fellowship (1990). *Report of Survey for Department of Health*. NSF News, May 1990, p. 1.

North, C., Ritchie, J. & Ward, K. (1993). *Factors Influencing the Implementation of the Care Programme Approach*. London: HMSO.

Nottingham Hostels Liaison Group (1991). *Mental Health Support Team for Homeless People.* Nottingham: NHLG.

Talbott, J. A. & Lamb, H. R. (1984). Summary and recommendations. In H. R. Lamb (ed.), *The Homeless Mentally Ill*, pp. 1–10. Washington, DC: American Psychiatric Association.

Department of Health (1992). *The Health of the Nation: A Strategy for Health in England.* London: HMSO. (Cm 1986).

Walker, J. (1991). Psychiatric problems of American cities. In M. Page & R. Powell (eds.), *Homelessness and Mental Illness*, pp. 35–8. London: Concern Publications.

16

Evaluating services for homeless people with mental disorders: theoretical and practical issues

Max Marshall

Introduction

This chapter is in two sections. The first section will be a survey of the types of evaluative studies that have been conducted on services for homeless people with mental disorders. The survey will pay particular attention to the problems that have arisen in carrying out these studies. This section will be illustrated throughout by examples of evaluative studies from the UK literature; where UK studies are lacking, examples will be taken from the world literature.

The second section will consider how far evaluative studies have provided evidence for the effectiveness of hostels for the homeless. As indicated in Chapter 9 the role of hostels in this area is increasingly controversial.

A SURVEY OF EVALUATIVE STUDIES

Evaluative studies of services for homeless people with mental disorders can be classified according to design. Such a classification produces the following broad groupings:

(1) Retrospective evaluations.
(2) Evaluations based on the impressions of a trained observer.
(3) Surveys.
(4) Follow-up evaluations.
(5) Before and after evaluations.
(6) Single case and 'action research' evaluations.
(7) Quasi-experimental evaluations.
(8) Randomized controlled trials.

Examples of evaluations from each of these groupings will be discussed below. The discussion will pay particular attention to the reasons for adopting particular designs and the problems that arise in implementing these designs with homeless subjects.

Retrospective evaluations

Description

Retrospective evaluations are based on the analysis of routine data collected during clinical work.

Uses of retrospective evaluations

Retrospective evaluations may usefully describe the structure of a new service and the activities of that service. Retrospective evaluations may also raise questions about the effectiveness of a service.

Examples

An example of a retrospective evaluation is the description by Ferguson & Dixon (1992) of a walk-in psychiatric service in a hostel for the homeless in Nottingham. An example of a retrospective evaluation that raised questions about the effectiveness of a service, is the study by Hamid & McCarthy (1989) of community psychiatric nurses (CPN) working with 'homeless' and 'home-based' clients in Bloomsbury. This study found that homeless clients were less likely to receive supportive care from the CPN service and were more likely than home-based clients to be referred elsewhere; even though the homeless group were more likely to suffer from schizophrenia.

Advantages

Retrospective evaluations are relatively cheap and fairly easy to carry out.

Disadvantages

Retrospective evaluations are usually based on poor quality information and are prone to many sources of bias. Whilst retrospective evaluation may highlight problems with a service, they are of little value in assessing the service's effectiveness.

Evaluations based on the impressions of a trained observer

Description

An observer is placed within a service for a time. The observer examines the activities of the service by, for example, attending management meetings or observing interactions between staff and clients. The observer then synthesizes his or her impressions into a report. Such reports are usually, but not invariably, backed up by interviews with consumers of the service (both clients and representatives of other interested parties), and with more objective data on the types of patients seen by the service.

Uses of evaluations based on impressions

Evaluations based upon the impressions of an observer can be used to identify problems with an existing service or problems that arise while setting up a new service. Such studies have also been used as the main means of assessing the effectiveness of a new service, but this use is problematic. A powerful, but uncommon, use of an observer, is to complement the findings of an empirical evaluation, such as a randomized controlled trial.

Examples

A good example of the use of an observer is provided by a study of the reaction of agencies to 'difficult to place' homeless clients in Oxford, most of whom were suffering from mental disorders (Vagg, 1992). The observer concluded that 'many of the most difficult problems were picked up by the voluntary sector, which might be characterized as the only place left to go when statutory agencies decided that individuals had become too difficult to cope with'. As a result of the observer's recommendations a care management team was set up to organize and supervise 'shared care' in the city, between voluntary and statutory agencies.

An observer was used to assess the effectiveness of a new service for the homeless as part of a controversial evaluation (Williams & Allen, 1989) of the work of two multi-disciplinary primary care teams in London (Tower Hamlets and Camden). The evaluation was based on observer's impressions, interviews with patients, general practitioners (GPs) and hostel staff, and data on the type of patients seen by the teams. The study concluded that the teams were ineffective and should be discontinued. It was suggested that specialized services would only serve to marginalize those homeless people already on the fringes of society.

Advantages

Evaluations based on impressions are relatively cheap, though not as cheap as retrospective studies. Perceptive observers may provide information that cannot be obtained from more formal empirical approaches. For example, observers can detect good or bad practices, or gain an understanding of the motivations or frustrations of staff and clients. The findings of observers may lead to hypotheses that can then be tested in empirical studies. Such findings may also be used to complement or 'explain' the findings of empirical studies. For example, a randomized control trial might establish that a new service was no more effective than usual treatment, whilst the findings of an observer might help explain why this was so.

Disadvantages

The study of primary care teams in London (Williams & Allen, 1989) illustrates well the problems of evaluating a new service by means of an observer. Without suitable empirical data to back up the impressions of the observer it is impossible to counter the argument that the observer's impressions were misleading or biased. The inevitable result of a negative report will be a wrangle between proponents and opponents of the service. Thus, observational methods, whilst of value in identifying problems with existing services, are not helpful when used as the sole means of assessing the effectiveness of a new service. This is not to say however that they should not be used to complement a suitable empirical approach, such as a randomized control trial.

Surveys

Description

Surveys are based on data collected from a cross-section of the users of a service. The subjects selected should be representative of the users of the service (but rarely are).

Uses of evaluations based on surveys

Surveys may be used to evaluate a service for the homeless either by (a) eliciting clients' opinions about the service, or (b) assessing the quality of care that the subjects are receiving. Subjects' opinions may be elicited using standardized instruments, such as satisfaction questionnaires, or simply by seeking opinions on specific aspects of care. Quality of care may also be assessed using standardized instruments, or more simply, by seeking the opinion of a panel of acknowledged experts. The findings of evaluative surveys are difficult to interpret unless there is some 'yardstick' against which the subjects' opinions or the quality of care can be assessed.

Examples

Eliciting clients' opinions

A study of women's hostels in London asked mentally disordered residents whether they wished to live elsewhere. The study found that only 16 out of 61 residents (26%) wished to remain in the hostels, and all of the 16 complained about lack of privacy (Marshall & Reed, 1992). Thus, a majority of the residents did not consider the hostel accommodation satisfactory.

Assessing the quality of care

The care provided to severely mentally disordered residents was assessed using the MRC Needs for Care Schedule in a study of two Oxford hostels for the homeless (Hogg & Marshall, 1992). Standardized instruments were used to measure the performance of 46 mentally ill residents in 20 areas of psychiatric and social functioning. Ratings of performance in each area of functioning were then compared with criteria provided by the schedule. If a subject's performance in an area fell below the standard set by these criteria then a problem was present. The authors determined whether the problem was a need using a list of suitable interventions supplied by the schedule for each problem area. A problem was identified as a need when there were one or more suitable interventions that had not been offered in the past year. Although the authors felt that the MRC Needs for Care Schedule had many limitations, the study indicated that there were high levels of need for psychiatric and social care amongst the residents, on average about two needs per resident.

Advantages

Surveys are useful in that they provide a good means of assessing the quality of care being provided by a service at one point in time. Surveys also permit us to evaluate a service indirectly by providing information about how the recipients of the service perceive it.

Disadvantages

Surveys can be difficult to conduct, particularly when representative samples are required and standardized instruments are used. Surveys do not allow us to assess the actual outcome for clients but only the quality of care at one point in time. Surveys cannot determine whether one approach is superior to another. Where quality of care is being assessed, it may be very difficult to find a suitable yardstick against which the care of the index group may be compared.

Follow-up evaluations

Description

A group (or cohort) of clients receiving a service is identified and assessed at one point in time and is then reassessed some time later.

Uses of follow-up evaluations

Follow-up evaluations may be used to determine the outcome for those using a service, and by implication the effectiveness of that service. They are most useful in finding out how clients fare within an established system of care.

Examples

A Bristol follow-up study reported a favourable outcome in 16 out of 48 homeless men who had attended a psychiatric clinic (Tomison & Cook, 1987). The study concluded that 'psychiatric intervention can achieve something'. On the other hand, the East London Homelessness Health Team (HHELP), a primary health care team, reported that only 8 out of 112 subjects of no fixed abode, and 12 out of 144 subjects in unstable accommodation, obtained stable accommodation during their period of contact with the team (Balazs, 1993).

Advantages

Follow-up evaluations are easier to conduct than randomized controlled trials and quasi-experimental designs. Such studies complement surveys because they assess the outcome of care rather than the process of care. Follow-up evaluations provide a reasonable indication of how far a service is achieving its goals, and may indicate when a service is performing poorly.

Disadvantages

Follow-up evaluations are difficult to carry out with homeless persons because the high mobility in this group leads to high drop out rates. Furthermore good outcome for clients cannot necessarily be attributed to the effects of the service, whilst a poor outcome may reflect factors outside the control of the service in question. Nevertheless such studies give some indication of how well homeless people are being served by the current system of care.

Before and after evaluations

Description

Before and after comparisons are similar to follow-up studies except that subjects are recruited and assessed *before* receiving a service and are then reassessed after a fixed period.

Uses of before and after comparisons

Before and after comparisons may be used to obtain a preliminary evaluation of the effectiveness of a service.

Examples

The Psychiatric Shelter Program of the Presbyterian Hospital in New York City was evaluated by comparing the social circumstances of 32 homeless mentally ill men before and after the men were placed by the programme in community housing (Caton *et al.*, 1990). Findings were a reduced level of criminal justice contacts and an increased utilization of psychiatric after care services.

Advantages

Before and after evaluations are a useful method of making a preliminary assessment of a new service when either: (a) more suitable designs are not possible, or (b) the investigator wishes to determine whether it is worth proceeding to a controlled trial. The simple design of before and after studies makes them relatively easy to conduct.

Disadvantages

There are likely to be high drop out rates in samples taken from homeless populations. Furthermore, before and after evaluations tend to over-estimate the effectiveness of an intervention because, without suitable control groups, it is impossible to rule out the possibility that changes in the index group were not due to natural improvements over time (regression towards the mean), or to other factors that changed during the study. This second confounding factor can be a particular problem in studies of the homeless because of the frequent policy changes that occur towards this group.

Single case and 'action research' evaluations

Description

In a single case study, data on some suitable index of the service's performance are collected over a long baseline. At the end of the baseline period a change in the service is implemented and the effects of the change on the index variable are observed over a further period of time. 'Action research' is a special variety of the single case approach. Action research attempts to achieve some specified goal by proceeding 'in cycles of evaluation, policy change, re-evaluation and further policy change' (Leach & Wing, 1978).

Uses of single case designs

Single case designs are particularly useful in situations where the investigator wishes to evaluate the effect of a change in the way a service is being provided. Single case designs can also, in principle, be used to evaluate the effectiveness of a new service.

Examples

One of the best known examples of action research was provided by a team of investigators working with the St Mungo's Community in London (Leach & Wing, 1978). From September 1971 to August 1976 the investigators monitored the effectiveness of the community in resettling homeless men. At intervals in the course of the research the investigators put forward recommendations as to how the Community's practices should be changed to improve resettlement rates. The researchers then observed the effects of the changes they had recommended on resettlement rates, and accordingly made further recommendations and so on. As described in Chapter 9 the investigators were ultimately successful in improving resettlement rates, though with unforeseen consequences for the Community.

Advantages

Single case designs are a fairly robust alternative to randomized controlled trials that may be used in many situations where the former design would not be possible or suitable.

Disadvantages

Single case evaluations of services may require baseline data to be collected for very long periods, as was the case in the study described above. Where it is important to establish that improvements have occurred due to the intervention in question, rather than extraneous factors, complex designs with multiple 'cases' may be required. Thus, for example, if a study were being conducted to assess the effect of a change in hostel policy it might be necessary to collect baseline data on several hostels and then implement the change at different times in each hostel in a random order.

Quasi-experimental evaluations

Description

In quasi-experimental evaluations the outcome for an index group of subjects (who receive a service) is compared with that for a control group of subjects (who do not receive the service). The allocation of subjects to index and control groups is not random.

Uses of quasi-experimental evaluations

Quasi-experimental evaluations can be used to assess the effectiveness of a service, or the relative effectiveness of one or more different types of service. They are most useful in situations where randomized controlled trials are not possible.

Examples

No examples from the literature on homelessness are known to this author, although such designs have been used in studies of home-based care (Dean *et al.*, 1993).

Advantages

Quasi-experimental evaluations avoid the need for randomization, with its attendant ethical and administrative problems.

Disadvantages

Failure to randomize subjects to treatment and control groups means that differences in outcome between groups may be attributed to factors other than the intervention. Quasi-experimental evaluations are prone to bias and their findings are therefore much less robust than the findings of randomized controlled trials.

Randomized controlled trials

Description

Subjects are randomly allocated to treatment and control groups. The outcome for subjects is usually assessed after a fixed period of time.

Uses of randomized controlled trials

Randomized controlled trials are the most suitable method for determining whether a service is effective. They are also the most suitable method for determining whether one service is superior to another.

Examples

In an evaluation of the effectiveness of a multi-disciplinary psychiatric team working with the homeless in Lewisham, 95 homeless men with psychiatric disorder were randomly allocated to receive either 'advice' or 'full case management' (Timms, 1990). After 1 year, 50% of the advice groups were lost to follow-up as compared to 20% of the treatment group. Such high drop-out rates make it difficult to interpret the other findings of the trial.

A more successful comparison of three different treatment approaches was carried out by Morse *et al.* (1992) in St Louis. A total of 150 homeless mentally ill subjects were randomly allocated to receive either: outpatient treatment, treatment at a drop-in centre, or assertive community treatment. At 1 year subjects in the assertive community treatment group had more contact with their treatment programme, were more satisfied with their programme, spent fewer days homeless and made use of more community resources than subjects in the other two groups.

Marshall *et al.* (1995) carried out a randomized controlled trial, in a medium-sized English city, to evaluate a social services case management team for people with long-term mental disorders.

Subjects were referred from: hostels for the homeless; night shelters; a GP clinic for the homeless; the City Council homelessness unit; and local voluntary sector group homes. Eighty subjects consented to be randomized to treatment or control groups. At 14 month follow-up there were no significant differences between treatment and control groups in number of needs, quality of life, employment status, quality of accommodation, social behaviour and severity of psychiatric symptoms. The authors concluded that social services case management was successful in reducing deviant behaviour, but otherwise made little difference to the lives of the subjects.

Advantages

The randomized controlled trial is the most robust way of producing definitive evidence for the effectiveness of a service or for its superiority over another service.

Disadvantages

Randomized controlled trials are difficult to organize under the most favourable conditions. Unfortunately evaluations of services for the homeless tend to take place under conditions that are particularly unfavourable to organizing a successful clinical trial. The greatest problem is caused by high drop-out rates, either because subjects have moved away from the area altogether, or have changed 'address' locally and therefore lost contact with the investigators. Even where an index intervention leads to low drop-out rates, a study may fail because of high drop-out rates in the control treatment, as was the case in the first trial described above. The second trial reported above, attempted to overcome the problem of high drop-out rates by replacing subjects who dropped out with other subjects randomly allocated to the three treatment groups (Morse *et al.*, 1992).

Further problems likely to face those attempting to organize randomized controlled trials with homeless mentally disordered subjects are: insufficient numbers of subjects; difficulties obtaining consent to randomization; and difficulties obtaining co-operation for randomization from voluntary organizations.

THE EFFECTIVENESS OF HOSTELS FOR THE HOMELESS IN CARING FOR PEOPLE WITH SEVERE MENTAL DISORDERS

Hostels are caring for large numbers of people with severe mental disorder. Not surprisingly many have questioned the suitability of hostels for this role. For example, in a report by a subgroup of the Working Party on Single Homelessness in London (SHIL, 1987), hostels were described as 'irrelevant' to the needs of many homeless people. The report concluded that hostels 'need to go, to be replaced with a range of ... facilities which can meet the real needs of their current users'. In view of this controversy this section will consider the role of hostels and will examine the evidence for their effectiveness.

The role of hostels for the homeless in caring for people with severe mental disorders

Hostels provide four distinct types of assistance to people with severe mental disorders:

1. Hostels act as a safety net.
2. Hostels provide a place to live.
3. Hostels provide a resettlement service.
4. Hostels are a place where care and support can be provided.

How good are hostels at providing each of these four types of assistance?

Acting as a safety net

Hostels are the last resort before the street corner for many people with mental disorders. The data presented in Chapter 9 leave little room for doubt about the effectiveness of hostels in this role as a 'safety net'. Further evidence is provided by hostel surveys demonstrating that many mentally disordered residents have been abandoned by or lost touch with, the statutory services (Marshall, 1989; Marshall & Reed, 1992). Over the past 40 years as 'care in the community' has been implemented, hostels have absorbed increasing numbers of people with severe mental disorders, many of whom are extremely socially disabled. Unfortunately, the loss of hostel beds in recent years

(7000 in London alone in the past 10 years) has greatly impaired the capacity of hostels to continue performing this vital role. This has led some to conclude, not unreasonably, that 'the increasing numbers of homeless people on the streets have been generated primarily by the disappearance of direct access accommodation' (Timms, 1993).

The success of hostels as a safety net appears to be for three reasons. First, large to medium hostels usually have beds immediately available. Secondly, they do not impose complex referral or assessment criteria before admission and thirdly, they are usually easily located by potential users.

Providing a place to live

Whilst conditions in some hostels are unacceptable, they are not invariably poor. Nevertheless the available evidence suggests that most mentally disordered hostel residents would prefer to live elsewhere. For example, in a study of women's' hostels in London 16 out of 61 women (26%) expressed a preference to remain in the hostel; moreover all 16 who wished to remain complained about lack of privacy (Marshall & Reed, 1992). The author's own work in Oxford hostels (unpublished results) indicates that less than one in three male residents with severe mental disorder would prefer to remain in the hostel. We must assume therefore that many hostel residents would prefer to live elsewhere.

Providing a resettlement service

There is considerable evidence to suggest that hostels are not successful at resettling residents with severe mental disorder in more suitable accommodation. For example, a follow-up of mentally disordered hostel residents in Oxford found that only 10 out of 48 residents were rehoused in an 18 month period. Those residents who were rehoused went either: back to their families, to private bedsits, or to accommodation provided by the hostels. No residents obtained accommodation supported by health, social services or housing associations (Marshall & Gath, 1992). In this respect there has been little improvement from the days of the Camberwell Reception Centre (Wood, 1976). It would appear however that this failure to resettle residents is not so much a failure of the hostels as a failure of the statutory services to support the hostels.

A place where care and support can be provided

There is evidence to suggest that hostels are not succeeding in providing the care and support that people with severe mental disorders require. The high levels of need in Oxford hostels have been described above (Hogg & Marshall, 1992). Other recent hostel studies have shown that only a minority of residents with severe mental disorder are in contact with the statutory services. Thus, in two women's hostels in London, less than half of those suffering from schizophrenia were in contact with the psychiatric services or receiving any form of treatment (Marshall & Reed, 1992); whilst in a representative sample of a London hostel for men (Timms & Fry, 1989) less than half of those with schizophrenia were in contact with the psychiatric services.

Findings such as these have led to suggestions that mentally disordered hostel residents have become 'isolated from mainstream community care'. It has even been suggested that hostels for the homeless may act as 'traps' for some mentally disordered people. Thus, a recent report described two cases of men severely disabled by schizophrenia who had lived in hostels for many years (Marshall & Sharpe, 1993). For years both had displayed complete incoherence in thinking and had been incapable of holding a conversation. Both were without friends or relatives. Neither resident could clothe or wash themselves and depended on hostel staff to perform these activities for them. Both residents showed considerable improvements in their ability to communicate and to care for themselves after admission to hospital and treatment with neuroleptic medication. These improvements were maintained after discharge.

The authors of the report felt that the case histories demonstrated a fundamental problem with hostel care. The problem is that whilst hostels have developed a remarkable capacity to tolerate deviant behaviour and to provide support to those incapable of self-care, they have only a limited capacity to assess the need for specialized treatment or to provide that treatment. Thus hostels end up 'containing' problems that could be cured or considerably alleviated by suitable treatment. This unfortunate situation is not the fault of the hostels; rather it is the fault of statutory services that have consistently failed to provide adequate liaison services.

CONCLUSION

The available evidence suggests that hostels for the homeless are successful in one major aspect of their role; that of acting as a safety net for mentally disordered people who would otherwise have nowhere to go. However, on the other three aspects of the hostels' role the evidence is not so favourable. On providing a place to live, the limited evidence suggests that only a minority of mentally disordered residents wish to remain in hostels, and few find that the accommodation provided is satisfactory. On acting as a resettlement service, the evidence suggests that hostels are largely unsuccessful. On acting as a place where care and support can be provided, the available evidence suggests that hostels are not succeeding.

The limited effectiveness of hostels is not, however, a strong argument for their immediate closure. By collecting and concentrating people with mental disorders in one place, hostels have provided, and continue to provide, a useful opportunity for statutory agencies to fulfil their obligations. The signal failure of statutory agencies to take up this challenge is hardly the fault of the hostels. What is required is a much more dynamic and aggressive effort by statutory agencies to identify, treat and especially resettle, mentally disordered hostel residents. Until this effort materializes and hostel beds are lying empty, we should leave the messenger unharmed.

References

Balazs, J. (1993). Health care for the single homeless. In K. Fisher (ed.), *Homelessness, Health Care and Welfare Provision*, pp. 51–93. London: Routledge.

Caton, C. L. M., Wyatt, R. J., Grunberg, J. & Felix, A. (1990). An evaluation of a mental health program for homeless men. *American Journal of Psychiatry*, **147**, 286–9.

Dean, C., Phillips, J., Gadd, E. M., Joseph, M. & England, S. (1993). Comparison of community based service with hospital based service for people with acute, severe, mental illness. *British Medical Journal*, **307**, 473–7.

Ferguson, B. & Dixon, R. (1992). Psychiatric clinics in homeless hostels – your flexible friend. *Psychiatric Bulletin*, **16**, 683–4.

Hamid, W. A. & McCarthy, M. (1989). Community psychiatric care for homeless people in inner London. *Health Trends*, **21**, 67–9.

Hogg, L. I. & Marshall, M. (1992). Can we measure need in the homeless mentally ill? Using the MRC Needs for Care Assessment in hostels for the homeless. *Psychological Medicine*, **22**, 1027–34.

Leach, J. & Wing, J. K. (1978). The effectiveness of a service for helping destitute men. *British Journal of Psychiatry*, **113**, 481–92.

Marshall, E. J. & Reed, J. L. (1992). Psychiatric morbidity in homeless women. *British Journal of Psychiatry*, **160**, 761–9.

Marshall, M. (1989). Collected and neglected: are Oxford hostels for the homeless filling up with disabled psychiatric patients? *British Medical Journal*, **299**, 706–9.

Marshall, M. & Gath, D. G. (1992). What happens to homeless mentally ill people? Follow up of residents of Oxford hostels for the homeless. *British Medical Journal*, **304**, 79–80.

Marshall, M., Lockwood, A. & Gath, D. (1995). How effective is social service case management for people with long-term mental disorders? A randomised controlled trial. *Lancet*, **345**, 409–12.

Marshall, M. & Sharpe, M. (1993). Untreated schizophrenia in hostels for the homeless: a cause for concern? *Bulletin of the Royal College of Psychiatrists*, **17**, 16–18.

Morse, G. A., Calsyn, R. J., Allen, G., Tempelhoff, B. & Smith, R. (1992). Experimental comparison of the effects of three treatment programs for homeless mentally ill people. *Hospital and Community Psychiatry*, **43**, 1005–10.

SHIL (Single Homeless In London) (1987). *Primary Health Care for Homeless Single People in London: A Strategic Approach*. Report of a Joint working party on single homelessness in London. London: SHIL.

Timms, P. W. (1990). Psychiatric care of the homeless – a domiciliary asylum service. *Abstracts for the Royal College of Psychiatrists Annual Meeting*, 12–13.

Timms, P. W. (1993). Origins of homelessness specific to the mentally ill. In K. Fisher (ed.), *Homelessness, Health Care and Welfare Provision*, pp. 100–16. London: Routledge.

Timms, P. W. & Fry, A. H. (1989). Homelessness and mental illness. *Health Trends*, **21**, 70–1.

Tomison, A. & Cook, D. (1987). Rootlessness and mental disorder. *British Journal of Clinical and Social Psychiatry*, **5**, 5–8.

Vagg, J. (1992). A little local difficulty: the management of difficult-to-place people in Oxford. *International Journal of Law and Psychiatry*, **15**, 129–38.

Williams, S. & Allen, I. (1989). *Health Care for Single Homeless People*. London: Policy Studies Institute.

Wood, S. M. (1976). Camberwell Reception Centre: a consideration of the need for health and social services of homeless single men. *Journal of Social Policy*, **5**, 389–99.

17

Future directions for homeless mentally ill

Dinesh Bhugra

The lessons from a literature review from around the world suggest that the definitions of homelessness vary but the association between homelessness and chronic severe mental illness is fairly well known. The health services also vary according to the local socio-economic and political structures, which means that the true assessment of actual numbers of the homeless and their needs presents a major problem. In the UK, localized catchment area based community services may enable a closer primary and secondary care interface as described in Chapter 11. In the USA, marked reduction in low-cost housing and deinstitutionalization of state and county mental hospitals have contributed to the problem of social construction of homelessness (Robertson & Greenblatt, 1992). The global view, not comprehensive by any means, outlined in this volume suggests that there are common themes for research, management and social policy change and that there are also differences in terms of definitions of poverty and homelessness, which may be inextricably linked, and also in terms of service provision. If any strategies for change in research, social policy and management are to succeed there have to be concentrated efforts on the part of the researchers, clinicians, policy makers and politicians. As the causes of homelessness are multi-dimensional, their management as well as social policy changes must be multi-factorial and multi-dimensional.

Commonalities across the globe

There are common confusions regarding definitions of homelessness, how people enter the spiral of homelessness and associations with mental ill-health and vulnerability factors for physical illness.

Definitions

Many policy makers seem to think that the homeless are a homogeneous group. Many sociologists and clinicians along with epidemiologists have struggled with the diversity of causes of homelessness, types
of homelessness complicating the presence of mental illness. There
needs to be an element of agreement in definitions of homelessness as
well as classification. Leach (1979) had urged a simple intrinsic versus
extrinsic divide – the former including those where the mental or
physical disability antedated their homelessness, whereas in the latter
their homelessness was attributed to situational factors. Leach went
on to propose that the subgroups would need different service
programmes. However, Morse *et al.* (1991) suggested that a
taxanomic system based on current impairment was superior to the
system based on past history. Obviously the roofless versus shelterless
definitions will vary across countries. Furthermore, the presence of
co-morbidity will affect the definitions and the outcomes. There need
to be multi-centred studies across the globe addressing the issues of
definitions, pathways and antedating factors.

Pathways into homelessness

Pathways into homelessness are many and vary dramatically according to the age of the individual, social support available, local health
and social services, gender as well as race. When the social services
benefits were cut down for the under eighteens in the UK, there was a
marked increase in the number of homeless youth on the streets. In
the past 10 years in the UK, over 1.25 million households have been
accepted as homeless by local authorities – bringing the number of
individuals up to a total of more than 3 million, half of them children
(Burrows & Walentowicz, 1992). The numbers do not tell the full
story – hence the suggestion by Koegel (1992) that longitudinal
life-history type of social anthropological approaches must be used.
Victor (1992) has used a model of pathways into homelessness in her
study in West London but more information is needed to identify the
crisis points in order to make appropriate changes in social policy. In
developing countries these crisis points may be different as the social
support would vary. However, with a change in social milieu
occurring rapidly, the processes of capitalism, industrialization and

urbanization and disintegration of family structures and reliance on nuclear family structures, may bring about changes that may be worth studying. In the developed countries, the mentally ill homeless are also likely to have less contact with family and friends and more barriers to employment even if it is readily available.

Numbers of homeless mentally ill

With co-morbidity of physical and mental illness and substance misuse becoming an important issue around the globe, the overall numbers are likely to increase. Outcome studies are rare for these groups and as the American experience demonstrates that if suitable programmes are in place that are multi-dimensional, need orientated and individual focused they are more likely to be successful (Leda & Rosencheck, 1992). As we know, mental illness, social dysfunction and homelessness are related problems that exacerbate one another. Looking at the information available from around the globe the absolute numbers of homeless individuals are likely to grow – the proportion of mentally ill in the homeless group may increase, too. There are no consistent explanations for the observations of increased numbers and visibility of the homeless mentally ill across the globe. Successful clinical intervention must target problem areas of social dysfunction, homelessness and mental illness.

As Leshner (1992) recommended, well-being of the homeless mentally ill is not the sole province of the mental health services and requires the co-ordinated efforts of many service systems working together.

This has to be seen as a starting point for successful mutual collaboration between the housing and social services on one side, and the statutory health services on the other.

Differences around the globe

Definitions of poverty and the basic poverty line will depend upon the Gross Domestic Product (GDP) and the Gross National Product (GNP) of each country so there may be an element of comparing oranges with apples. There needs to be an international perspective on this very important issue.

Definitions of poverty

In the developed countries, where social services exist, the official
poverty line may determine the social services support and benefits.
In less developed countries, these basic supportive networks may not
be present and a combination of poverty, overcrowding and industrialization may lead to child labour as well as to large scale
migrations into urban areas producing large areas of shanty towns.
Here, houses may have nothing more than a basic structure with
walls and a roof, but no availability of basic amenities for clean water
or sewage disposal. Furthermore, the truth behind the definitions
may be used by the policy makers to hide the extreme poverty or
exaggerate it to fulfil certain aims. The men, women and children
who must live on the streets and shelters may find little privacy and
less support. The homeless are only the most visible of the poor. The
much greater number of very poor who cling to vermin-infested
rooms or live doubled and tripled up with relatives are otherwise little
different in the USA (Hilfiker, 1989). Although Hilfiker (1989) goes
on to observe that in the USA the poor and marginalized must fend
for themselves – this is true of most of the globe – certainly from
countries where information is openly available. A lack of resources
and denial of access to these resources compound the problems of
poverty and its impact on people of different ages, ethnicity and
gender. These factors need to be studied in relationship to homelessness.

Relationship of patterns of poverty, homelessness and mental illness

Poverty and unemployment may be linked although the two states
can exist separately. However, poverty can be defined objectively and
applied consistently only in terms of the concepts of relative depriva-
tions where members of the community lack the resources to obtain
the type of diet, activities of the community and living conditions
approved by the society (Townsend, 1979). Specific psychological
impacts of poverty have been mentioned including a different
conceptualization of time restriction of linguistic code and poor
self-esteem, which are well known. Individual differences in the
development and maintenance of low self-esteem are important

factors and these would need to be assessed along with the other vulnerability factors. Lower educational attainments and lack of financial savings have been suggested to be related to inability to postpone gratification (see Bhugra, 1993 for a review). The estimates of psychiatric morbidity in the homeless vary. Co-morbidity of physical illness, psychiatric illness and substance misuse although well described does not always translate into an understandable structural model. In developing countries, for example, physical illness and chronic infections may lead to poverty, unemployment or homelessness. However, it is fair to say that the evidence of a correlation between homelessness and alcoholism or mental illness and homelessness does not mean that either factor is a cause or consequence of homelessness (Wright, 1989). In the UK disorganized schizophrenia is common in homeless populations, it is not clear whether this is true elsewhere as well. The social substrate of health perceived by the homeless individual will also affect the relationship with the therapist.

Patterns of help-seeking

Patterns of help-seeking depend upon the type of illness, the explanatory model used for that particular illness, the types of service available and accessibility to those services. It would thus make sense that homeless mentally ill across the globe may have different patterns of help-seeking. This, when combined with the perception of social substrate for health, affects help-seeking. The individual may display a limited trust in statutory services. Furthermore, in the UK, sectorization and emphasis on catchment area services along with a perceived rigidity and inflexibility of the health services, especially secondary care, mean that the homeless mentally ill may not always be booked into health services. In addition, the theoretical model of money following the patient after the National Health Service (NHS) reforms means that any definition of last home may prove difficult and unacceptable, thereby stopping the 'follow the patient flow' of the money. If the individuals are not registered with general practitioners, a hand-over and subsequent continuity of care will prove impossible. Some homeless individuals blame their non-registration on their own mobility and the inflexibility of services. The innovative outreach services can therefore prove to be more accessible, approachable and therefore successful. In other countries, the access to services may be more difficult especially if health care is totally or even largely private.

Socio-political factors

It is apparent that the patterns of help-seeking as well as types and definitions of homelessness and poverty depend upon the health structures. The health care system in any country is decided by social, economic, political, geographical and historical factors. The health demands of the population along with the epidemiological factors determine the needs of the whole population along with those of the special groups. The control by the government over the health service in the UK was one of the factors in the development of the NHS and the state became more involved in the health of the population and the regulation of the medical profession throughout the nineteenth and early twentieth centuries. The 1834 Poor Law was the first acknowledgement that government had some responsibility towards the care of the population (Burns & Bhugra, 1995). These changes led to a clear identification of the functions of the NHS, which was meant to provide preventative and curative health care. Similarly in latter contexts although the so-called NHS reforms have not made it difficult to seek help for chronic disabling conditions, they have added further layers of bureaucracy and management.

Structures

The physical and political structures of the health and social services provide help for the homeless mentally ill individual. These structures of the health care systems also include personal/social and complementary health sectors, which may be used by those needing health care. In the USA it was estimated that between 70% and 90% of all illness episodes are treated within the personal/social sectors, which may be a reflection of the general health care system available. In other countries, including the UK, such information is not readily available, but another possible area of investigation across various centres may well be the extent of use of alternative therapies and other options. Nevertheless, not having any fixed, easily available, approachable social support, the homeless individual may have to rely more on personal resources. This may also produce extra stress if these resources, especially physical and emotional, are not good enough. The structures of existing family and community networks would need to be studied.

Future directions

There remain several avenues in research that can be followed. There are two areas that could immediately be researched fruitfully – these include age-related differences and special needs groups within the broad mentally ill homeless category. In addition, some further suggestions are made below.

Impact of urbanization

In less developed countries the impact of urbanization on numbers of homeless mentally ill individuals as well as social and psychological stressors and functioning needs to be studied. Although initial welcome steps have been taken in Latin America, the Far East, Middle East and South East Asia still need to be studied (for a discussion on Latin America see Harpham & Blue, 1995). As Harpham (1993) had previously cautioned, risk factors such as poverty and poor environmental conditions have been repeatedly identified as having an independent association with ill-health among the urban poor in general, but their impact across various cultures and in various settings is not always very clear. Maternal education, maternal age, parity and marital status for the women have been shown to be key features associated with ill-health, and have already been demonstrated by Harpham in Brazil. Another additional factor that needs to be assessed is that of intra-urban differences. Social drift and social residue have been shown to be two possible factors for the intra-urban differences (Ekblad, 1990). The pull towards the bright lights of the city and push factors from the rural poverty need to be studied. It will be worth investigating which of the two factors plays a more important and sustained role in the genesis and perpetuation of mental disorders.

European models and their significance

As shown by the European perspectives, the varieties of homelessness and the state's response to the needs of the mentally ill homeless individual vary a great deal but there is a lot that can be adapted by other countries. For the young homeless for example, the model demonstrated by Van der Ploeg (1989) in the Netherlands suggests various dimensions of negative family backgrounds, past history of professional help along with negative school experiences, low self-perception and lack of friends, although reports from elsewhere also suggest that there may be generalities that are common across countries and cultures and there are specifics that must be taken into account. Similarly the models presented in this volume suggest that not only is there an accumulation of severely mentally ill in the lodging houses, there is also a possibility of reduction in numbers due to availability and government commitment to providing low-cost accommodation to those in need, as demonstrated by reports from Denmark. Similar numbers in Eire suggest various social factors at play.

Anthropological approaches

Koegel (1992) argues that the dearth of rich qualitative descriptions of lives in the processes of homelessness, together with an emphasis on preoccupation with pathology and disaffiliation, a failure to view the homeless in the broader socio-economic and situational contexts of their lives and the absence of longitudinal perspectives make it more difficult to provide relevant social policy information. He goes on to observe that the danger in using epidemiological techniques when focusing on homeless individuals is that such individuals are isolated from the broader socio-economic contexts that are crucial in shaping the characteristics, behaviours and choices. Thus, the explanatory models highlighting critical influences of broader factors, settings and other people rather than an individual deficit model can give an insight into the processes of homelessness. Furthermore, studying individuals over a period of time in an ethnographical context means that processes and insights into their experiences of double jeopardy of mental illness and homelessness can work. In addition, the anthropological method of participant observation moves beyond an exclusive reliance on self-report by working on the principle that behaviour is being studied using a blend of both interviewing and observation (Koegel, 1992).

Summary

For service provision, the gap between the needs of the homeless mentally ill and the available resources and services have to be matched. The multi-dimensional problem needs multi-dimensional solutions and any medical interventions planned will have to be highly tailored. Furthermore, housing, welfare benefits and service delivery have to be interlinked. Joint planning between the statutory health services and voluntary services may produce unique innovative models of assessment and management. As Craig *et al.* (1995) recommend, the needs of the newer subgroups within the homeless population (younger, ethnic minority and women) should be targeted. There is no doubt that preventative work, especially if it is multi-disciplinary, will prove to be fruitful.

References

Bhugra, D. (1993). Unemployment, poverty and homelessness. In D. Bhugra & J. Leff (eds.), *Principles of Social Psychiatry*, pp. 355–84. Oxford: Blackwell Scientific Publications.

Burns, A. & Bhugra, D. (1995). History and structure of the National Health Services. In D. Bhugra & A. Burns (eds.), *Management for Psychiatrists*, pp. 3–17. London: Gaskell.

Burrows, L. & Walentowicz, P. (1992). *Homes Cost Less Than Homelessness*. London: Shelter.

Craig, T., Bayliss, E., Klein, O., Manning, P. & Reader, L. (1995). *The Homeless Mentally Ill Initiative*. London: DOH.

Ekblad, S. (1990). Family stress and mental health during rapid urbanisation. In E. Nordberg & D. Finer (eds.), *Society, Environment and Health in Low-income Countries*. Stockholm: Karolinska Institute.

Harpham, T. (1993). Urbanisation and mental disorder. In D. Bhugra & J. Leff (eds.), *Principles of Social Psychiatry*, pp. 346–54. Oxford: Blackwell Scientific Publications.

Harpham, T. & Blue, I. (1995). *Urbanisation and Mental Health in Developing Countries*. Aldershot: Avebury.

Hilfiker, D. (1989). Are we comfortable with homelessness? *Journal of the American Medical Association*, **262**, 1375–6.

Koegel, P. (1992). Through a different lens: an anthropological perceptive on the homeless mentally ill. *Culture, Medicine and Psychiatry*, **16**, 1–22.

Leach, J. (1979). Providing for the destitute. In J. K. Wing & R. Olsen (eds.), *Community Care of the Mentally Disabled.* pp. 90–105. Oxford: OUP.

Leda, C. & Rosencheck, R. (1992). Mental health status and community adjustment after treatment in a residential treatment program for homeless veterans. *American Journal of Psychiatry,* **149,** 1219–24.

Leshner, A. (1992). A new system of care for the homeless mentally ill. *Hospital and Community Psychiatry,* **43,** 865.

Morse, G., Calsyn, R. & Burger, G. (1991). A comparison of taxanomic systems for classifying homeless men. *International Journal of Social Psychiatry,* **37,** 90–8.

Robertson, M. & Greenblatt, M. (1992). Homelessness: a national perspective. In M. J. Robertson & M. Greenblatt (eds.), *Homelessness – A National Perspective,* pp. 339–49. New York: Plenum Press.

Townsend, P. (1979). *Poverty in the United Kingdom.* London: Allen Lowe.

Van der Ploeg, J. D. (1989). Homelessness: a multidimensional problem. *Children and Youth Services Review,* **11,** 45–56.

Victor, C. (1992). Health status of the temporarily homeless population and residents of North West Thames Region. *British Medical Journal,* **305,** 387–91.

Wright, J. (1989). *Address Unknown: Homeless in America.* New York: Aldine de Gruyter.

Index

numbers and characteristics of
     residents 143–7
older homeless 158
rehousing 141
residents
  psychiatric characteristics
     146–7
  social characteristics 145–6
  social disability caused by
     mental disorder 146
role in caring for people with
     severe mental disorders
     292–4
  acting as a safety net 292–3
  place where care and support
     can be provided 294
  providing a place to live 293
  providing a resettlement
     service 293
schizophrenia
  higher prevalence 139–41
  possible explanations 140–1
  see also schizophrenia
separating hostel studies from
     shelter studies 135–6
social and psychiatric
     characteristics 145–7
studies 137
trends in prevalence of mental
     disorder amongst users 139
unclassified studies 138
hotels, Germany 205
'houselessness' 231
houses of correction 12–13
  first workhouses 13
houses of religion, relief to the poor
     12
housing
  associations 268
  benefits 268
     problems 268–9
  Germany 200
  for homeless, likely to deteriorate,
     Australia 245
  mentally ill vulnerable 245–6

lack, and definition of
     homelessness 232
low-cost
  decline, London and NYC
     160
  and homelessness, Ireland 211
  reduction of availability 4, 31,
     34, 160, 267–8
policies, co-ordination 275
provision, mentally ill homeless
     affected by lack of funds and
     treatment 254–6
securing for the mentally ill 267–8
shortage, as reason for
     homelessness 4
special needs of mentally ill
     235–6
stable, as goal 234–6
see also accommodation; residential
     planning
Housing Act 1967 268
Housing Act 1985 160, 268
Housing Act 1988 268
Housing and Homeless Person's Act
     1976 268
humiliation at circumstances 174

income benefits (support) for the
     mentally ill 268
older homeless 159
  London and NYC 154
problems 268–9
see also statutory health services
incontinence amongst mentally ill
     hostel residents 147
Indo-Pakistani women, homeless
     66–7
inner cities, homelessness 245–6
  origin 31–3
redevelopment and
     'gentrification', contribution
     to homelessness 34, 268
Inner London Homeless Mentally
     Ill (HMI) initiative (1990)
     275–6